# THE MEDICAL MESSIAHS

# THE MEDICAL MESSIAHS

*A Social History of
Health Quackery
in Twentieth-Century America*

JAMES HARVEY YOUNG

PRINCETON, NEW JERSEY
PRINCETON UNIVERSITY PRESS

Published by Princeton University Press, 41 William Street,
Princeton, New Jersey 08540
In the United Kingdom by Princeton University Press, Oxford

Library of Congress Card No. 67-21031

*Library of Congress Cataloging-in-Publication Data*
Young, James Harvey.
The medical messiahs: a social history of health quackery in
twentieth-century America / James Harvey Young.—Expanded pbk. ed.
p.  cm.
Includes bibliographical references and index.
ISBN 0-691-00579-6 (pbk: alk. paper)
1. Quacks and quackery—United States. I. Title.
[DNLM: 1. Quackery—history—United States. WZ 310 Y73m]
R730.Y68  1992
616.8′56′0973—dc20
DNLM/DLC
for Library of Congress     91-45700

First Princeton Paperback printing, 1975
Expanded paperback edition, 1992

Princeton University Press books are printed on acid-free paper,
and meet the guidelines for permanence and durability of the
Committee on Production Guidelines for Book Longevity of the
Council on Library Resources

10  9  8  7  6  5  4  3  2  (pbk.)

Printed in the United States of America

*To the Memory of*
*Blanche DeBra Young*
*and*
*William Harvey Young*

*Bertha Shirley Goode*
*and*
*Galen McGregor Goode*

# CONTENTS

CONTENTS

# PREFACE

IN *The Toadstool Millionaires* I sought to describe the origin, development, and criticism of patent medicines in America from the importation of British brands during colonial days to the enactment in 1906 of the first federal restraining statute, the Pure Food and Drugs Act. This present book is a sequel to the former one: The medical messiahs are the 20th-century successors of the toadstool millionaires.

Many reformers who worked diligently to secure the 1906 law would not have thought that a sequel would ever be required. The editor of the *Nation* greeted the new law by asserting that medical quackery had now been dealt a death blow. The *New York Times* and the American Medical Association's *Journal* also predicted the imminent doom of harmful nostrums.

In our own day, when we consider some of the trends since 1906, we too may be surprised that a sequel has proved necessary. For in the six succeeding decades the arsenal of anti-quackery weapons has been vastly augmented. The rigor of legal controls has been increased. Standards of medical education have been upgraded, licensing laws improved, hospital regulations tightened. Scientific knowledge about the human body and illnesses that assail it has progressed so far that 1906 seems by comparison a dark age. In that year there was but the merest hint of the coming revolution in chemotherapy. The educational level of our citizenry has been markedly raised. Surely, if not in 1906, at least in 1966, amid all this enlightenment and law, quackery should be dead.

But of course it is not. Indeed, it is not only not dead; never in previous history has medical quackery been such a booming business as now. A reasonable guess as to the "overall annual quackery take," estimated John W. Miner, a lawyer in the district attorney's office of Los Angeles County who specializes in medicolegal crimes, speaking in October 1966, would be two or more billion dollars. "It exceeds," Miner went on, "the research total expended on disease."

[ ix ]

*The Medical Messiahs* is concerned with this paradox, the concurrent rise in 20th-century America of modern medical science and of pseudo-medical nonsense. Thus the setting within which quackery has been viewed is necessarily broad. Trends in quackery, for example, are seen within the wider compass of self-medication. Laws have not sought to abolish self-medication but to make it safe and to ensure honesty in the promotion of self-dosage wares. Where lie the legitimate limits of autotherapy has been a question for continuing debate, with no firm consensus as to the exact border between quackery and non-quackery.

An effort has been made also to interpret quackery and self-medication in relation to trends in science, marketing, and government. Medical, pharmaceutical, and nutritional sciences have been revolutionized during the 20th century. Advertising has acquired a calculated psychological sophistication merely blundered upon occasionally in earlier days. Legislation to protect the consumer has expanded enormously during several waves of 20th-century reform. All of these major forces have influenced the stage upon which the quack has played his wily role.

Laws to curb quackery, indeed, form such a central part of the whole enterprise that they provide a major structuring principle for this book. The 1906 law—How did it succeed? How did it fail? How did promoters innovate to elude its modest restraints?—furnishes a key early theme. When Congress provides the Food and Drug Administration with more stringent laws, these questions are repeated. The Post Office Department, striving to restrain fraudulent use of the mails, and the Federal Trade Commission, seeking to keep advertising honest, also receive major attention. So too do the educational efforts to combat quackery of such groups as the American Medical Association, the National Better Business Bureau, and writers of books and for the press.

Case examples of medical messiahs from various important areas are given—the mail-order male-weakness treatment, the alleged tuberculosis-curing liniment, the potent weight-reducer, the vitamin and iron tonic ballyhooed at gargantuan medicine shows, the complex array of nutritional products vended by an itinerant "lecturer," the diabetes and the cancer "clinic." In such various ways did shrewd operators sometimes make fortunes that their 19th-century predecessors would have envied. It should perhaps be said that my concern has been with the promotion of drugs, food supplements, and devices, either direct to lay users, or to practitioners who in turn use these wares and machines in treating patients. I am not concerned with medical cults or sects as such.

Any individuals, societies, or organizations discussed in this book are mentioned without malice. To the best of my knowledge I am reporting the truth, not with the intent to harm but to inform to the best of my ability as a scholar who has devoted years of research to this significant social theme. The common good requires that such a major hazard to health be given public comment. All interpretations of the evidence are, of course, my own.

The major research for *The Medical Messiahs* was done during a sabbatical year while I held a fellowship from the Social Science Research Council. My research and writing also have been supported, over a span of several years, by Public Health Service Research Grant GM 07199 from the Division of General Medical Sciences. I am most grateful for this generous help. Also I greatly appreciate the courteous and valuable aid given me during the course of my research by officials, archivists, and librarians at various agencies, organizations, and repositories. Some of these debts are indicated in my Note on the Sources. Indispensable to the accomplishment of my task was permission from the Food and Drug Administration to consult archival records not barred to me by law and from the Post Office Department to study fraud order manuscripts.

I wish to thank Miss Ruth Walling, Emory reference librarian, for coming up with answers to my difficult questions; Mrs. John Lyon for serving as my research assistant for a year under the Public Health Service Grant; and Mrs. James Shaw for typing the manuscript.

Valuable suggestions were given me by three friends who

graciously yielded to my request that they read the manuscript: Thomas W. Christopher, Dean of the School of Law, University of New Mexico; Harry F. Dowling, Chairman of the Department of Medicine, College of Medicine, University of Illinois; and Winton B. Rankin, Deputy Commissioner of the Food and Drug Administration. Abraham Levine, an attorney in the Office of the General Counsel of the Post Office Department, kindly read and commented on Chapters 4 and 13.

I am grateful to R. Miriam Brokaw and Dorothy Hollmann of Princeton University Press for their continuing interest in my project and expert help with the manuscript.

Most of all my thanks go to my family. My wife, Myrna Goode Young, my sons, Harvey Galen and James Walter, all took notes for me that found their way into the pages of my book. And, as for my earlier writing, my wife continues first reader and key critic.

JAMES HARVEY YOUNG

*Emory University*
*November 1966*


In an afterword written for this new edition, I have sought to summarize what has happened regarding health quackery in America during the nearly quarter century that has elapsed since I sent the original manuscript to press. The paradox there chronicled continues: while scientific medicine has made marvelous discoveries, pseudomedicine has continued to expand, rather than to decline. Between them, indeed, the battle for the allegiance of the people rages more bitterly than before.

For their help in getting this new edition to press, I should like to thank Deborah Tegarden and Timothy Mennel of Princeton University Press.

*July 1990*                                                                J.H.Y

# ACKNOWLEDGMENTS

QUOTATIONS from the Franklin D. Roosevelt Papers are used by permission of the Franklin D. Roosevelt Library, Hyde Park, New York. The letter from H. L. Mencken to Morris Fishbein, found in the Department of Investigation of the American Medical Association, is quoted by permission of Dr. Fishbein and of the Mercantile-Safe Deposit and Trust Company of Baltimore. Quotations from Arthur Kallet and F. J. Schlink, *100,000,000 Guinea Pigs*, are used by permission of Vanguard Press, Inc., New York.

Credit for material used in the section of illustrations is given in the captions.

Permission has also been given me to use in this book in revised form material which I have published previously, as follows: "The Hadacol Phenomenon," *Emory University Quarterly*, 7 (June 1951), 72-86; "The 'Elixir Sulfanilamide' Disaster," *ibid.*, 14 (December 1958), 230-37; "The 1938 Food, Drug, and Cosmetic Act," *Journal of Public Law*, 13 (1964), 197-204; "Social History of American Drug Legislation," in Paul Talalay, editor, *Drugs in Our Society* (Baltimore: The Johns Hopkins Press, 1964), 217-29; and "Device Quackery in America," *Bulletin of the History of Medicine*, 39 (March-April 1965), 154-62.

# THE MEDICAL MESSIAHS

# 1

## BRANE-FUDE

*"The lesson to be learned is that the law must be obeyed."*

—PHARMACEUTICAL ERA, 1908[1]

THE first court trial under the Pure Food and Drugs Act,[2] pitting the federal government against the maker of a remedy with the inspired and inspiring name of Cuforhedake Brane-Fude, got under way during February 1908. This was nearly twenty months after Theodore Roosevelt had signed the pioneering statute and more than thirteen months after the law's effective date.

In the meantime Harvey Washington Wiley, chief of the Bureau of Chemistry in the Department of Agriculture, had not been idle. Wiley, whose crusading zeal had been of central significance in the enactment of the law, was now charged with its enforcement. Recruiting a staff of scientists and inspectors took time. The task of regulation-making proved equally demanding. For such a complicated subject, the 1906 law was very short. General statements required elaboration with more specific meanings. Hearings, conferences, addresses, conversations, correspondence kept every hour busy. Since the passage of the law, wrote Wiley, "we have been absolutely flooded with work."[3]

---

[1] Editorial, 39 (Apr. 23, 1908), 513.
[2] Act of June 30, 1906, ch. 3915, 34 Stat. 768.
[3] Secy. of Agric. James Wilson to Wiley, July 24, 1906, Wiley Papers, box 60, Manuscripts Div., Library of Congress; *1907 Report of Bureau of Chemistry*, 4 [this and subsequent *Reports* are cited from the reprinted versions in Food Law Institute Series, *Federal Food, Drug and Cosmetic Law, Administrative Reports, 1907-1949* (Chicago, 1951)]; Wiley to American Medical Association, Jan. 2, 1907, Letterbook, General Corres., Bur. of Chem., Record Group 97, National Archives. Hereafter RG and NA.

[ 3 ]

At long last the Bureau, with staff and regulations ready, sought to determine which of the many violations of the law should be tackled first. They decided on a patent medicine case that bade fair to make a significant precedent. To protect the public in its right of self-medication, the law forbade statements on the labels of proprietary remedies that were "false or misleading in any particular." Wiley and his aides chose a nostrum with several possible misbranding particulars: the percentage of a key ingredient, the nature of the exhortations to would-be purchasers, the very name itself, Cuforhedake Brane-Fude. The remedy, moreover, was manufactured within the District of Columbia. This had two advantages: busy Bureau officials could better participate in helping the district attorney's office to work up the case, and the law set heavier penalties for District than for interstate violations. In addition to all this, the manufacturer was not an ignorant nobody, but a trained pharmacist and a prominent citizen.[4]

Robert N. Harper had begun making his headache remedy back in about 1888. He was then a student at the Philadelphia College of Pharmacy, at the same time gaining practical experience by working as a chemist for the pharmaceutical manufacturing firm, John Wyeth & Brother. Synthetic pain-killers and fever-reducers, derived from coal tar and imported from Germany, were still in the early exciting stages of their impact upon American medicine and pharmacy. In 1886 two German physicians, by sheer accident, because a young pharmacist erred in filling a prescription, had discovered that one such derivative, acetanilid, could bring down fever and deaden

[4] The primary sources for this case are the records filed in Seizure No. 28, Record File Interstate Office, and Hearing No. 49, I. S. 8751, RG 88, NA; Food and Drug Case 3, Office of the Solicitor of the Dept. of Agric., RG 16, NA; and the printed Notice of Judgment 25, issued Nov. 25, 1908. Biographical information on Harper and data on the trial have also been found in the *Oil, Paint and Drug Reporter,* 73 (Feb. 3, 1908), 25-26; (Feb. 17), 9; (Feb. 24), 40-41; (Mar. 2), 28D, 29, 30; (Mar. 9), 9-10; (Mar. 16), 9, 16, 17, 40; (Mar. 23), 7-8, 28B; (Mar. 30), 8-9; (Apr. 6), 22; (Apr. 20), 15-16; the *Wash. Herald,* Mar. 17, 18, 19, Apr. 16, 1908; *Wash. Post,* Mar. 6, 13, 19, Apr. 16; *Wash. Star,* Mar. 16, 17; and in the Harper's Cuforhedake Brain Food folder, Dept. of Investigation, Amer. Medical Assoc., Chicago.

pain.[5] Their report was quickly confirmed, and the news crossed the Atlantic. Harper, running across this information, gave acetanilid the central role in a formula he concocted, tried out on himself and his friends, and then—as any ambitious citizen had a perfect right to do—put on the market. He called it Cephalgine. Upon graduating, Harper had transferred his base of operations to the nation's capital. A ready seller, Harper's mixture of acetanilid, antipyrine, caffeine, sodium and potassium bromide, and alcohol continued to do well after 1905, when he changed the name because of a possible trademark violation of which he had been unaware up to that point. By 1908, indeed, some two million bottles of the remedy had been sold. As Harper's market grew, so did his stature in the community. He was elected president of the Retail Drug Association. He served for several years as a Commissioner of Pharmacy for the District. He became head of a bank. He was chosen president of the Chamber of Commerce. A Virginia Democrat, Harper swung some political weight.

When the Pure Food and Drugs Act became law, Harper went by the office of the Bureau of Chemistry to ask how he should change his Cuforhedake Brane-Fude label. He was told the same thing that Wiley and Lyman Kebler, head of the Bureau's drug division, told all inquirers, that they could not give positive instructions on this point. It was up to the manufacturer to read the new law and make his labeling conform. Harper modified his label to show that his remedy contained 30 per cent alcohol and 16 grains of acetanilid (the law demanded that the proportion of these two ingredients be indicated) but otherwise left things the same.

These changes, Wiley and Kebler believed, were not enough. For one thing, analysis showed the percentage of alcohol to be not 30 but 24 per cent. For another, the descriptive matter on the label and in a pamphlet packed with each bottle contained statements that struck the Bureau officials as false and misleading. No such mixture of ingredients could truly claim that it was "a most wonderful, certain and harm-

[5] Martin Gross, *Acetanilid: A Critical Bibliographic Review* (New Haven, 1946), 1-2.

less relief," or that it contained "no . . . poisonous ingredients of any kind." Extensive use of acetanilid might be fraught with hazard. One of the terrifying blasts aimed against patent medicines during the battle that led to the new law had been directed against headache mixtures loaded with acetanilid. Samuel Hopkins Adams in the pages of *Collier's* had printed a box enclosing the names and addresses of 22 victims, allegedly brought to death by acetanilid poisoning.[6] Dr. Kebler and his aides, after combing medical literature and querying physicians, believed that there might be a great many more, in addition to numerous cases of chronic poisoning and habituation to the drug.[7] Thus acetanilid was deemed a major threat to the public health, and it was an act of misbranding when Harper assured the public that this remedy contained "no . . . poisonous ingredient." Wiley was also persuaded that Harper's trade name was misleading. Cuforhedake certainly looked like an evasive spelling for headache cure. And none of the nostrum's ingredients was food for the brain.

Going to a Washington drugstore, a representative from the district attorney's office, acting in accordance with the procedures of the new law, seized some bottles of Cuforhedake Brane-Fude by a process of libel for condemnation. Later the Bureau gave the druggist a hearing. Harper showed up too. Wiley and Kebler explained their objections to the Brane-Fude labeling. Harper debated some of the criticisms, noted that he had recently made new modifications, and asserted that many users—including two Senators—had testified to the therapeutic value of his remedy. This defense did not persuade the Bureau of Chemistry officials. Convinced that they had a winning case, they submitted their evidence to the Department of Justice. Not only was a civil action needed against the seized medicine itself, Wiley argued, but also a criminal action against its manufacturer. In January 1908 an information was

[6] *Collier's*, 36 (Dec. 2, 1905), 16-18.

[7] L. F. Kebler, F. P. Morgan, and Philip Rupp presented the results of their study in *The Harmful Effects of Acetanilid, Antipyrin and Phenacetin*, Bulletin 126, Bur. of Chem., 1909, and in the less technical *Harmfulness of Headache Mixtures*, Farmers' Bulletin 377, Dept. of Agric., 1909. Gross offers a recent critique of this work, 58-103.

[ 6 ]

filed against Harper in the Police Court of the District. A
month later the case came to trial.

The proceedings presented a 16-day debate over the definition of terms.[8] Were Harper's key ingredients "poisons" or
were they not? Could they be considered food for the brain?
Was it proper to give to a drug which relieved a headache
the name of "cure"? A handful of prosecution witnesses, especially Dr. Reid Hunt, a pharmacologist from the Hygienic
Laboratory of the Marine Hospital Service, expounded on the
dangerous nature of acetanilid and antipyrine. Too much acetanilid taken over too long a period, Dr. Hunt testified, could
destroy up to four-fifths of the red blood cells. In cross-examination, the defense attorney slyly got the doctor to admit that
little of his research had been done with people, most with
rabbits, guinea pigs, and mice. Hunt and other government
witnesses asserted that acetanilid benumbed the nerves rather
than treating the basic ailments of which headaches were one
symptom. It was inaccurate, therefore, to term acetanilid a
headache cure.

Dr. Wiley himself took the stand. Alcohol, he said, might
in small quantities furnish the body "a modicum of food." But
alcohol provided no special nourishment for the brain, indeed,
might do it serious injury.

"In what way, Doctor?" he was asked.

"It tends to harden all the cells with which it comes into
contact," he answered, "and to coagulate their contents."

There was a simplicity, almost a casualness, about the prosecution case that suggests either inadequate preparation, perhaps from the pressure of other work, or, more likely, the feeling that Harper's misbranding was prima facie and needed
little more than pointing out. The Harper defense which
followed must have surprised Bureau of Chemistry officials,
it was so massive, so vigorous, so telling.

The reason a government chemist found that Cuforhedake
Brane-Fude contained 24 per cent of alcohol instead of the labeled 30 per cent, testified a chemistry professor from George-

---

[8] The fullest account of the trial itself is in *Oil, Paint and Drug Reporter*, 73 (Feb. 3–Apr. 20, 1908, *passim*).

town University, was that he did not seem to realize that not
absolute alcohol but commercial alcohol was used in the
remedy's manufacture. The commercial grade, reckoned at
94.9 per cent pure, was the standard ingredient for proprietary remedies requiring alcohol. Not only was the Bureau of
Chemistry careless, the defense insisted, its officials were too
literal-minded in their definition of terms. Acetanilid was
not a poison. The nation's leading authority on coal tar products came down from New York to say so. Virgil Coblentz,
professor of pharmacy at Columbia University, had sat at the
feet of the German professor who discovered acetanilid's medical properties.

"Professor," he was asked, "what is a lethal, or fatal dose,
of acetanilid?"

"There is no such thing," he answered. Doses as large as
an ounce—437⅓ grains—had been taken without harmful results. A whole bottle of Cuforhedake Brane-Fude contained
only 24 grains of acetanilid. Moreover, Coblentz added, whatever depressant effect the acetanilid might have was to some
degree counteracted by the caffeine present in the mixture.
Harper's formula was harmless. "The dosage is very, very moderate. . . ."

Presumed cases of acetanilid poisoning, the professor testified, were often caused by impurities not removed from the
coal tar starting product during manufacture. Also, some people displayed an idiosyncrasy to acetanilid, but this was no
reason to label the drug a poison. Some people developed a
rash from eating strawberries.

Coblentz's statements were echoed by several Washington
physicians, who stoutly denied that there was anything poisonous in Harper's formula. It was indeed, they testified, a
mixture of ingredients very like ones they themselves often
prescribed for patients. Pharmacists from the District were
called to the stand to demonstrate the truth of this assertion.
Bringing prescriptions which they had filled during the last
year, the pharmacists showed that from 9 to 10 per cent of the
total had been for formulas similar to that which Harper had
been marketing, the acetanilid in the prescriptions varying

from considerably less to a little more than in Cuforhedake Brane-Fude. In all their experience, the druggists added, they had never heard the Brane-Fude blamed for bringing harm to anyone.

In this judgment by the pharmacists the defense physicians concurred. The coal tar pain-killers were not only not harmful, they were a positive blessing. Their increasing use had cut down on reliance upon opium with all its attendant dangers. Moreover, the doctors argued, contrary to what government witnesses had said, acetanilid really "cured" a headache. To throw an impressive weight of evidence behind this definition of "cure," the defense put more than a score of satisfied customers on the witness stand, many of them prominent citizens of the District. One was an editor of the Washington *Times*, another an official of the National Baseball League. The United States Senators did not testify. But two of Harper's witnesses (like Dr. Wiley) worked for federal agencies—the Census Bureau and the ICC. The prosecuting attorney protested against this evidence: laymen could have no understanding of the effect of drugs upon their bodies. The judge, however, let them testify how they had suffered misery with headaches, had taken Cuforhedake Brane-Fude, and the headaches had vanished.

Harper himself was final witness in his own defense. Poised and confident, he recounted his autobiography and insisted that through 20 years and 2,000,000 bottles no word had reached him of any harmful effect upon any user of his remedy.

The judge charged the jury forthrightly. The prosecution need not prove all its points, he said, but merely one, for the law used the phrase "false or misleading in any particular." Unless there was a distinct kind of food that nourished the brain as distinct from a food that nourished the whole body, the judge stated, and unless Harper's Brane-Fude was such a food, then he must be found guilty. In evaluating the labeling, the jury must consider how statements would influence the average citizen. "This law was passed," the judge said, "not to protect experts especially, not to protect scientific men who know the meaning and value of drugs, but for the purpose

of protecting ordinary citizens, like the jury and like counsel...."⁹

One private observer guessed that the prosecution expected
to be beaten. But the twelve ordinary citizens promptly found
Harper guilty of misbranding his Cuforhedake Brane-Fude.
There was some hint that they had reached their verdict on
the "brain food" point alone, not going into the other issues,
so hotly argued between prosecution and defense, as to
acetanilid's alleged curative properties and poisonous character, a debate destined to rage on for many years.¹⁰

Between the rendering of this verdict and the sentencing,
the case of United States v. Harper took a dramatic turn. A
message reached the prosecuting attorney that he should hurry
to the White House. There he had an interview with Theodore
Roosevelt. "It is your duty," the President told the lawyer,
according to a newspaper account, "to make an example of this
man, and show to the people of the country that the pure food
law was enacted to protect them. He has been convicted after
a fair and impartial trial, and you should use every argument
in your power to convince the judge to impose a jail sentence.
To a man of his wealth, a fine as the penalty . . . would be little
less than ridiculous."¹¹

Some newspapers railed about violation of the separation of
powers. Harper resigned his bank presidency. But the lawyer
took the President's advice and urged the judge to send Harper

⁹ Judge Kimball's charge is reprinted in Mastin G. White and Otis H.
Gates, compilers, *Decisions of Courts in Cases under the Federal Food
and Drugs Act* (Wash., 1934), 11-18.

¹⁰ *Oil, Paint and Drug Reporter*, 73 (Mar. 16, 1908), 9; (Mar. 23),
7. Early debate about acetanilid, as during the Harper trial, has been
seen in retrospect as "a welter of polemics," with the critics unduly
harsh and the proponents much too optimistic. *Dispensatory of the U.S.*
(25th ed., 1955), 5. If the sinister reputation acetanilid had with Wiley
and Kebler was too extreme, and based in some measure on erroneous
judgments, time was to confirm some of the hazards and reveal others;
this plus the development of safer analgesics was to bring the virtual
displacement of acetanilid in pain-killers sold direct to the American
laity. Torald Sollmann, *A Manual of Pharmacology* (8th ed., Phila.,
1957), 723, 728-30.

¹¹ *Wash. Herald*, Mar. 17, 1908. Roosevelt made his statement at the
urging of officials of the Departments of Agriculture and Justice. *Oil,
Paint and Drug Reporter*, 73 (Mar. 23, 1908), 28B.

to prison. "This is a new law," he argued. "To a certain extent the court is blazing the way. It now remains to be seen whether this law is to be enforced, so that every manufacturer, every druggist—not merely in the District of Columbia, but in the whole land—will know that they must obey this law, that was made for the benefit of the people of the United States."[12]

Harper's attorney protested. "The request of the district attorney," he said, "is absolutely unprecedented in the annals of jurisprudence in this District, unless my friend is compelled to make this request by an influence which it is unnecessary for me to mention here."

The judge did not sentence Harper to jail. Prison was not necessary, he explained, for the medicine maker's reformation. Harper had changed his labeling after his medicine was seized, and he was not likely to err again. Nonetheless, the manufacturer had not been "an innocent, technical violator of the law, but knew what he was doing." So the judge fined Harper on one count the maximum money penalty under the law, $500, and added a fine of $200 on another count. He had made up his mind, the judge noted, immediately after the jury's verdict, and before "any controversy in the newspapers." Representatives of drug trade associations had attended the trial, the judge observed, for the purpose of reporting the proceedings all over the nation. News of the maximum fine, he hoped, would exercise a deterrent effect on potential violators of the law.[13]

Harper was not unduly chastened. The well-wishing he had been receiving after his castigation by the President, he smilingly told a reporter, made him feel not at all in "the jail bird class." Wiley was not as elated as he might be. "I thought the judge was going to send him to jail," the chemist said later. Harper "had made two million on the product. He was fined $700 . . . and was just $1,999,300 ahead." Many reformers rejoiced that the first court trial under the law was at least a victory. Harper's "money, position, and influence," editorialized a drug magazine, "were unable to save him from the

12 *Wash. Herald*, Apr. 16, 1908.
13 *Ibid.*

stigma of conviction. This phase of the suit and decision is very gratifying." "The lesson to be learned," another drug editor wrote, "is that the law must be obeyed."[14]

[14] *Wash. Star*, Mar. 17, 1908; [*Decatur* (Ill.) *Herald*, Jan. 21, 1913], clipping, Wiley Papers, box 237, Library of Congress (Wiley exaggerated Harper's income from the headache remedy); *Midland Druggist*, cited in *Eclectic Medical Gleaner*, ns 4 (1908), 317; *Pharm. Era*, 39 (Apr. 23, 1908), 513. Harper initiated an appeal from his defeat, but later withdrew it, saying he felt confident of winning, but that victory would require a retrial under the same unsatisfactory conditions as had prevailed before. With label modified, Harper continued to vend his remedy. *Druggists' Circular*, 52 (Nov. 1908), 582; *Oil, Paint and Drug Reporter*, 73 (Apr. 6, 1908), 22.

# 2

# THE LAWLESS CENTURIES*

---

*"For many years, a vast system of medical empiricism, sustained by popular credulity and the sanction of government, has prevailed in this country, to the serious detriment of the public health and morals. . . . The increase of empiricism and of patent medicines within the 19th century, is an evil over which the friends of science and humanity can never cease to mourn."*
—HOUSE REPORT NO. 52, 30TH CONGRESS, 2ND SESSION, 1849

---

IN 1908 Robert Harper of Washington paid a fine for misbranding Cuforhedake Brane-Fude. In 1708 Nicholas Boone of Boston paid a fee for placing the first patent medicine advertisement in an American newspaper. At the Sign of the Bible near the corner of School-House Lane, noted apothecary Boone in the *News-Letter*, he would sell "DAFFY'S Elixir Salutis, very good, at four shillings and sixpence *per* half pint bottle."[1] In the two centuries between the Elixir and the Brane-Fude, patent medicines in America had flourished mightily.

Daffy's Elixir was the first of a score or more of packaged remedies shipped over from the mother country which dominated the American nostrum market during the late colonial years. From Boston to Charleston, from New York to Savannah, merchants advertised Bateman's Pectoral Drops, Turlington's Balsam of Life, Dr. Benjamin Godfrey's Cordial, and other therapeutic wonders. This American advertising was drab, a mere listing of the patent medicine brands just arrived on the latest ships from London and now for sale by apothecary, postmaster, grocer, printer, or physician. More vivid was

---

* This chapter owes its being mainly to the author's *The Toadstool Millionaires: A Social History of Patent Medicines in America before Federal Regulation* (Princeton, 1961).
[1] *Boston News-Letter*, Oct. 4, 1708.

the English prose crowded on the paper wrapper, sealed with wax over the vial of distinctive shape which contained each brand of medicine. Here the proprietor let himself go, boasting of the curative merits of his product, both in his own glowing adjectives and in testimonials from customers who had used his remedy with success.

Some of the English medicines—like Turlington's Balsam—had actually been patented. This proud fact was heralded on the wrapper, indeed, was even molded into the glass. The distinction, however, between patented brands and unpatented ones, like Daffy's Elixir, grew fuzzy in the trade. All brands, patented or not, sat side by side on the same shelf, were listed indiscriminately in the same ads, were spoken of in common parlance as "patent medicines." In time, this lack of distinction was to lead to some confusion. Patenting a nostrum, in England and later in America, required revealing its ingredients, so all might know its composition. But unpatented "patent medicines" made a virtue of their very secrecy. Since most nostrums in the American future were to be unpatented and secret, the term "patent medicine" became increasingly inappropriate. Misnomer though it was, the term stuck tenaciously, despite much criticism.

The American Revolution, disrupting trade as well as other ties between mother country and colony, ended the dominance in America of the old English patent medicine brands. Even before the war, American apothecaries had begun to imitate a flourishing English custom, that of imitating the noted proprietary packages. Importing empty vials (or refilling used ones), importing printed wrappers (or having facsimile versions printed), venturesome Americans marketed their own counterfeit versions of Daffy's Elixir and other British brands. A recent diving operation at old Fort St. Marks has retrieved a lead seal used to affix the wax on wrappers around bottles of Godfrey's Cordial during those days between the French and Indian War and the Revolution when the British owned the Florida peninsula.[2] Neither there nor farther northward was

[2] Correspondence during May and June 1962 with S. J. Olsen of the Florida Geological Survey, Charles H. Fairbanks of Florida State University's Department of Anthropology and Archeology, and George B. Griffenhagen of the American Pharmaceutical Association.

the problem difficult as to what to put in the various vials. Formulas for some of the patent medicines had become official in the London and Edinburgh pharmacopeias, and versions had been included in many popular medical handbooks for laymen, like *Primitive Physic* compiled by the founder of Methodism, John Wesley. Patent medicine formulas were blood brothers of preparations prescribed in the orthodox medicine of the day. The 18th-century physician knew little about the precise action of drugs in relation to given ailments. Polypharmacy was in vogue, and Robert Turlington, in the patent specifications for his Balsam, reflected prevailing orthodox standards in naming 26 botanicals, some from the Orient and some from the English countryside.

In America much deviation occurred from the original formulas, as the practice of filling empty bottles went on apace, booming during the war. But the customer was seldom aware, since bottle shape and wrapper looked familiar, that his English healing draught was being brewed on American shores. After the war British proprietors again dumped their therapeutic wares on the American market, but it was too late for them to regain their pre-Revolutionary ascendancy. American imitations were too widespread and too cheap. The old English medicines came to play a different, a sort of generic, role. Their proprietary status gone, they now were formulas in books, ready for concocting by any wholesale or retail druggist. As such they were much used during the 19th century, nor are they yet completely gone.

Why did not some shrewd colonial, observing the steady sales of British proprietaries, and sensing the gold that might lie at the end of such a rainbow, launch a competitive homegrown remedy? The answer is that there were indeed fumbling efforts heralding the day of native American nostrums. Yet, prior to the Revolution, no American entrepreneur managed to offer a real challenge to Bateman's Pectoral Drops or Hooper's Female Pills. Many mountebanks wandered about the colonies, persuading the gullible to purchase their panaceas: one Francis Torres showed up in Philadelphia selling something called Chinese Stones to cure toothache, cancer, and the bites of mad dogs and rattlesnakes. Moreover, humble men and women, most of them no doubt sincere, went into the marketplace with remedies borrowed from folk medicine, and occasionally advertised them. So Benjamin Franklin's mother-in-law, the Widow Read, promoted "her well-known Ointment for the ITCH."[3] But such commercial efforts were local, sporadic, and limited.

Not until the cultural nationalism accompanying and following the Revolution did the British proprietary example take firm root in American therapeutic soil. Imbued with the pride of victory, the United States gloried in new American text-books, American maps, American inventions, and American drugs. Reputable medicine as well as pseudo-medicine was quickened by the upsurge of patriotism. American physicians sought diligently to discover American herbs which could relieve the American sick of unrepublican dependence on European remedies. Benjamin Rush, a signer of the Declaration of Independence and the new nation's most distinguished physician, proclaimed that there were twenty times more intellect and a hundred times more knowledge in America than there had been before the Revolution.[4] In such a spread-eagle mood, made-in-America patent medicines really began.

Colonial reticence gave way. Some of that shrewdness and boldness that had characterized the English medicine wrappers began to appear in American advertising. The localism of prewar pitches also was abandoned, as several proprietors anxious to sell their products far and wide began to insert column-long advertisements in scores of the ever more numerous newspapers. Few colonial products had borne distinctive names. New Sovereign Ointments, Grand Restoratives, and Damask Lip-Salves came on the market. Congress enacted a patent law under the new federal Constitution, and a few medicine makers looked to government to protect their inventive genius represented in such wonders of medical science as Bilious Pills.

Samuel Lee, jun., of Windham, Connecticut, got the first patent, in 1796. The specifications for his "Bilious Pills" were

[3] *Pa. Gazette*, Aug. 19, 1731.
[4] Rush cited in Oliver Wendell Holmes, *Medical Essays, 1842-1882* (Boston, 1892), 192.

burned in a Patent Office fire, but a later dispensatory gave the ingredients as gamboge, aloes, soap, and nitrate of potassa. Guarded by an American eagle, Lee's remedy went forth to battle bilious and yellow fevers, jaundice, dysentery, dropsy, worms, and female complaints.[5]

This pioneering nostrum maker is a shadowy figure, but some of Lee's character may be deduced. He had ingenuity, as the priority of his patent attests. He possessed vigor, for he made a success of his patent by marketing techniques scarcely yet exploited by American entrepreneurs. He was equipped with imagination, as the cleverness of his advertising attests. One more trait is evident from the scanty record. Samuel Lee had an abundant capacity for indignation, and he had occasion to use it, for three years after he had begun selling his Bilious Pills another Samuel Lee began to trespass on his preserve.

Samuel H. P. Lee was a physician who also lived in Connecticut. In 1799 this New London doctor secured a patent, and the name of his medical invention was also "Bilious Pills." The coincidence seemed too great. The original Samuel, obviously angry, addressed the public on the subject of his upstart rival. After the launching of his own pills, he wrote, "the demand soon became so great and benefits . . . so amply demonstrated" that the New London scoundrel, thinking to "take advantage of the similarity of names and of the credit of my Pills," obtained a patent. The public needed a warning. "If people incautiously purchase his pills for mine," Samuel, jun., cautioned, "I shall not be answerable for their effects."[6]

The national appetite for Bilious Pills was obviously enormous. Drug catalogues listed both varieties, and the Connecticut rivals fought each other from nearby newspaper columns with an acerbity worthy of their English ancestors. The vigor of the competition may have boosted the sale of both brands. When 14 years had expired, each patent was renewed, and on the contest raged. Nor was it limited to Connecticut and sur-

[5] Lyman F. Kebler, "United States Patents Granted for Medicines during the Pioneer Years of the Patent Office," *Jnl. Amer. Pharmaceutical Assoc.*, 24 (1935), 486-87; *Dispensatory of the U.S.* (10th ed., Phila., 1854), 75n.

[6] *Columbian Museum & Savannah* [Ga.] *Advertiser*, Sep. 29, 1802.

rounding states. Early in the 19th century Bilious Pills were being sold in Georgia to the south and in the newly acquired territory west of the Mississippi River. And numerous other aspiring promoters throughout the nation had entered the battle against biliousness.

A critic of nostrums observed sadly as early as 1800, "The venders of patent medicines in almost every capital town in the United States are fattening on the weakness and folly of a deluded public."[7] This was just the first fruits of cultural nationalism applied to the nostrum field.

Patent medicine promoters also profited from the state of regular medicine. During the early 19th century, from the patient's point of view, the arduous impact of disease was aggravated by the arduous impact of therapy. Both as to science and as to ethics, medicine yet rested on unsure foundations. The prevailing American vogue in therapy, owing much to the influence of the patriotic Dr. Rush, stressed extreme bleeding and purging. It was medicine's "heroic" age. Not every sick man felt like being a hero, and irregular practitioners appealed to the cowards with promises of mild medication. Many nostrum makers—like Samuel Lee, jun.—boasted that there was no harsh mercury in their formulas. They pictured regular doctors, armed with scalpels and mercurial purges, as heartless brutes. Physicians, wrote Samuel Thomson, a self-taught botanical irregular, learned nothing about the true nature of the medicines they prescribed except "how much poison [could] be given without causing death."[8]

Suspicion of the regular doctor because of his heroic therapy deepened with the rise of Jacksonian democracy. The upsurge of democratic sentiment in the West and in the poorer sections of cities had its anti-intellectual aspects, and to many citizens the plain man of common sense seemed superior to the trained expert. "The priest, the doctor, and the lawyer," charged Thomson, were all guilty of "deceiving the people." A committee of the New-Hampshire Medical Society reported "so strong an antagonistic feeling" between physicians and the public that

7 *N.Y. Daily Advertiser*, Sep. 18, 1800, citing *Gazette of the U.S.*
8 Cited in Wilson G. Smillie, "An Early Prepayment Plan for Medical Care," *Jnl. Hist. Med. and Allied Sciences*, 6 (1951), 253.

the people considered "their reliance upon nostrums and quack administrations of medicine more valuable than any dependence upon a learned profession." This sentiment was bolstered by the emotional power of popular religion, which opposed the use of male physicians in obstetrical cases and condemned the dissection of cadavers for anatomical study. The judicious might grieve, but the people had their way. In a pioneering report on the public health in Massachusetts, Lemuel Shattuck wrote, "Any one, male or female, learned or ignorant, an honest man or a knave, can assume the name of physician, and 'practice' upon any one, to cure or to kill, as either may happen, without accountability. It's a free country!"[9]

In such an atmosphere of self-reliance, nostrum brands on the market doubled and doubled again. A New York drug catalogue in 1804 listed some 80 or 90 names; by 1857 a Boston catalogue included 500 to 600. Regional and local brands swelled the number. A list compiled in 1858 from newspaper advertising totaled over 1,500 patent medicine names. It took no real medical knowledge to launch a new nostrum. "Any idle mechanic," as an Ohio editor pointed out, could do it. He "by chance gets a dispensatory, or some old receipt book, and poring over it, or having it read to him . . . he finds that mercury is good for the itch, and old ulcers; that opium will give ease; and that a glass of antimony will vomit. Down goes the hammer, or saw, razor, awl, or shuttle—and away to make electuaries, tinctures, elixirs, pills, plasters, and poultices."[10]

The expanding market for patent medicines owed much to the expansion of American newspapers, since a popular press proved a good medium for promoting the sale of popular remedies. At the beginning of the century, there had been 200 papers, some 20 of them issued daily. By 1860 there were nearly 4,000 papers, almost 400 of them dailies. Among the dailies were many examples of the penny press. First begun in the

[9] Samuel Thomson, *New Guide to Health . . . to Which Is Prefixed a Narrative of the Life and Medical Discoveries of the Author* (Boston, 1835), 201; New-Hampshire Medical Society, *Transactions, 1856* (Concord), 36; Shattuck, *Report of the Sanitary Commission of Massachusetts, 1850* (Cambridge, 1948), 58.

[10] *Portsmouth* [Ohio] *Journal*, cited in Madge E. Pickard and R. Carlyle Buley, *The Midwest Pioneer: His Ills, Cures, and Doctors* (N.Y., 1946), 286.

1830's, these were newspapers for the urban masses, flamboyant in both news and advertising. Almost every village had its weekly gazette. Whether in city or village, these papers secured their greatest revenue from advertising, and patent medicine advertisers were the first and most extensive national advertisers. "Nothing can be done without the press," wrote the physician-author of *Quackery Unmasked*. "Enterprise must stop here, and the skill of the wizard be hushed in darkness, unless the Press will publish it to the world."[11] At least one pill man, according to a Congressional committee in 1849, was spending $100,000 a year in advertising his purgative.[12]

Promoters were assisted in other ways by the workings of Jacksonian democracy. The expansion of public elementary education in the North and West better equipped the common man to read the gory symptoms, the glorious cures, the glowing testimonials, of nostrum advertising. Provision for free delivery of newspapers, if published in the county of the subscriber's post office, gave the manufacturer readier access to potential customers. Internal improvements, effected in part through popular pressures, helped the nostrum proprietor convey his wares by wagon, steamboat, and eventually rail to the ailing throughout the nation.

Urbanization, during these same years, brought changes in the disease pattern which offered new opportunities to quackery. After 1815 mortality began to rise, largely as a result of the increase of tuberculosis and the dread typhoid, typhus, and yellow fever. In 1831 cholera appeared. Pulmonic syrups and pectoral lozenges abounded on the nostrum shelf, and remedy makers brazenly promised cures for the worst scourges.

City eating habits aggravated the widespread biliousness—renamed dyspepsia—which had prompted the Lees to market their patented pills. For the dietary dark ages still prevailed and developed a deeper gloom among the urban poor. The belief was widespread that all foods contained one "universal element" which kept life going, so quantity and not quality was stressed. Over-eating was a national habit, an evil com-

[11] Dan King, *Quackery Unmasked* (Boston, 1858), 249.
[12] *Patent Medicines*, 30 Cong., 2 ses., House Rep. 52 (1849), 31.

pounded by a diet stressing starchy dishes, salt-cured meats, and fat-fried foods. Especially lacking in urban diets were fresh fruits and vegetables and milk.

Purges of various potencies were a popular prescription by regular physicians. The quacks, too, as a New York doctor pointed out, fastened on the "almost universal prevalence of indigestion." But no one who read the advertisements needed to be told. There were scores of remedies on the market "whose chief mission," as a pharmacist put it, "appear[ed] to be to open men's purses by opening their bowels."[13]

The unabated suffering from countless ailments, rapid growth in the population of the expanding nation, the spirit of therapeutic laissez-faire in a democratic age, the constant growth in media for advertising, legislation that could be turned to good account—all these were factors broadening the market for vendors of packaged remedies. And the big-scale patent medicine maker, during the first half of the 19th century, blazed a merchandising trail. He was the first American manufacturer to seek out a national market. He was the first producer to help merchants who retailed his wares by going directly to consumers with a message about the product. He was the first promoter to test out a multitude of psychological lures by which people might be enticed to buy his wares. While other advertising in the press was drab, his was vivid; while other appeals were straightforward, his were devilishly clever. The patent medicine promoter was a pioneer, marching at the head of a long procession of other men with ships and shoes and sealing wax to sell.

During the great boom of American industrialism after the Civil War, the nostrum promoter continued in some ways to pace the field. In total money spent for national advertising, the proprietary medicine industry held on to top place throughout the 19th century. Advertising media expanded mightily. The craving for news from the fighting fronts during the Civil War had enlarged the size of daily papers and inflated their circulations. The Sunday edition had been born. Pressure for newsprint hastened the discovery of wood pulp

[13] David M. Reese, *Humbugs of New-York* (N.Y., 1838), 121; George D. Coggeshall, "Address . . . ," *Amer. Jnl. Pharm.*, 26 (1854), 205.

paper, introduced in the seventies. This cheaper paper and technical improvements in the printing process permitted newspaper size and advertising volume to grow. The war years also saw the real beginning of magazine advertising. During the year 1860, for every person in the United States, there had been issued 29.5 copies of daily, weekly, or monthly periodicals. As a result of the revolution launched by the war, the figure had grown to 107.5 by 1900.[14] In almost every case each separate issue was larger in size. There was no limit to the advertising space the venturesome nostrum maker might fill.

In prewar days a purgative proprietor had awed his rivals by achieving a total annual advertising outlay of $100,000. In the closing years of the century, many major nostrum vendors spent two, four, or six times this sum. To carry the messages of Scott's Emulsion and Lydia E. Pinkham's Vegetable Compound to the American people required the expenditure in behalf of each remedy of about $1,000,000 a year.[15]

With the boom in advertising, in the war years and after, the advertising agency, an antebellum infant, passed through a stormy adolescence. Nostrums, as one executive put it, provided the "backbone" of the typical agency's business. Medical advertising "offered the ad.-writer his greatest opportunity," wrote Claude Hopkins, who had himself been through that mill, and "the greatest advertising men of my day were schooled in the medicine field."[16] Thus nostrums were deeply involved in the growing sophistication of business life.

They shared too in another major economic trend of the late 19th century, that toward the concentration of business ownership. Not all of the patent medicine fortunes amassed during these years were a pot of gold at the end of a rainbow that began with a poor man and his recipe. Many of the mightiest entrepreneurs had never mixed a formula, but were men who bought and sold medicines as other men might buy and sell mills or railroads. Charles Crittenton of New York was a merchant-manufacturer of this type, keeping 12,000

[14] George B. Waldron, "What America Spends in Advertising," *Chautauquan*, 38 (Oct. 1903), 156.
[15] *Scientific American*, 73 (Oct. 5, 1895), 214; Jean Burton, *Lydia Pinkham Is Her Name* (N.Y., 1949), 230.
[16] Claude C. Hopkins, *My Life in Advertising* (N.Y., 1927), 73.

proprietary articles in stock, constantly acquiring and launching new brands of his own. The same trend toward concentration, on a smaller scale, went on regionally. In 1904 an Atlanta druggist, Joseph Jacobs, was able to turn over to his pharmacy 82 proprietaries which he had been assembling for nearly 20 years, among them Jacobs' Antikink, Aunt Fanny's Worm Candy, and Palmer's Hole in the Wall Capsules.[17] The trademark for a medicine was a highly marketable commodity, a fixed star in a universe of flux. The formula might change from time to time; the diseases for which medicines were advertised might vary; but the trademark, protected first by common law and then by federal statute, endured forever. Skillful merchandisers like Crittenton amassed whole galaxies of proprietary trademarks.

In this new day of ever-bigger business, the small-time operator found the going hard. Yet the would-be maker of medicines was better off than the beginner in petroleum or steel. Costs of raw products were scarcely higher than before the war, even if promotion was both more expensive and more complex. Certainly formulas were as cheap as ever. Hundreds of hopeful men and women kept coming to the market with their wares. The number of nostrums, it seemed, was almost as "formidable . . . as were the frogs of Egypt." In 1905 a leading drug journal listed the names of over 28,000, and the next year a witness before a Congressional committee estimated that there were 50,000 patent medicines made and sold in the United States.[18] Thus, while there was a trend toward concentration in the proprietary field, it by no means came even within shouting distance of absolute monopoly.

Another form of economic consolidation, characteristic of the times, brought the major medicine manufacturers together in a trade association. Early in the Civil War a group of New York proprietors, hearing that a patent medicine tax was being

[17] *Pharm. Era*, 16 (1896), 968-70; the Jacobs' contract, Aug. 9, 1904, was given to the author by Jerome A. Conner.
[18] William Brewer, "Reminiscences of an Old Pharmacist," *Pharm. Record*, 4 (1884), 326; Philip L. Allen, "Dosing the Public as a Business," *Leslie's Monthly Mag.*, cited in *Druggists' Circular*, 49 (1905), 124; *Hearings before the Committee on Interstate and Foreign Commerce . . . on H.R. 13086* (Wash., 1906), 7.

considered as an emergency revenue measure, sent a delegation to Washington to protest this action. Their journey was in vain. Thaddeus Stevens, chairman of the House Ways and Means Committee, told them, "Gentlemen, you must respond. The country is in peril. We must have money. When this exigency is past, your showing will be considered."[19]

Twenty years later the exigency was long since past, but the 4 per cent tax on the retail price of all proprietary medicines still hung on. Individual protests had been made by medicine manufacturers who believed it unjust to tax the people's right of self-dosage, at least in times of peace. But these had come to nought. To a group of proprietors who had begun meeting informally from time to time in New York, organized pressure seemed to offer greater hope of success. During November 1881, in the office of Charles Crittenton, there was established The Proprietary Medicine Manufacturers and Dealers Association. Immediately they sent off a memorial to Congress urging repeal of the tax. In March 1883 the deed was done.

Right from the start the growing Proprietary Association found other duties to perform. It represented the manufacturers in protracted and vain attempts with trade associations of drug wholesalers and retailers to stabilize nostrum prices. It vented its wrath on certain drug journals that printed formulas purporting to be those of remedies made by Association members. It sought to restrict the infringement of trademarks and the counterfeiting of labels. It lobbied against a tax on grain alcohol used in manufacturing and the arts. It sought to keep another emergency tax, when the Spanish-American War came, at as low a rate as possible. It took quick and decisive action whenever any measure restricting patent medicines was even hinted at in the corridors of state legislatures or the national Congress. In short, the Proprietary Association did those things in the interest of the trade which other trade

[19] Herbert D. Harding, "The History of the Organization among Manufacturers and Wholesale Dealers in Proprietary Articles," *Amer. Druggist*, 36 (1900), 190-93; Frederick Humphreys, "Origin and History of the Association," *Pharm. Era*, 16 (1896), 900-905; Frank A. Blair, "The Proprietary Association, Its History Since the Founding in 1881," *Standard Remedies*, 19 (June 1932), 4-7, 24-26; Frederick J. Cullen, "The First Twenty-Five Years," mimeographed copy of address delivered in May 1956.

associations were doing in the turbulent business economy of the late 19th century.

On the eve of the Civil War, in 1859, the proprietary medicine industry had an output valued in census figures at $3,500,000. By 1904 the sum had multiplied by more than 20 times. An observer reckoned that the value of cocoa and chocolate, blacking and bluing, flavoring extracts and axle grease, beet sugar and glue, castor oil and lard, kindling wood and cosmetics could all be added together, and still the total sum would not bulk so large as the $74,500,000 which was the manufactured value of American patent medicines.[20] At retail prices, the nostrum-taking public paid many millions more.

This great growth in products for self-dosage had taken place during the same decades that saw a revolution in the science of medicine. The "heroic" age of massive interference by the physician with nature's effort to heal the patient had been succeeded, at least on the part of America's most advanced doctors, by therapeutic nihilism, a theory that gave nature the primary role and urged upon the physician extreme caution. Then, in the 1870's, came word from Europe that some interference with nature might be resumed, and for the first time in history on genuinely scientific grounds. For the researches of Louis Pasteur and Robert Koch and their fellow scientists had not only demonstrated that bacilli could cause disease, but that weakened bacilli introduced by inoculation could promote immunity. American physicians had played only a very small part in establishing the germ theory, nor did all of them accept it as valid before the new century. It took time for the separate details of the new medical knowledge to be comprehended, evaluated, coordinated, and applied. The old killers were still the big killers in 1900: influenza and pneumonia, tuberculosis, and gastrointestinal complaints. And the level of education among practicing physicians was discouragingly low. With respect to drugs they received less training than had once been the case, since therapeutic nihilism had weakened the emphasis in the medical curriculum upon pharmacology and the materia medica.

[20] Bureau of the Census, *13th Census of the United States* . . . , VIII, *Manufactures, 1909* (Wash., 1913), 452; Allen, 123.

Being the chameleon-like creature that it is, quackery continued growing during the late 19th century by taking advantage of orthodox medicine's promising prospects as well as its persisting weaknesses. For one thing nostrum makers began to simulate the methods by which medical and pharmaceutical science kept the profession informed of new developments, turning the doctors themselves into unwitting allies in the campaign to reach the public. Articles were planted in medical periodicals reporting exciting therapeutic advances. The names of the new remedies had a scientific lilt, and complex (if non-sensical) formulas were revealed. Reprints were mailed to doctors, who soon were visited by detailmen, talking as knowingly as did the agents of reputable pharmaceutical manufacturers. The truth was, however, that the first prescription which a doctor wrote for products like Fellows' Syrup of Hypophosphites was apt to be the last. When the sufferer looked at the printing on the carton and the pamphlets packed within it, he found enough medical advice in vigorous, down-to-earth, and frightening prose to let him dispense with a doctor. As late as 1915 Fellows' proprietary syrup was still being promoted exclusively to physicians, with not a cent spent on direct advertising to the consumer, but 90 per cent of its sales were over the counter without a prescription.[21]

As to the germ theory itself, many Americans got their first inkling of this signal scientific advance through the distortions of patent medicine advertising. Long before most American physicians had been persuaded of the theory's soundness, a rash of germ-eradicating nostrums had assailed the mass market. One of the boldest was the Microbe Killer invented by a Texas gardener named William Radam. He was willing to credit Pasteur and other titans of natural science with discovering, slowly and laboriously, that a few diseases were caused by bacteria. But these inquirers had been halting and short-sighted, Radam said, and it had been left for him to discover the whole truth, that all diseases were caused by microbes.

[21] Solomon Solis Cohen, "Shall Physicians Become Sales-Agents for Patent Medicines?" Phila. County Med. Soc., *Proceedings*, 13 (1892), 213-16; George H. Simmons, "Work of the Council on Pharmacy and Chemistry," *Southern Med. Jnl.*, 8 (1915), 259-65.

Killing microbes was like killing bugs on plants, and Radam's pale pink liquid, he asserted, killed all microbes and hence cured all disease. The Microbe Killer contained, according to governmental analysis, 99.381 per cent water.[22] The rest—what rest there was—was hydrochloric and sulphuric acids and red wine. The liquid was nonetheless potent enough to float Radam from his Texas acres to a New York mansion overlooking Central Park.

Quacks were just as quick to exploit advances in the physical sciences as they were to pervert biological achievements. The discovery of radium by the Curies gave a cue to Dr. Rupert Wells, though even his name was a fake. He called his medicine Radol, labeled it as "radium impregnated," and advertised that it would cure all cancer. The liquid was really an acid solution of quinine sulphate with alcohol added, and such a product could be expected to exhibit the bluish fluorescent glow which Wells attributed to radium. But Radol, as a critic said, contained "exactly as much radium as dishwater" did and had the same therapeutic powers when treating cancer.[23]

Thus the glamor of new science was twisted to benefit the unscrupulous promoter and to injure poor, suffering humanity, ill equipped to differentiate between the valid and the specious in the realm of health. Nonetheless, even with respect to quackery, the public was gaining by the advance of scientific discovery. For never before in history had there been so firm a foundation of medical and pharmaceutical knowledge on which to build a sound critique of quackery.

On commonsense grounds, medical quackery had long been assailable. Judicious men had, of course, always known that many advertising boasts could not be true. During the heroic age critics had often pointed out that nostrums promoted as

[22] The American Medical Association issued three volumes on *Nostrums and Quackery*, all published in Chicago. The first volume appeared in 1911 with a 2nd ed. in 1912; the second volume, edited by Arthur J. Cramp, was published in 1921; the third volume, also edited by Cramp, was published in 1936 and bore the longer title, *Nostrums and Quackery and Pseudo-Medicine*. In references below, the titles of all three volumes are abbreviated as *N&Q*, and the 2nd ed. of the first volume is used. The Microbe Killer analysis is at i, 447.

[23] *Ibid.*, 68-75; Samuel Hopkins Adams, *The Great American Fraud* (Chicago, 1906), 91.

cures for mercurial poisoning were themselves loaded with mercury. As part of the humanitarian wave accompanying Jacksonian democracy, there had occurred the nation's first major campaign against medical quackery. Perceptive physicians, like Oliver Wendell Holmes, had written and spoken out against dishonest therapeutic claims, faked statistics, fabricated testimonials, hazardous ingredients, and other disreputable features of the nostrum game. But so long as the causes of disease were a mystery even to physicians, and their own curative attempts were mistakenly bold—as with heroic treatment —or circumspectly hesitant, their critique of quackery could not be completely persuasive.

In 1889 a physician-pharmacist named R. G. Eccles exposed the watery formula of William Radam's Microbe Killer and termed the ex-gardener a "misguided crank" intent on "outquacking the worst quacks of this or any other age" while earning profits of 6,000 per cent. "A universal microbe killer," the doctor asserted, "would necessarily be a universal life destroyer."[24] Dr. Eccles represents a new and sounder type of attack on quackery: the Microbe Killer and other specious nostrums could be measured against the yardstick of the new bacteriology and the new chemistry. The yardstick was not yet as precise a tool as it would become, but it was already capable of measuring many of quackery's weaknesses with considerable precision.

The Eccles critique had appeared in a trade paper, the *Druggists' Circular*. Similar exposures were printed in medical journals, although reforming doctors were so concerned with the Fellows' Syrup of Hypophosphites type of racket within their own ranks that their attacks on old-fashioned patent medicines promoted directly to consumers were only sporadic. The lay public, of course, did not read either the *Druggists' Circular* or the *Journal of the American Medical Association*. Nor did they see in any great number the occasional antinostrum bulletins coming from the pens of a new type of scientist, the agricultural chemist. The Civil War had launched a boom in canned and packaged foods. Greater remoteness of producer from consumer, with complicated processing in be-

[24] *Druggists' Circular*, 33 (1889), 195-96.

tween, coupled with new chemical techniques, led many manufacturers to sophisticate the foods they packaged. Farmers were aroused at the use of chemistry to revive rancid butter and recolor aged peas. What chemists had learned to disguise, the farmers began to realize, chemists could learn to detect. On state payrolls there began to appear agricultural chemists, men interested not only in exposing fraud in food, but intrigued by any crookedness involving chemistry. From Connecticut to North Dakota, these chemists began to issue official pamphlets reporting the real ingredients in nostrums and denouncing the falsity of label claims. Valuable as these bulletins were, their circulation was slim.

Nor was there much else that the layman might read, in the waning years of the 19th century, wherein he might find patent medicines questioned. An occasional farm journal assumed a skeptical stance; *Popular Science Monthly* was steadily hostile; the *Ladies' Home Journal* took a stern view of nostrums that were liquor in disguise. Most magazines and newspapers, however, were a haven for the patent medicine advertiser, not for his critic. Indeed, the remedy proprietor developed a technique to try to make sure that this continued to be so. He invented a "red clause" to insert in advertising contracts. "It is mutually agreed," the red type read, "that this Contract is void, if any law is enacted by your State restricting or prohibiting the manufacture or sale of proprietary medicines." This clause, boasted the maker of Hall's Catarrh Cure to his fellow members of the Proprietary Association, was "pretty near a sure thing." It could be pointed to explicitly, from time to time, when danger threatened from some legislative proposal.[25] During the 1890's, therefore, the newspaper reader saw columns of patent medicine advertising, but almost no questioning of patent medicine efficacy.

With the dawn of the new century came the Progressive period, and with the Progressive period came a vigorous crusade against patent medicines that reached fruition in the anti-nostrum provisions of the 1906 Pure Food and Drugs Act. Voices of reform, hitherto muted and isolated, gained strength

---

[25] Mark Sullivan, *The Education of an American* (N.Y., 1938), 188-91; *Collier's*, 36 (Nov. 4, 1905), 13-16, 25.

and cohesion during the Progressive years and reached the ears of most Americans, who now, alarmed at the evils threatening the nation's institutions, were anxious to control them. Malefactors of wealth—and the patent medicine proprietor could be made to fit this category—were placing in jeopardy ancient virtues like freedom, honesty, cleanliness, the integrity of the political process.

The "muckraking" of nostrums was a collaborative effort, now possible because of the Progressive climate of opinion, dependent for its raw data on the new knowledge in medicine and chemistry. The American Medical Association at long last purged its journal of questionable advertising, and the Council on Pharmacy and Chemistry, created to supervise this effort, made its investigations known to other foes of nostrums. Drug journal editors did likewise, and state chemists pooled their knowledge of nostrum analyses. Most important, all of these scientists were eager to furnish specific information on proprietary articles to lay reporters.

For an increasing number of newspaper editors, the "red clause" lost its deterrent force during the Progressive years. William Allen White's *Emporia Gazette* led a procession of papers willing to point out to readers the hazards of self-dosage with patent medicines. But the main medium through which the broad public learned of nostrum evils was the popular magazine. The *Ladies' Home Journal* broadened its attack to other types of quackery besides high-alcoholic bitters, especially after losing a libel suit. In an editorial, Edward Bok had listed the ingredients of various nostrums, citing a document some quarter of a century old that had been issued by the Massachusetts State Board of Health. One of the medicines did not contain the ingredients Bok had mentioned, and the careless mistake proved costly. But it spurred Bok to greater relentlessness in his anti-nostrum efforts, using fresh and accurate information gathered for him by a young, Harvard-trained journalist and lawyer named Mark Sullivan.[26]

The most provocative and exciting muckraking effort aimed at patent medicines was the Samuel Hopkins Adams series

[26] *Ladies' Home Jnl.*, 21 (May 1904), 18, and (July 1904), 18; Bok, *The Americanization of Edward Bok* (N.Y., 1923), 342-43.

that began in late 1905 in the pages of *Collier's,* then under the enlightened editorship of Norman Hapgood. Adams was a free-lance journalist, who rendered his judgment of nostrums in his series title, "The Great American Fraud." He had done sleuthing as a crime reporter and had written articles on medical developments. This background helped him in his investigations, and he also relied on counsel from agricultural chemists and editors of pharmaceutical journals. The result was a series crammed with facts and imbued with moral passion.[27]

"Gullible America," Adams began, "will spend this year some seventy-five million dollars in the purchase of patent medicines. In consideration of this sum it will swallow huge quantities of alcohol, an appalling amount of opiates and narcotics, a wide assortment of varied drugs ranging from powerful and dangerous heart depressants to insidious liver stimulants; and, far in excess of other ingredients, undiluted fraud. For fraud, exploited by the skilfulest of advertising bunco men, is the basis of the trade."

After this sweeping introduction, Adams got down to cases. He rebuked Pond's Extract for "trading on the public alarm" by running an advertisement baldly headed "MENINGITIS" while New York was suffering an epidemic. Next to his criticism was a reproduction of the offending ad. Adams reported on the institution of the "red clause" and demonstrated his words with a picture of the contract offered by a proprietary company to the *Emporia Gazette.*

The whole series was equally explicit and vivid. Adams exposed the boozers and bracers that did a brisk business in prohibition territory. He examined the fake antiseptics, like Radam's Microbe Killer. His bitterest venom Adams reserved for catarrh powders that contained cocaine and soothing syrups that contained opium. It was a "shameful trade," he asserted, "that stupefies helpless babies and makes criminals of our young men and harlots of our young women." He attacked the pain-killers overloaded with acetanilid—like Cuforhedake Brane-Fude—and condemned all nostrums, whether they contained active ingredients or were inert, which preyed on the

[27] The series ran in *Collier's* between Oct. 7, 1905, and Feb. 17, 1906; a second series ran between July 14 and Sep. 22, 1906.

incurables, offering false hope to men and women suffering from consumption, epilepsy, and heart disease.

The only effective method of curtailing patent medicine abuses, Adams believed, was the enactment of a national law. Efforts to secure such a law from Congress were at high tide when "The Great American Fraud" series went to press. For a quarter of a century, from time to time, food and drug bills had been before Congress, seldom reaching a vote in either House. Proprietary manufacturers had been wary but not worried through most of these years, since the proposed national bills specifically excluded their medicines from control. State formula disclosure bills had been the grave threat. By 1903, however, the Proprietary Association was much concerned. In the atmosphere of Progressivism, successful passage of a national law seemed close at hand. Could patent medicines preserve the favored exempt status they had in earlier bills? The prospect did not look promising. Many critics demanded that legislation extend to proprietary remedies. The voice of one man in particular worried the proprietors. He was the generalissimo of the pure food crusaders, Harvey Washington Wiley.

Wiley was a state chemist who had gone to Washington.[28] Born in southern Indiana, he had been trained as a doctor, though he never practiced. It was the nutritional side of health that interested him. In 1874, after study at Harvard, Wiley became professor of chemistry at the newly opened Purdue and, simultaneously, state chemist of Indiana. One of his tasks was to reveal the extent to which cane sugars and syrups sold in the state were adulterated with glucose. In 1883 Wiley became chief chemist of the Department of Agriculture. With him to Washington went his antipathy to adulteration. Enlarging upon the modest beginnings of his predecessor, Wiley launched a continuing analysis of America's food and drink, revealing in 1,400 pages published over 16 years how nearly every item on the family dinner table was being modified by "creative" chemistry. When the first Congressional hearings

[28] An excellent biography of Wiley is Oscar E. Anderson, Jr., *The Health of a Nation: Harvey W. Wiley and the Fight for Pure Food* (Chicago, 1958).

were held on a pure food bill, in 1899, Wiley was scientific adviser to the Senate committee, first witness, and chief draftsman of the bill presented in the Senate.

Wiley also undertook to arouse public opinion to the need for a law. Raised in an evangelical home, the chief chemist applied his moral fervor to the pure food crusade. The science of his bulletins was buttressed by the passion of his oratory. Like an itinerant preacher, he stumped up and down the country, and every women's club rostrum was a pulpit. Like most Progressives, his sense of righteousness was offended by fraud, and he inveighed against adulterators as economic cheats.

"Dr. Wiley is built on large lines," a journalist wrote of him. "He is tall and massive of stature, with a big head firmly poised above a pair of titanic shoulders. His hair never stays in order, but masses itself forward on both sides of the forehead, giving him at times a somewhat uncouth appearance. The penetrating glance of his rather small eyes, the large and roughly modeled nose, and the severe lines of his mouth add to this impression."[29] Wiley had a light touch and a warm heart. His wit was the talk of the banquet circuit, and he had a flair for clever doggerel. A bachelor, he was free to move about, and he was an ardent clubman, an eager dinner guest. Wiley had the knack of eliciting tremendous loyalty, and his personal associations, tending toward the conspiratorial, were as important as his public speaking in creating organized pressure for a food and drug bill. Endowed with tremendous energy, he could operate without tiring on several fronts at once.

Wiley's main interest was fraudulent food; this had monopolized his research time and oratory. Of course, he abominated medical quackery, but it had held a low priority among his concerns. As chief chemist he had collected "bales of advertising of fraudulent remedies," and his bureau had tested "lost manhood" treatments for the Post Office Department. In 1903 he got around to expressing himself forthrightly in public on

[29] Edwin Björkman, "Our Debt to Dr. Wiley," *World's Work*, 19 (1910), 12,443.

the nostrum issue. The new law that soon would come, he said, should contain "stringent" controls over patent medicines "especially."[30]

Since Wiley had hitherto gone along with draft bills that exempted proprietary medicines, his call now for tight controls sounded especially ominous to the remedy makers. It came at a time of increasing tempo of anti-nostrum publicity, and it was shortly followed by a Senate bill that defined drugs in a sweeping way and stated that any drug was adulterated which fell below the professed standard under which it was sold. For the first time in a Congressional hearing, proprietary remedies were extensively debated. This particular bill did not pass. But the pressure on proprietors was great enough to jar their intransigence. They forsook their adamant opposition to a national bill that controlled proprietary remedies in any way and centered on versions sponsored by the Wiley-led reformers. At a special secret meeting in December 1905, the Proprietary Association called for an end to nostrums containing narcotics and remedies overloaded with alcohol. They urged their committee on legislation to work for a law that would exercise restraint in these respects. It was close to the midnight hour. Samuel Hopkins Adams' "Fraud" series was in full swing, and President Theodore Roosevelt, somewhat tardily, had just spoken out in behalf of a national law.

A Senate bill was passed in February 1906, with a moderate set of nostrum controls, weakened from the stronger initial version after considerable floor debate. The House bill, containing more rigorous provisions, seemed for a time destined to suffer the fate of earlier bills, death by inaction. Then the shocking impact of Upton Sinclair's novel, *The Jungle,* with its incidental description of the horribly unhygienic way in which American meat was processed, made a pure food law inevitable.

The House debate in June made clear how much wider was the awareness of the nostrum menace than it had been five years, even a year, before. To be sure, no attention need be given meat, for a separate inspection bill had already been

[30] Wiley, "Drugs and Their Adulterations and the Laws Relating Thereto," *Washington Medical Annals,* 2 (1903), 205-28.

swept through the House. There was discussion of the food, whiskey, and administrative provisions of the bill, themes which had dominated debate in earlier Congresses. But the main theme was the patent medicine evil. "Of all the great civilized nations of the earth," stated a Texan, "the United States is about the only one that has not a strict law on the subject." Even Russia did, he added. For every illness caused by unclean meat, insisted another member, there were a hundred cases of poisoning and death from nostrums. More than that, tainted meat was not habit-forming. Congressmen were chided for giving testimonials to proprietary concerns. "Indeed," jibed a member, "Peruna seems to be the favorite Congressional drink." The anti-nostrum provisions, asserted the Congressman from Adams' home district, were "the most important subjects of the bill." Others expressed the same sentiment, and the name of Adams came frequently into the debate. Congressman James R. Mann acknowledged with appreciation that the list of dangerous drugs which must be named on medicine labels had been drawn up with the journalist's help. Wiley, too, had been at Mann's elbow throughout the final stages of House consideration, supplying clippings, nostrum analyses, and advice on strategy. Women's organizations and the American Medical Association exerted significant pressure for a rigorous bill.[31]

The House bill passed on June 23, and from the House and Senate conference to reconcile their different versions, nostrum provisions emerged somewhat stronger than they had been in either bill. On June 30 Theodore Roosevelt put his signature to the Pure Food and Drugs Act, a measure often spoken of at the time and since as Dr. Wiley's law.

Almost all segments of opinion greeted the new law with approval. The most ardent champions of the pure food and drug cause were too optimistic in their appraisal. As a result of the act, editorialized the New York Times, "the purity and honesty of the food and medicines of the people are guaran-

[31] Cong. Record, 59 Cong., 1 ses., 8,889-9,801; Wiley, "The Value of the Food and Drug Act to the Consumer," Chautauquan Daily, July 29, 1908, clipping in box 191, Wiley Papers, Library of Congress; James G. Burrow, AMA, Voice of American Medicine (Baltimore, 1963), 74-83.

teed." The patent medicine provisions, predicted the *Nation,* would deal a "death-blow" to harmful nostrums. The law was "far better in every respect," asserted the *Journal of the American Medical Association,* than its most ardent supporters could have hoped. "Certainly the powerful Proprietary Association of America has not proved to be so powerful after all."[32]

Yet the Proprietary Association was not unhappy. Frank J. Cheney, its president, thought it was "silly" to require him to put a new label on Hall's Catarrh Cure just because it contained "a trifling amount of alcohol." But the general effect of the law, he said, would be good. "People generally will reason, and reason correctly, that preparations which come up to the requirements of a congressional enactment must be all right, or, certainly, that they are not harmful or dangerous." Even the *National Druggist,* most acrimonious foe of legislation, termed the final result "not such a terrible thing after all." "But let it not be supposed," the editor added, "that the law would have been enacted in its present rather innocuous form but for hard, intelligent and most tactful work on the part of the representatives of the interests it is intended to regulate."[33]

As to proprietary remedies, the new Wiley law required that the labels which manufacturers put upon their medicines must tell the truth—not the whole truth, but the truth in certain significant respects. The presence and amount of certain dangerous drugs—alcohol, the opiates, chloral hydrate, acetanilid, and several others—must always be stated on the package. Other ingredients need not be named unless the proprietor wished to, but if he chose to indicate that certain substances were present, they must indeed be there, and in the quantity claimed. If he asserted that certain ingredients were not present—denying that a nostrum contained opium was a favorite promotional device—then they must in fact be missing. As the law put it, a remedy was adulterated "if its strength or purity fall below the professed standard under which it is sold." If a proprietor could not beguile consumers

[32] *N.Y. Times,* July 1, 1906; *Nation,* 82 (1906), 523; *JAMA,* 47 (1906), 42, 116.
[33] *Ntl. Druggist,* 36 (1906), 210, 372.

with respect to ingredients, neither could he deceive in other respects or be guilty of misbranding. He could not misinform about the state, territory, or country in which his product was made. Nor, indeed, could he put upon his label "any statement, design, or device" regarding the medicine or its ingredients which was "false or misleading in any particular."[34]

Keep quiet on the label or do not lie, the law said. Respecting the listed dangerous ingredients, silence was forbidden. Thus the law did not strike a blow against self-medication, but sought to make it safer. It was based on a favorite Progressive assumption, an assumption as old as American independence, that the average man was intelligent enough to plot his own course and would avoid risks if he was aware of them.

The Pure Food and Drugs Act represents a new Progressive assumption as well, that the national government can and must deal directly with aspects of natural science imbued with great public concern. Science and democracy were not, to the progressive, incompatible. The objectivity and dedication to truth which science represented were needed for the securing of economic and political justice. And the fruits of science must be used by government for the general welfare. The National Bureau of Standards was established in 1901, and the Bureau of the Census, giving permanence to what had been a makeshift decennial venture, was created in 1902.[35]

In the realm of public health, the urgency was especially great. It was more than a matter of humanitarian concern: the national interest was vitally involved. Health was a valuable American asset subject to extravagant waste. "If we appraise each life lost," wrote Irving Fisher, chairman of the Committee of One Hundred on National Health, in 1909, "at only $1,700 and each year's average earnings for adults at only $700, the economic gain to be obtained from preventing preventable disease, measured in dollars, exceeds one and a half billions."

[34] Ch. 3,915, 34 Stat. 768.
[35] A. Hunter Dupree, *Science in the Federal Government: A History of Policies and Activities to 1940* (Cambridge, Mass., 1957), 279, 291-92, 300-301, 385. Dupree, 296-97, suggests that, during the Progressive years, government science was marked by practicality, utility; basic research was not deemed a proper function of government, but of the universities.

Governmental as well as private action was mandatory to preserve this indispensable natural resource. Thus did Progressivism link its passion for conservation to the public health.[36]

With respect to health, the national government took many concrete steps during the Progressive years. It set up the Yellow Fever Board in Cuba (1900), transformed the Hygienic Laboratory of the Marine Hospital Service into the Public Health Service (1902 to 1912), established tests and licensing for manufacturers of serums and vaccines (1902), and participated in the first effort aimed at international control of narcotics (1909), as well as seeking to regulate narcotics within the nation's borders (1914). Thus the food and drug law was part of a much broader pattern.[37]

Both despair and hope, a characteristic Progressive mood, marked the atmosphere in which these federal actions took place. Irving Fisher and other commentators could, with much justice, bemoan the needlessly high death rate, the tardiness in applying hygienic knowledge already learned, the inadequate training of many physicians. The very fact of the lamentations, however, was an optimistic sign, indicating that America had ceased to take for granted its second-rate status in medical science. The future was bright. "The world is gradually awakening to the fact of its own improvability," wrote Fisher. "Hygiene, the youngest of the biological studies, has repudiated the outworn doctrine that mortality is fatality, and must exact a regular and inevitable sacrifice at the present rate year after year. Instead of this fatalistic creed we now have the assurance of Pasteur that 'It is within the power of man to rid himself of every parasitic disease.'"[38]

If expectations of a millennium of health soared too high, Pasteur and his successors were indeed providing health reformers with legitimate grounds for hope. Besides new biologi-

[36] Fisher, *Report on National Vitality: Its Wastes and Conservation* (Bull. 30, Committee of One Hundred on National Health: Wash., 1909), 1; Richard H. Shryock, *The Development of Modern Medicine* (N.Y., 1947), 403-405.

[37] Dupree, 264-69; H. J. Anslinger and William F. Tompkins, *The Traffic in Narcotics* (N.Y., 1953), 29-30.

[38] Dupree, 299; Fisher, 14.

cal vaccines and antitoxins, the new century brought to the United States from Germany the first results of modern chemotherapy, especially Paul Ehrlich's salvarsan for treating syphilis. During the same years, sanitation techniques that could virtually eliminate insect-transmitted yellow fever and malaria and curtail epidemics of typhoid fever spread by water and milk were being proved and improved. A better understanding of nutrition arrived with the new century; the first years of the food and drug law's operation coincided with animal experiments demonstrating the need for minerals and vitamins in the diet. In 1911 the word "vitamine" was coined.[39]

Cities and states, as well as the national government, accelerated their application of health research to the welfare of the citizenry. So likewise did private philanthropy, as represented by the Rockefeller Foundation and the Carnegie Institution, and so did national voluntary societies, pioneered in 1904 by the National Tuberculosis Association, each aiming its activities against a major disease. The American Medical Association employed the yardstick of the new science not only to exclude nostrum advertising from its journal, but also to elevate the standards of medical practice, education, and hospitals.[40]

Much might be done for the American by governments and private organizations, but the citizen in a democracy possessed great personal responsibility for his own health. Progressivism conjoined corporate and personal endeavor for desirable ends. Popular magazine articles, large traveling exhibits, courses in the school curriculum, all were used to alert Americans to a properly hygienic mode of life.[41] Skepticism with respect to patent medicines was one part of this mode, but only one. Children also marched about singing, to the tune of the Battle Hymn of the Republic, this didactic ditty:

[39] Dupree, 269; Shryock, *Development of Modern Medicine*, 438-49; Julius Stieglitz, ed., *Chemistry in Medicine* (N.Y., 1928), 123-40, 333-35, 397, 464-66, 485; Glenn Sonnedecker, "The Concept of Chemotherapy," *Amer. Jnl. Pharmaceutical Education*, 26 (1962), 1-3; David L. Cowen, "Ehrlich the Man, the Scientist," *ibid.*, 4-11.

[40] Stieglitz, 333-35, 653-54; Dupree, 297-99; Shryock, *National Tuberculosis Association, 1904-1954* (N.Y., 1957), Preface; Burrow, 27-53.

[41] Shryock, *Development of Modern Medicine*, 317, 330; Shryock, *National Tuberculosis Association*, 100-103.

The filthy fly is flying in a flight that's strong and fleet;
He carries germs and microbes in his mouth and on his
feet;
Let us swat the dirty insect with a blow that's swift and
neat,
While he is flying on.[42]

The effort, therefore, to punish a prominent citizen of the nation's capital for mislabeling his Cuforhedake Brane-Fude was not an isolated incident. It was one event in a great campaign to improve the public health. If, during the Progressive years, the great campaign, and, within it, the anti-nostrum crusade, were pursued with too great expectations, they nonetheless both were worthy and both made significant gains in behalf of American health.

[42] Gary Webster [Webb B. Garrison], *Codfish, Cats and Civilization* (Garden City, N.Y., 1959), 135.

# 3

# A DECADE OF ENFORCEMENT

*"Half success is the best that can be claimed for the Pure Food Law insofar as it affects nostrums. The reason is that we who fought to get the law passed aimed at the wrong side of the bottle. We should have attacked the advertisements in the newspapers. That is where the real damage is done."*
—SAMUEL HOPKINS ADAMS, 1915[1]

THE Cuforhedake Brane-Fude case was a dramatic victory but not an accurate harbinger of the fate of nostrum makers under the 1906 law. The nature of Harvey Wiley's interests, the shrewdness of proprietors, the decisions of judges, all joined to hold enforcement of the patent medicine provisions to a very modest level indeed.

Dr. Wiley's dominating passion was pure food, and it controlled his enforcement decisions as it had earlier influenced his crusading. Of the first 1,000 judgments rendered under the law, covering cases up to mid-1911, only 135 actions concerned proprietary medicines. Food adulteration, to the Bureau chief, constituted a greater threat to the public than patent medicines and, considering the limited personnel available, must be given top priority.[2]

This policy meant no abatement in Wiley's hostility to quackery. Right from the start, he sought to make the law as effective an anti-nostrum weapon as he could. The job of regulation-making was imposed by the act upon the Secretaries of Agriculture, Commerce, and the Treasury, and these cabinet

[1] *Harper's Wkly.*, 60 (1915), 155.
[2] Anderson, *The Health of a Nation*, 197-259; James C. Munch and James C. Munch, Jr., "Notices of Judgment—the First Thousand," *Food Drug Cosmetic Law Jnl.*, 10 (1955), 219-42 [Hereafter cited as FDC Law Jnl.].

officers delegated the responsibility to three subordinates, Wiley serving as chairman. Announcing a tentative set of rules, the three-man commission held hearings in New York. Representatives of the food and drug industries came to question and to protest. The proposed regulations, in the words of one pharmacist, hit the drug trade with "the shock of a volcanic explosion."[3]

What bothered the proprietary manufacturers was the way in which the regulations stretched the law. The law did not precisely define "label"; the commission wanted "label" to include pamphlets packed in the carton. The law forbade a false statement with respect to place of manufacture; the commission insisted that the true place of manufacture be given. And so it went, even to the size of type required in labeling. Proceedings were "friendly and courteous," but there were tensions held in check. The main points of the commission's draft, accepted by the three cabinet secretaries, struck many in the drug trade as "so comprehensive as greatly to supplement the act."[4]

This sort of protest did not deter Wiley at all. He went even further in tightening the screws through interpretations of the regulations which he began to draft for the Secretary of Agriculture to promulgate. Intent on vigorous protection of the consumer, Wiley would sometimes brush aside the suggestion by his associates that some prospective step was not countenanced by the law. The chief would answer: "We must read it into the law!"[5]

At the same time, Wiley was interested in securing as much voluntary compliance as possible by informing the trade as to the law's provisions. There were deputations to consult with, speeches to deliver, correspondence to read and answer. Scores of letters flowed into the red-brick Bureau of Chemistry build-

[3] Secy. of Agric. James Wilson to Wiley, July 24, 1906, Wiley Papers, box 60, Library of Congress; John Uri Lloyd, "The National Pure Food and Drug Act," reprint from *Eclectic Medical Gleaner*, May 1907, 5.

[4] *Amer. Druggist*, 49 (1906), 158, 173-78; *Bull. Pharmacy*, 20 (1906), 441-42; the regulations were reprinted in 59 Cong., 2 ses., Sen. Document 252.

[5] Fred B. Linton, "Federal Food and Drug Laws—Leaders Who Achieved Their Enactment and Enforcement," *FDC Law Jnl.*, 4 (1949), 462.

ing, from the lawyers of major medicine concerns, from Congressmen in the interest of their constituents, from small-time proprietors themselves, begging for information. "I can't find out from any one what is what about the new law that takes effect," wrote a druggist who made a skin ointment, "and perhaps I will never know. . . . I am not looking for trouble and if your department will help me, will avoid it. The law is too complicated for poor devils to understand it."[6]

Wiley and Dr. Kebler, chief of the drug laboratory, responded patiently to the poor devils who sought help.[7] They assigned them guaranty numbers in return for a promise that their products were not adulterated or misbranded within the meaning of the law. This regulation was a way of absolving retail druggists of responsibility for wares on their shelves that might prove to be illegal. "It should be distinctly understood, however," Wiley and Kebler warned proprietary manufacturers, "that the filing of a guaranty and the securing of a serial number does not in any way mean that the Government guarantees your products." The chief chemist and his aide advised against use of the word "cure" on labels, except in cases beyond medical dispute. "The term 'corn cure,'" Wiley observed drolly in one instance, "is in itself a misnomer, because it is not the corn that is ill and needs to be cured." They raised questions about the appropriateness of nostrum names. "You ask," a Kansas promoter responded, "what connection Mexican has to do with my [Barb Wire] Liniment. Nothing whatever only a name."[8]

[6] *Amer. Druggist*, 50 (1907), 35-37, 48-50; numerous letters in Incoming Corres. of the Bur. of Chem., RG 97, NA; the quote from Leopold Kusnick, Cincinnati, Dec. 6, 1906. Congressman W. C. Adamson inquired Dec. 21, 1906, about Horn of Salvation, made by a Newnan, Ga., constituent.

[7] The Drug Laboratory was organized Mar. 1, 1903, and was renamed the Division of Drugs Jan. 1, 1908. Lyman F. Kebler, its chief, had come to the Bureau after a decade's experience as chief chemist at a Philadelphia pharmaceutical manufacturing concern. "Division of Drugs," ms. by Kebler in folder "Drug Lab" (243), Bur. of Chem., General Corres., 1909, RG 97, NA; *Who's Who in America, 1914-1915*, 285-86.

[8] Wiley to Indian Black Vegetable S. & R. Co., Dec. 26, 1906, and Wiley to Amer. Druggist Publishing Co., Dec. 21, 1906, from Letterbooks, General Corres., Bur. of Chem., RG 97, NA. Harry Leonard to

Many proprietors wrote in that they were voluntarily modifying their labels, and some admitted to making changes in ingredients. The changes might be slight and they might be grudging, but they were detectable. "So far as I have gone," Samuel Hopkins Adams wrote to Wiley in 1907, "I find a general disposition to obey the law in the letter, though to evade it as far as possible in the spirit." "Our experience," Wiley answered, "is in accord with yours."[9]

One token of voluntary change was a marked reduction in the narcotic content of patent medicines, especially those marketed by large-scale manufacturers. The composition of Mrs. Winslow's Soothing Syrup, for example, a particular whipping boy of the nostrum muckrakers, was modified, first to cut down on the percentage of morphine present, then to eliminate it altogether. The Harrison Narcotic Act of 1914 accelerated this trend by placing a ceiling—considered low at the time—on the amount of such drugs which proprietaries could contain. The proportion of alcohol in patent medicines also declined after 1906, although voluntaryism was supported by pressure from the Commissioner of Internal Revenue, who taxed proprietors whose wares seemed to exist mainly to satisfy the thirsty in the ever-expanding prohibition territory. To avoid the tax, the makers of Hostetter's Bitters reduced their alcohol from 39 to 25 per cent and "decidedly" increased the amount of cinchona and serpentaria in their remedy. "The demand for these new Bitters," the president told the stockholders, "is entirely problematical."[10]

The "before" and "after" picture, that ancient promotional technique among nostrum proprietors, now furnished the cue for their opponents. Many famous American labels did not

James Wilson, Dec. 3, 1906, Incoming Corres., Bur. of Chem., RG 97, NA.

[9] For example, Erso Proprietary Co. to Secy. of Agric., received Dec. 29, 1906, and The Herpicide Co. to Bur. of Chem., Nov. 8, 1906, Incoming Corres., Bur. of Chem., RG 97, NA. Adams to Wiley, Mar. 26, 1907, and Wiley to Adams, Apr. 1, 1907, Gen. Corres., RG 97, NA.

[10] John P. Street, "The Patent Medicine Situation," *Amer. Jnl. of Public Health*, 7 (1917), 1037-38; *Jnl. Amer. Pharmaceutical Assoc.*, 7 (1918), 71; *Bull. Pharmacy*, 22 (1908), 332-34, 444; President's reports, 1908 and 1909, Minute Book of the Hostetter Company, examined in the Hostetter Corporation archives, Pittsburgh, 1956.

look the same after 1906 as they had looked before. A good deal of the change was voluntary, to avoid trouble with the law. The labeling sections, noted a journal representing the interests of the major proprietors, "caused some serious introspection . . . and many abuses which had crept into the business were remedied." Manufacturers, this journal explained, had made exaggerated claims through ignorance on the part of their medical or chemical advisers or through the excessive enthusiasm of their advertising or sales managers. Whatever the reasons, the situation required change, and change there was. Nostrum critics were not averse to reproducing for the consumer these "before" and "after" views, or to picturing side by side labels used on the same proprietaries prepared for sale in America and in England, where labeling restrictions were as yet not so severe. Piso's Cure for Consumption, for example, had become Piso's Remedy, A Medicine for Coughs and Colds.[11]

Occasionally, when the letter of the law was violated, the government went to court, and it won the vast majority of cases. In one way the Brane-Fude case did prove to be a precedent: convictions did not bring imprisonment. If Wiley hoped that the Harper decision would establish a tradition of maximum fines for those proved guilty, he was destined to be disappointed. Only rarely were fines levied at the top figure, which was $200 for interstate violations. More often the sums assessed were very low, from $50 down to one cent. Only rarely did a company with an annual advertising budget of hundreds of thousands fall afoul of the law. Proprietary Association spokesmen asserted that some of these cases doubtlessly would have been won by the manufacturers, except that it was cheaper to plead guilty and pay a nominal fine than to go to all the trouble of a court trial.[12]

Egregious violations by small-scale proprietors made up the bulk of criminal cases involving nostrums in the early years of the law. Numerous other headache "cures" besides

[11] *Standard Remedies*, 4 (Jan. 1918), 8-10; *N&Q*, I, 671-80; II, 101, 162.
[12] *Reports of Bureau of Chemistry*, 1907-1911; Munch, "Notices of Judgment—the First Thousand," 219-42; *Hampton's Mag.*, 27 (1911), 393; *Standard Remedies*, 1 (Sep. 1915), 809.

Harper's fell under Dr. Wiley's ban. Campaigns were also conducted against broad-gauge tonics (one was Humbug Oil), male-weakness remedies (like Sporty Days Invigorator), "cures" for cancer (including the radium-imitating Radol), alleged germicides, and "cures" for narcotic addiction. Some of this work was done in cooperation with the Post Office Department. Seldom did a proprietor see fit to offer the Bureau a serious contest in the courts. Pleas of "not guilty" were few and far between. Besides criminal action against the proprietor, the law gave federal district attorneys another type of legal action to bring on the basis of evidence provided by the Bureau of Chemistry. This was the seizure of the adulterated or misbranded article itself and a suit for its condemnation. In the early years of enforcement, few seizure actions were directed against proprietary remedies.[13]

Success in these limited campaigns against the most dangerous types of nostrums prompted the Bureau of Chemistry to issue now and then an optimistic assertion. In 1910 Wiley reported that, as a result of cooperation between the Bureau and postal authorities, "the mail-order 'cancer-cure' business" had "to a very large extent, been suppressed in this country." Drug-addiction cures were also yielding to the pressure.[14]

These advances in a limited sector of the patent medicine front, plus what improvement had been brought about by voluntary modifications in formulas and labels, were not the overwhelming victory which the more hopeful food and drug reformers had predicted when they rejoiced at the enactment of the law. Many manufacturers continued to defy its provisions, willfully or out of ignorance. New abuses, indeed, were arising, ironically enough out of the very circumstances of enforcement. Despite reiterated warnings, nostrum makers told their would-be customers that the phrase "Guaranteed under the Pure Food and Drugs Act"—really intended to protect retailers from the misdeeds of manufacturers—meant a governmental certification of healing potency. And, if this

[13] *Reports of Bureau of Chemistry*, 1907-1911; Munch, 219-42. On Post Office anti-quackery efforts see ch. 4 below.
[14] *1910 Report of Bureau of Chemistry*, 19, 35.

distortion was not bad enough, Wiley had to suffer the personal indignity of finding his warnings against the misuse of pain-killers distorted in advertisements in such a way as to make him sound like a testimonial-giver to their efficacy.[15] In 1911 a new blow fell, a blow which badly crippled the modest controls over remedy labeling which the law had seemed to contain. The Supreme Court ruled that the law's prohibition of false labeling did not apply to therapeutic claims.

The misbranding section of the law did not explicitly refer to curative promises. A food or drug article was misbranded, the law stated, "the package or label of which shall bear any statement, design, or device regarding such article, or the ingredients or substances contained therein which shall be false or misleading in any particular." Wiley and Kebler, in their initial regulations, had aimed this general clause directly at unwarranted assertions that promised relief or cure. At the time questions were raised about the Bureau's interpretation. In view of the differences of opinion prevailing over matters therapeutical, a drug editor suggested, "it will be interesting to know who is to be judge of the truth or falsity of the therapeutical claims which may be made."[16] Certainly among medical practitioners an ancient therapeutic debate had reached a new and bitter stage. In the American Medical Association's effort to improve standards, Association spokesmen were condemning the healing practices of various sects and cults.[17] These groups fought back with vigor, defending their therapies and opposing the AMA's effort to enforce therapeutic monopoly. While such a debate was going on, could Wiley and Kebler, perusing nostrum labels, find firm scientific grounds on which to approve or reject? They themselves took this for granted and, during the first years of the law, so did the trade. Many manufacturers toned down their therapeutic claims. Others did not, but when hauled into court

[15] John Uri Lloyd to Wiley, Dec. 2, 1908, Wiley Papers, box 65, Library of Congress; typescript copy of Tarrant's Seltzer-Aperient poster in Falls Church Railway Car, *ibid.*, box 60; Orangeine ad in *Chicago Tribune*, Feb. 17, 1907.
[16] *Amer. Druggist*, 49 (1906), 234.
[17] Burrow, *AMA*, 2-6, 33, 100-101, 317-18.

admitted Wiley's view of the law's applicability by pleading guilty.[18]

Out in Kansas City an eclectic physician named Johnson decided on a different legal course. He had been vending an assortment of tablets and liquids as "Dr. Johnson's Mild Combination Treatment for Cancer." For this purpose, of course, the concoctions were worthless. Johnson fulfilled the law's requirements as to the accurate labeling of his ingredients. It was solely against his false curative promises that the government brought its suit. The medicine man's lawyers moved to quash the indictment, pleading that Congress had not intended the law to forbid such practices. When the case had run its course, the Supreme Court had agreed. Oliver Wendell Holmes delivered the decision, a tortuous exploration of grammatical construction that could find no proper link between the prohibition of false labeling and assertions of healing potency. Congress was not apt to legislate, Holmes argued, in the debatable realm of what could cure and what could not. This would "distort the uses of its constitutional power to establishing criteria in regions where opinions are far apart."[19]

Charles Evans Hughes wrote a vigorous dissent. His study of the grammar of the law revealed the connection Holmes could not see. He cited the act's legislative history to show that Congress had indeed intended a prohibition of therapeutic nonsense on nostrum labels. Even the makers of medicines had generally assumed the law to be so written, Hughes pointed out, since so many had promptly entered pleas of guilt. Holmes had "impressively described," the dissenting justice said, the conflict that did indeed exist between schools of medicine and the difficulty of legislating in such an uncertain area. "But granting the wide domain of opinion," he added, "and allowing the broadest range to the conflict of medical views, there still remains a field in which statements as to the curative properties are downright falsehoods and in no sense expressions of judgment. This field I believe this

[18] Message from President Taft, *Cong. Record*, 62 Cong., 1 ses., 2380 (June 21, 1911).

[19] White and Gates, in *Decisions of Courts in Cases under the Federal Food and Drugs Act*, cite the District Court decision, 85-88, and the Supreme Court decision, including the dissent, 267-73.

statute covers." This type of downright falsehood was what Johnson had placed on the labels of his cancer cure.

But Holmes had the majority with him. The decision, wrote an incensed George Creel, was "first aid to fraud and murder," leaving the nostrum provisions of the law with "as much bite as a canton flannel dog." Wiley was angry. Maybe Holmes understood his opinion, the chief chemist said. "I don't. All I can make out is that it gives anyone the right to lie about drugs whenever he feels like it." Wiley preferred to stand with Hughes. "He disagreed," the chemist added bitterly, "probably, because he had not been on the bench long enough to know better."[20]

The decision in the Johnson case, said President Taft, meant that over 150 cases of the same type pending in the courts, "involving some of the rankest frauds by which the American people were ever deceived," would have to be dismissed. He urged the Congress promptly to pass a law to plug the hole. Holmes had made clear—and Hughes had agreed—that "any attempt to legislate against mere expressions of opinion would be abortive." Thus the new law should proscribe only "knowingly false misstatements of fact as to the effect of the preparations." Such a measure, the President was persuaded, would control "the greater part of the evil."[21]

Congressman Swagar Sherley of Kentucky introduced a bill, and it was passed by Congress "without any blare of trumpets." The amendment to the food and drug law declared an article misbranded "if its package or label shall bear or contain any statement, design, or device regarding the curative or therapeutic effect of such article or any of the ingredients or substances contained therein, which is false and fraudulent."[22]

In view of the Johnson decision, "false and fraudulent" was as strong a phrase as Congress could very well enact. But

[20] *Harper's Wkly.*, 60 (Jan. 2, 1915), 60; *Chicago Tribune*, Dec. 9, 1911.

[21] *Cong. Record*, 62 Cong., 1 ses., 2379-80.

[22] *Ibid.*, 11,322-23, 11,352, 11,744; the Amendment was passed Aug. 23, 1912, ch. 352, 37 Stat. 416; *Outlook*, 101 (1912), 993. There had been a brief hearing: *The Pure Food Law*, Hearings before the Committee on Interstate and Foreign Commerce, House of Representatives, 62 Cong., 2 ses. (Wash., 1912).

would proving fraud be such an impossible task as to offer quackery an open road? Congressman Sherley acknowledged this hazard: "very frequently," he said, the government would have difficulty "in convicting the guilty man." A fellow Congressman, James Covington of Maryland, foresaw no untoward danger. "The proof of intention in the criminal law," he said, "does not mean the metaphysical reading of a man's mind. Specific proof of intent is not necessary; it may be established by evidence of attending facts and circumstances, and therefore the Government can easily show that a false statement on a label regarding a drug is one from which fraudulent intent may be implied. Conviction in all proper cases will be consequently comparatively sure."[23]

Wiley was less cheerful. The dangers Congressman Sherley saw as likely, Wiley viewed as certain. The word "fraudulent" in the amendment, he said, was a "joker" which would nullify the law's intent. Congress had "given the manufacturers of fake cure-alls another lease on life and enabled the roots of fraud and corruption to sink deeper into the soil of protective legislation—protective to vested interests, not to public welfare." But enforcing the Sherley Amendment was not to be Harvey Washington Wiley's responsibility. Five months before Taft signed the law, Wiley had resigned his post as chief of the Bureau of Chemistry. The decision had been, perhaps, impending since 1906. The talents required for crusading in behalf of a law are not the same talents required for enforcing it. The measure was a pioneering one, and weaknesses in drafting became apparent, especially a lack of clarity as to enforcement responsibilities. Wiley's categorical stand against food preservatives antagonized industries with great political power, and this power they brought to bear. President Roosevelt, becoming unsure of Wiley's science, created checks upon his single-handed action within the Bureau which hamstrung the chief chemist. Bitter internecine warfare developed which, in Taft's administration, led to a charge of malfeasance against Wiley. Although he was vindicated by the President, Wiley felt that Taft should then have proceeded to oust his enemies and restore his authority. This the President did not

[23] *Ibid.*, 16; *Cong. Record*, 62 Cong., 1 ses., Appendix, 676.

do. Embittered, tired of fruitless fighting, and anxious to increase his income because of his recent marriage, Wiley quit.[24]

In the whole protracted struggle, patent medicines played almost no part at all. One of Wiley's opponents within the Department of Agriculture had chided the chemist for working up weak food cases when so many strong cases might be developed against vicious nostrums sold within "the shadow of the National Capitol." Granted that the complaint possessed some merit, it has all the earmarks of a blow aimed at embarrassing Wiley in the continuing battle. At any rate, the Johnson case had already been decided against the government in the District Court.[25]

Although patent medicines were not a real issue in the fight, Wiley's resignation was an important factor in rekindling the anti-nostrum crusade. The controversial chemist had been much in the press during the contest with his enemies, especially since a Congressional committee had investigated the misconduct charge against him. Pure food advocates were outraged at this charge and tended to view Wiley's departure from government as, in effect, a firing. Widespread publicity about the law's main architect was accompanied by a revived attention to the various facets of the law. In this renewed public interest, patent medicines shared. The Johnson decision and the Sherley Amendment also helped direct attention to the theme. Concerned observers began to conclude, moreover, that truthful labeling—even if the Bureau of Chemistry really had the will and the funds to secure it—was not enough. Granted there had been improvement. Granted—though this was uncertain—there might be more improvement under the Sherley law. The situation was still appalling. From the per-

[24] Wiley cited in *Rural New Yorker*, Sep. 14, 1912, clipping, Wiley Papers, box 236, Library of Congress; Wiley, "The Public Tricked Again," *Good Housekeeping*, 55 (1912), 694. Wiley's account of his struggles is given in his *The History of a Crime against the Food Law* (Wash., 1929). An impartial and excellent appraisal is Oscar E. Anderson, Jr., "The Pure-Food Issue: A Republican Dilemma, 1906-1912," *Amer. Hist. Rev.*, 61 (1956), 550-73, and the matter is treated at length in Anderson, *The Health of a Nation*, 197-258. See also Dupree, *Science in the Federal Government*, 179-80.

[25] George R. McCabe to Wiley, Jan. 29, 1910 (copy), Wiley Papers, box 200, Library of Congress; Anderson, *The Health of a Nation*, 233-34.

spective of the medicine maker, as the *National Druggist* had predicted in 1906, the law had proved "not such a terrible thing after all."[26] From the viewpoint of the ardent reformer, therefore, something was needed.

In the renewal of patent medicine muckraking, the famous writer-editor team of Samuel Hopkins Adams and Norman Hapgood again took the lead. Now, however, they were not harnessed together as in 1905. Hapgood, having moved from *Collier's* to *Harper's Weekly*, got George Creel to write a series of hard-hitting attacks on the "Poisoners of Public Health." Adams aimed his shots mainly from the pages of *Collier's* and the *New York Tribune*. He also wrote a novel about the nostrum business. With a proprietor based on the old German who made Peruna and a plant modeled on the Swamp Root factory, *The Clarion* depicted details of nostrum production and promotion so critically as to bring anguished protests from real medicine makers. Adams' picture of the industry, charged the editor of the Proprietary Association's journal, was "as wide of the truth as anything ever set down in English," and Adams himself was "like a certain nasty breed of wooly dogs that delight to roll in filth and then sit down and rapturously smell themselves."[27]

Dr. Wiley himself became a muckraker. Upon resigning from the Bureau, he joined the staff of *Good Housekeeping* to keep its readers posted on the continuing food and drug crusade. Food still interested him most, but Wiley's column and correspondence contained frequent items of evidence to buttress his general thesis, asserted in the title of an article, "The Inherent 'No-Accountness' of Patent Medicines."[28]

---

[26] 36 (1906), 210.

[27] Creel had eleven articles in *Harper's Wkly.*, between Jan. 2 and Apr. 24, 1915. Adams published *Collier's* articles during 1912 and 1913 and the *Tribune* series was reprinted as *Some of the Adams Articles on Fraudulent and Deceptive Advertising. Published in the New York Tribune during Nineteen-Fifteen and the First Half of Nineteen-Sixteen* (N.Y., 1916). *The Clarion* (Boston, 1914); interview with Adams, Apr. 5, 1955; *Standard Remedies*, 1 (Mar. 1915), 7-10.

[28] Wiley's *Good Housekeeping* correspondence makes up boxes 163-173 of his Papers, Library of Congress; the magazine from late 1912 on contains his monthly contributions. "The Inherent 'No-Accountness' " article he wrote with Anne Lewis Pierce, 59 (1914), 384-92.

Wiley was a doctor, and in the new assault, the main artillery was fired by physicians. The American Medical Association took the lead, making an increasing effort not only to inform its own members about the hazards of quackery, but also to reach the laity. At their 1915 meeting, the AMA's House of Delegates addressed a petition to President Woodrow Wilson and the Congress. Despite the law, the petition asserted, "fraudulent and deceitful practices" with respect to proprietary medicines still abounded. The President should recommend that Congress establish a commission to investigate the evils and make them widely known. The next year a deputation from the Association waited upon Wilson to reiterate the request. Despite improvements resulting from enforcement of the law, the doctors told him, the patent medicine "problem as it affects the people of the whole country has scarcely been touched." Wilson expressed his sympathy with the Association's objectives, but made no promises.[29]

Physicians, journalists, and bureaucrats agreed that, despite the optimism with which it had been greeted and the integrity with which it had been enforced, the 1906 law had not eliminated quackery. There were some who argued that, quantitatively, the patent medicine evil was worse than it had been. "The passing of these sordid rascals [through the activity of the Bureau and the Post Office]," wrote Creel, ". . . made no more than a ripple on the surface of fraud. For every one that has been put out of business, a score has arisen to take the vacant places." In 1909 a President's commission had made the same point: "In spite of solemn protests and ostracism, the frightful list of . . . harmful . . . [secret and proprietary medicines] increases at the rate of about 200 a year."[30] The hope that an honest—though not fully revealing—label would warn an alert public away from danger had not been vindicated. Why not?

For one thing, the job was too big. There were too many patent medicines, too small a regulatory staff. "The Bureau

[29] *JAMA*, 65 (1915), 120, 122; 66 (1916), 974. On the AMA anti-quackery campaign, see ch. 7 below.
[30] *Harper's Wkly.*, 60 (1915), 5; William H. Baldwin, *Reports of the President's Homes Commission*, 60 Cong., 2 ses., Sen. Doc. 644 (1909), 246.

. . . ," wrote Creel, "is in the position of one who tries to mop up water on the floor while the spigot is still turned on." Each case was costly to try, if contested, running from $30,000 to $50,000. Penalties were too light to serve as deterrents. Fines, small as they were, were often remitted. Although the law permitted one-year sentences for second offenders in interstate commerce, no one went to jail. Upon learning that a man had been sentenced to four months of hard labor for imitating a trademark, the *Journal of the American Medical Association* editorialized, "Some day, possibly, a court may be found that will consider the crimes of making drug fiends of young people, of poisoning babies with opium mixtures or of killing women with headache powders as more serious offenses than the counterfeiting of the label of a fraudulent 'patent medicine.' Apparently, that time is far off."[31]

Some forms of quackery, the critics pointed out, could not be moved against at all. The 1906 law defined "drug" in such a way that mechanical devices promoted as sure cures for dread diseases had a clear field. So did quack concoctions promising to put flesh on the skinny or take it off the fat. Face creams, hair dyes, and other cosmetic preparations, although they might pose serious hazards to health, could avoid conflict with the law if their proprietors resisted the urge to put therapeutic claims upon the labels. This state of affairs, Wiley's successor felt, was one of the "serious limitations" of the law.[32]

The new Bureau chief, Carl L. Alsberg, also grieved that the law failed to include "any restriction whatever upon the use of many of the most virulent poisons in drugs." So long as the label announced the presence and proportion of the eleven dangerous drugs included in the law, things were legal. This list of poisons had been found to be woefully short. There were many others—Dr. Kebler compiled a list of 46—just as hazardous, which could be included in any quantity without a word of warning to the customer.[33]

[31] *Harper's Wkly.*, 60 (1915), 135-36; *JAMA*, 58 (1912), 706.
[32] *1917 Report of the Bureau of Chemistry*, 16; *Harper's Wkly.*, 60 (1915), 136.
[33] *1917 Report of the Bureau of Chemistry*, 16; *The Pure Food and Drugs Act*, Hearings before the Committee on Interstate and Foreign Commerce, House of Representatives, 62 Cong., 2 ses. (Wash., 1912), 68.

More important, the general theory behind the labeling provisions seemed, after a decade's experience, not quite so sound as it had seemed in 1906. How many Americans, reading a proprietary label, would understand the hazardous meaning of "heroin, alpha or beta eucaine, chloroform, cannabis indica," or, at any rate, would know how large a dose of any one of these drugs might be ingested with safety? How many Americans, indeed, seeking out proprietary remedies, paid much heed to labels at all? Pharmacists testified that most customers asked for nostrums by name and carried them off with scarcely a glance at the cartons. Thus, asserted Creel, the law as it stood failed to safeguard "the large percentage of ignorant, careless or reckless purchasers." Not until "the public is afforded a protection that does not rest upon the initiative of the individual," he believed, would "the ultimate goal" be reached. This would require a flat prohibition of certain dangerous ingredients in remedies offered for public sale. It would likewise require control of nostrum advertising.[34]

The very therapeutic claims on labels which the Sherley Amendment had forbidden, for the second time as it were, continued boldly in the advertising columns of much of the nation's press. The nostrum buyer who did not look at the label did not need to. He went into the drugstore with the promise of a cure "burned into" his mind from frequent re-reading of patent medicine advertising. "Printer's ink," wrote Creel, "in the last analysis, is the net that catches the victims of quackery. . . . The Food and Drugs Act cannot be anything but a circling of Robin Hood's barn as long as the patent medicine liar has the daily press at his disposal." Samuel Hopkins Adams might not be quite so discouraged, but he concurred in the basic point. "Half success is the best that can be claimed for the Pure Food Law insofar as it affects nostrums," he wrote. "The reason is that we who fought to get the law passed aimed at the wrong side of the bottle. We should have attacked the advertisements in the newspapers. That is where the real damage is done." The same judgment was rendered by Kebler and his new chief, by Wiley and his old superior. "I believe," wrote ex-President Roosevelt, "that legislation could be framed to forbid such advertisements."[35]

At the time the Sherley Amendment was being considered, Congressman William Richardson of Alabama had introduced a bill that would have brought advertising under some restraint and tightened the control of drugs in a number of other ways. Kebler from within the Bureau and Wiley from without urged a House committee to support the legislation. Kebler displayed reams of advertising and scores of offending bottles, stark exhibits to demonstrate that the 1906 law needed toughening to cope with quackery. But spokesmen both for proprietary manufacturers and for the prescription drug industry condemned the measure. The committee did not report it back to the House.[36]

The Proprietary Association was dead set against governmental control of advertising. Aware that there were excesses that needed curbing, the Association began to take steps to improve the standards of its members. This was one of several moves made in an effort to rehabilitate an organization that had been greatly demoralized by the events of 1906. In the month that the new food and drug law became effective, a drug periodical reported on the Association's moribund condition. "At present the proprietary association's meetings do not exhibit the old time éclat. The industry is being generally attacked by the independent magazine press, the retail trade is growing stronger in opposition to it, legislation restricting it and removing much of its secrecy is being enacted, and its influence is waning. Several of the manufacturers of so-called 'ethical' goods have resigned from its membership, as have also some of the leading 'patent' medicine manufacturers. The meetings . . . are paid very little attention to by the other branches of the trade nowadays, and, as a rule, the sessions are secret."[37]

From this rout there had been a slow rally. Proprietors

[35] Ibid., 136, 155, 158; 1917 Report of the Bureau of Chemistry, 14; Wiley, "The Public Tricked Again," Good Housekeeping, 55 (1912), 694; Roosevelt, "Applied Ethics in Journalism," Outlook, 97 (1911), 807-809; Kebler cited in The Pure Food and Drugs Act, Hearings . . . , 62 Cong., 2 ses., 81, 119.
[36] Ibid., passim; Cong. Record, 62 Cong., 1 ses., 2492, 2656; 2 ses., 12.
[37] Druggists' Circular, 51 (1907), 114.

found that by exercising a little diligence they could easily live with the new law. Brushes with the law were few, fines not unreasonable. Sales, instead of falling off, kept booming. In the decade between 1902 and 1912, the Association's president said, total production in the industry had increased 60 per cent. Census figures bore him out, with the future looming brighter still. And as the Bureau of Chemistry eliminated small fly-by-night promoters, the big proprietors got an increased proportion of the total volume. By 1915, members of the Proprietary Association were producing some 80 per cent of American proprietaries sold. Proponents of the 1906 law "who hailed it as the 'end of the patent medicine business,'" noted an industry spokesman, were "sorely disappointed. It was rather the beginning than the end."[38]

By 1913, members of the Proprietary Association felt enough at ease under governmental control to invite Lyman Kebler to address them. He urged the group to strengthen self-imposed restrictions on proprietary labeling and to develop its own code of ethics to cover advertising. Two years later the Association took steps to follow Kebler's advice. They sent a committee to confer with a special commission on proprietary medicines of the American Pharmaceutical Association. This commission, after long and diligent inquiry, had devised "Minimum Requirements with Which Proprietary Remedies Should Comply in Order to Render Them Safe for Direct Sale to the General Public," a set of standards which the parent body had formally approved. Out of the discussion between delegates of the two drug organizations came a somewhat revised version of the "Minimum Requirements," which was adopted by the Proprietary Association to govern its members. The law was to be obeyed. Narcotics for children and abortifacients were completely taboo. Narcotics in adult medicines should not exceed the Harrison Law ceiling. No other ingredient should be put in a medicine that would "endanger life

[38] *Standard Remedies*, 1 (Mar. 1915), 26; 4 (Jan. 1918), 8-10; 5 (July 1919), 8-10; Bureau of the Census, *13th Census of the United States* . . . , VIII, *Manufactures, 1909* (Wash., 1913), 40; Bureau of the Census, *Census of Manufactures: 1927, The Drug Industries* (Wash., 1929), 6; Leonard L. Minty, *The Legal and Ethical Aspects of Quackery* (London, 1932), 194.

or health if used in accordance with instructions accompanying the package." Alcohol should be kept at a minimum, no more than enough to keep the active ingredients in solution and to prevent freezing. "Statements [on the package] regarding therapeutic effects must neither be obviously unreasonable nor demonstrably false." As to advertising, the Proprietary Association rule was less stringent than the American Pharmaceutical Association standard, which recommended that advertising and labeling meet the same tests. The Proprietary Association version stated, "The preparation must not be advertised or recommended as a cure for diseases or conditions which are generally recognized as incurable by the simple administration of drugs."[39]

To enforce the requirements, a committee was created to scrutinize labeling—but evidently not to check advertising copy —used by members of the Association. By 1919 this committee could report that only 19 members had not yet met its approval on this score. A number of applicants for membership in the Association had been turned down.[40]

The code of ethics was only one part of the Proprietary Association's effort at rehabilitation. It made a determined and successful attempt to increase its membership. It set up a journal, *Standard Remedies*, to keep its members alert to common problems and aware of dangers. In this magazine, the Association counterattacked its critics with a vigor and bitterness not seen since pre-law days. When Norman Hapgood began to publish George Creel's sharp attacks in *Harper's Weekly*, *Standard Remedies* saw the purpose as "To Raise H--L and Sell Newspapers." The American Medical Association, the medicine makers charged, used "Hun methods" and the ethics of "the journalistic prostitute" in its anti-proprietary campaign. When the House of Delegates petitioned for a national commission of inquiry, *Standard Remedies* termed

[39] *Standard Remedies*, 1 (Dec. 1915), 17-18; 2 (May 1916), 11-12, 17-19; 5 (Apr. 1919), 30-31; 6 (Feb. 1920), 21-22; *Jnl. Amer. Pharmaceutical Assoc.*, 2 (1913), 1469-71; 4 (1915), 1148-67; 5 (1916), 1374-89; 7 (1918), 67-76. The American Pharmaceutical Association "Minimum Requirements" are listed *ibid.*, 4 (1915), 1165-66, and the Proprietary Association "Requirements for Membership," 5 (1916), 1374-75.
[40] *Standard Remedies*, 5 (Apr. 1919), 30-31.

the resolution "smug, . . . conceited, . . . impertinent," and inquired, "Is this a free country, or are we to be Russianized?"[41]

Despite the weaknesses in the law as it applied to nostrums, despite the revival of muckraking and constant pressure from the medical profession, no new national legislation was enacted. The alertness of the Proprietary Association and its efforts at good behavior were no doubt in some part responsible. Two other factors also seem important. Food and drug legislation had been one aspect of the Progressive movement, and the Progressive movement, sustained for more than a decade, was on the wane. Then, too, with the European War, public attention began to shift from domestic to foreign affairs.

No man better knew the need for a new law than Wiley's successor as chief of the Bureau of Chemistry, Carl L. Alsberg. No summary of the loopholes in the 1906 measure was more admirably succinct than that which Alsberg included in his 1917 annual report. Since no new law seemed forthcoming, however, Alsberg set out to enforce the Sherley Amendment as rigorously as he could.[42]

Like Wiley, Alsberg was a scientist. His degrees—including the M.D.—were all from Columbia, and he had engaged in postgraduate study at several German universities, taught chemistry at Harvard, and worked as a biologist in the Bureau of Plant Industry before Taft elevated him to head the Bureau of Chemistry. Wiley, on the outside, thought one of his own aides should have been promoted to the post. "Doctor Alsberg," the ex-chief wrote, "appears to me to be a very promising kind of young man if he can just keep under the right influence."[43]

[41] Ibid., 1 (Jan. 1915), 1, 5-6; (Apr. 1915), 7; (Aug. 1915), 3; 4 (Jan. 1918), 13; 5 (Jan. 1919), 13; (May 1919), 12-13; 6 (May 1920), 22; (Dec. 1920), 26. Standard Remedies began Jan. 1915 as the "baby" of the Proprietary Association. In May 1915 it was incorporated under private ownership, although intended to remain an organ of the major manufacturers of proprietary medicines. Until his death in 1934, Ervin F. Kemp, General Representative of the Proprietary Association since 1905, served as the editor. Ibid., 1 (Jan. 1915), 1; (May 1915), 3; 21 (Nov. 1934), 3.

[42] 1917 Report of the Bureau of Chemistry, 14-16.

[43] Alsberg discussed his background on the witness stand in the

The two men made a striking contrast in appearance and temperament. Whereas Wiley was "big-faced, big framed, bald-headed, large limbed, deep voiced and pugnacious," wrote a reporter, the new chief was of medium height, modestly dressed, possessed of plenty of hair and a black mustache, and imbued with the air of a man of leisure, imperturbable even under great pressure. When he walks, the newsman noted, no floorboards squeak.[44]

Dr. Alsberg believed his objectives were bound to be different from Wiley's mission. "I hope to sink my personality in the work," he said several months after his appointment. "My predecessor was a man of great strength of character and in the work of attacking the food adulterators and starting the fight, he necessarily came into the limelight. If I can knock out the food fakers and get the bureau down to hard constructive work as well that is all I want to do. I have no desire to be known as a great personage, a fighting character or a man who has killed a dragon."[45]

To make the Sherley act rapidly effective, Alsberg transferred as many chemists as could be spared from other work to a crash program against nostrums. Hundreds of patent medicines were analyzed within a few months' time. In this campaign the first seizure to be contested in court involved a product long known to patent medicine customers and critics, the Microbe Killer, that wondrous draught which had transformed an impoverished Texas gardener into a prosperous resident of New York. By now William Radam was dead, but his trademark lived on. Vended in stone jugs of three strengths, the Microbe Killer had lost none of its vaunted self-assurance. When the potent liquid was imbibed, the labeling said, Microbe Killer's healing gases were released by the heat of the stomach, from whence they went forth to disinfect the entire

Radam's Microbe Killer trial. Transcript of testimony in Food and Drug Case 4910, Office of the Solicitor of the Dept. of Agric., Notice of Judgment [NJ] 3004, RG 16, NA. Wiley to Albert B. Matthews, Apr. 11, 1913, Wiley Papers, box 112, Library of Congress. See also Fred B. Linton, "Federal Food and Drug Laws—Leaders Who Achieved Their Enactment and Enforcement," *FDC Law Jnl.*, 5 (1950), 103-15.
[44] *Minneapolis Journal*, Oct. 12, 1913.
[45] *Ibid.*

system, in the process curing headache and worms, measles and malaria, consumption and yellow fever, small pox and leprosy. The Microbe Killer was also effective preventive medication: added to drinking water, it acted as a safeguard against disease.[46]

A carload lot of this preposterous proprietary had been shipped from the New York manufacturer to his agent in Minneapolis. Dr. Alsberg arranged for federal authorities to seize 539 wooden boxes and 322 pasteboard cartons of the stuff, worth at retail prices some $5,166, although government chemists estimated the cost of making it at $25.82.

When the Microbe Killer agent contested the seizure, Alsberg and his key aides went west to help with the trial. "We have several hundred cases like this," the bureau chief said, "and if we lose here I do not know just what we will do. . . . On it practically hangs our pure food and drug law."[47]

The case pitted medical science against testimonials from the untutored. No mixture that was essentially 99 per cent tap water and 1 per cent sulphuric acid, Dr. Alsberg told the jury, could cure the diseases mentioned. The greatest therapeutic action the Microbe Killer might possess would be as a mild laxative. And for many people it would irritate the stomach and upper intestine.

"Then all your complaint . . . ," Alsberg was asked by the defense attorney, "is the inflammation which is caused by this medicine as it passes through the alimentary tract?"

"What we are complaining of is more than that," the bureau chief answered. "It is the fact that a man may be very sick and use this medicine until it is too late to use something else."

[46] *1913 Report of the Bureau of Chemistry*, 2. On the origins of the Microbe Killer, see Young, *The Toadstool Millionaires*, ch. 10. The discussion here is mainly based on the files of the Bureau of Chemistry (Interstate Office Seizure File, Seizure No. 1628, F&D No. 4910, RG 88, NA) and of the Office of the Solicitor of the Dept. of Agric. (F&D 4910, RG 16, NA.) Satisfied user testimony is from *Minneapolis Morning Tribune*, Oct. 11, 1913. White and Gates, 511-19, cite Judge Willard's charge. In 1909, during Wiley's regime, a shipment of the Microbe Killer had been seized in Washington state and condemned without contest (Office of the Solicitor, F&D 603, NJ 205, RG 16, NA).

[47] *Minneapolis Morning Tribune*, Oct. 10, 1913.

"Then it is the time he loses?"

"The time he loses may be sometimes the difference between life and death."

A District of Columbia bacteriologist testified. "I don't know of anything," he said, "in which sulphuric acid of that strength could be used as a therapeutic agent." Local physicians, one an old-timer who had practiced in Minneapolis for years, the other a University of Minnesota medical professor, supported the government's case.

The defense relied on testimony by satisfied users of the Microbe Killer. During a hearing in Washington that preceded the trial, an attorney for the manufacturer had told Alsberg about 47 bound volumes of letters in the company's possession, written by men and women grateful for their cures. To the witness stand in Minneapolis went a number of such champions: a woman who had vanquished cancer with five bottles of the Microbe Killer; a man who had rid himself of tuberculosis in three months; a woman who had knocked out her son's diphtheria in half a night. The Minneapolis agent was himself a devoted user. Twenty doctors had told him they could not help his throat trouble, he testified, but 20 to 30 gallons of the Microbe Killer, taken in the course of seven months, cured him completely. The most he had ever taken at one time, he said, was two whole bottles in one day.

Despite the earnestness of such testimony, the jury decided against the Microbe Killer. "If you believe," the judge had charged them, "that this remedy is so absolutely worthless, for example, for leprosy or for catarrh or for consumption or for diphtheria, that the manufacturer must have known that, then you would be justified in finding that the statements made with reference to these diseases upon the labels are false and fraudulent." So believing, the jury condemned the 539 boxes and 322 cartons of the Microbe Killer to destruction. "I favor," said the district attorney, "using an ax."[48]

Bolstered by a court decision indicating that fraud could be deduced from a nostrum's label, Alsberg accelerated his campaign against the most obnoxious patent medicines. Two years later the Supreme Court, with Justice Hughes delivering the

[48] White and Gates, 517; *Minneapolis Morning Tribune*, Oct. 14, 1913.

opinion, affirmed the constitutionality of the Sherley act. Eckman's Alterative, a "cure" for all throat and lung diseases, Hughes said, had been properly restrained by governmental action. Alsberg increased still more the pressure on quack labeling. To take charge of Sherley Amendment activity, he added to his staff a physician, M. W. Glover, from the Public Health Service. To give legal victories a greater impact for public education, the Bureau began to issue press notices. To prevent the distortion of the guaranty system, the guarantee of compliance was taken off the label, where the public could see it, and shifted to the bill of sale.[49]

Dr. Glover sought and secured wide support from state and local food and drug officials in screening sources of sale for mislabeled nostrums. This help was crucial in the first major effort employing the seizure provisions of the law to drive hazardous patent medicines from the market. Worried by baby soothing syrups, the Bureau engaged in multiple seizures, taking legal action wherever the nostrums might be found. Some 123 lots of one brand, Sirop D'Anis Gauvin, were acted against from Maine out to Michigan and the dangerous medicine destroyed. Some makers of similar soothing syrups stopped their manufacture.[50]

Most of Dr. Glover's work was aimed at remedies purporting to grapple with the uncontrollable diseases. "Our experience has taught us," he wrote, "that the appearance on the label of the name of a disease usually conveys to the user the impression that the preparation is all that he needs to get permanent relief from that trouble." Therefore more attention was given, in studying labels, to the names of diseases than to "associated wording." Those diseases about which there was no conflict

[49] Munch, "Notices of Judgment—Nos. 1001 to 5000," *FDC Law Jnl.*, 11 (1956), 17-34; *1916 Report of the Bureau of Chemistry*, 351. Press notices began in 1915, with a great many devoted to proprietaries through 1919; Press Notice file in Food and Drug Administration. A 1915 press notice notes the change in the guaranty system. White and Gates give the Jan. 10, 1916 Supreme Court decision (239 U.S. 510) in the Eckman's Alterative case.

[50] *Food and Drug Review*, 4 (Aug. 1920), 16-18. This journal was begun as a restricted private organ of the Bureau of Chemistry to keep its staff, in Washington and in the district offices, as well as state food and drug personnel, posted on matters of concern. Hereafter cited as *F&D Rev.*

of medical opinion, diseases which virtually all doctors would deem incurable, were those to which the Bureau was most alert. "We hold," Dr. Glover stated, "that a manufacturer of a medicine, when he tells people what diseases it is a treatment for, assumes a position of superior knowledge; of one who knows all about drugs and their relative value as therapeutic agents, and when he promises that a certain combination will do certain things, which it will not, that he is guilty of fraud." Untruthful statements, the Bureau held, "made with a reckless or wanton disregard as to whether they were true or false," thereby revealed their fraudulency.[51]

Scores of vicious nostrums were driven from the market, or made to modify their labeling. Campaigns were pushed against throat and lung proprietaries of the Eckman's Alterative type, against kidney and liver remedies, against mineral waters sold with cure-all claims, against abortifacients and male rejuvenators. During the years of the first World War an old quack practice quickly rose to threatening proportions. After testing many medicinal products offered the Surgeon-General's Office for treating sick soldiers, the AMA's Council on Pharmacy and Chemistry asserted that "it would seem unbelievable that such a variety of fakes would be offered in earnest to the government." Many medicines equally unworthy, especially concoctions promising to cure venereal disease, were offered for direct sale to the troops. The Bureau of Chemistry set out in hot pursuit.[52]

The result of the Bureau's anti-nostrum crusading, from the Microbe Killer decision into the early postwar years, amounted to a revolution. There was, in proprietary labeling, "a notable change for the better," in that flagrant and flat-footed claims to cure the dread diseases were markedly reduced. Fines for violation were generally higher than in the Wiley years.[53]

[51] M. W. Glover, "The Administration of the Sherley Amendment," *F&D Rev.* 4 (Oct. 1920), 17-19.

[52] Press Notice file, 1915-1920, FDA; Munch, "Notices of Judgment— Nos. 1001 to 5000," *FDC Law Jnl.*, 11 (1956), 17-34; Munch, "Notices of Judgment—Nos. 5001-15,000," *ibid.*, 196-211; *JAMA*, 72 (1919), 1741; *Reports of the Bureau of Chemistry*, 1918-1921.

[53] *F&D Rev.*, 7 (Jan. 1923), inside back cover; (Dec. 1923), 10; Munch, "Notices of Judgment—Nos. 5001-15,000," 206.

But what was the effectiveness of the revolution in protecting the public against quackery? Not very great. Subtle and devious label claims, too vague for Sherley Amendment action, continued—indeed, increased. These claims the ordinary man could interpret, if he bothered to read them at all, as an echoing of the nostrum maker's completely unrestricted boasting in his advertising, whence the old categorical claims had migrated. Thus the Sherley Amendment was a useful but not a decisive weapon for combatting quackery. Suddenly it became an even weaker weapon than it had seemed to be.[54]

[54] See ch. 5.

# FRAUD IN THE MAILS

*"There is something wrong with my testicles and I don't know what to make of it. I noticed for some time that they don't hang even and that the left one hangs lower. I ain't got the nerve to ask our doctor about it. Please use plain envelope."*

—TEST LETTER FROM POSTAL INSPECTOR TO THE INTERSTATE REMEDY COMPANY, 1913[1]

THE first federal agency to combat medical quackery was the Post Office Department. Before Dr. Alsberg sought to test the Sherley Amendment, even before Dr. Wiley began to enforce the Pure Food and Drugs Act, the Postmaster General had aimed a powerful weapon at unscrupulous medical promoters who used the mails.

Back in 1872, during the widespread chicanery of the Gilded Age, Congress, in revising the postal statutes, had devised a new way of fighting fraud. Promoters of get-rich-quick schemes involving securities, mining rights, counterfeit currency, and the like depended on the mails, especially the conveyance of money in registered letters, for the success of their shady transactions. Gullible people fleeced by such schemes usually lived too far away from the site of the crime to seek reparation by the usual legal remedies. So Congress proposed a means of protection. If the Postmaster General should become persuaded, "upon evidence satisfactory to him," that a person or corporation was operating a "scheme or device for obtaining money through the mails by means of false or fraudulent pretenses, representations, or promises," then the

[1] Cited in Hearing 80, Interstate Remedy Company, Mar. 12, 1914, Transcripts of Hearings of Fraud Order Cases, Records of the Post Office Dept., Office of the Solicitor, RG 28, NA.

cabinet officer could take a drastic step. By issuing a "fraud order," he could direct that all registered letters addressed to the crooked enterprise be intercepted, stamped "Fraudulent," and returned to their senders. In 1895 Congress extended the same procedure to cover all other types of mail arriving for an illegal promoter. It all was stopped, stamped "Fraudulent," and sent back. Letters with no return addresses went to the dead letter office, for even fraud was not sufficient grounds for violating the mail's sanctity. No postmaster or any other person, the 1872 law read, could open a letter not addressed to him.[2]

It is not clear when the first mail-order medical quack felt the heavy hand of the Postmaster General upon his shoulder, but probably not until the very end of the century. Up to that point, the Post Office Department sought to restrain fraud involving finance but not fraud involving health. Not until 1901 did the Postmaster General refer in his annual reports to "quack medicines." Two years earlier, however, the Bureau of Chemistry began a collaboration destined to continue for decades, when Dr. Wiley analyzed some "medicinal tablets" for the Post Office Department, finding them "wholly and intentionally fraudulent." Similar services were performed by the Bureau with increasing frequency during the next several years. Over from the Postmaster General came pills to restore "lost manhood," powders to turn black skin white, lotions to straighten kinky hair.[3]

One of the purported skin whiteners, Wiley discovered, was

[2] 17 Stat. 322-23 (June 18, 1872); 28 Stat. 963 (Mar. 2, 1895). The basic phraseology remains almost identical in current law. 39 U.S. Code, 259 (1958). In 1878 the words "firms or corporations" were omitted in a revision of postal statutes, so the law applied only to persons until 1890, when "company" was included. 26 Stat. 466. Dead letter office personnel are permitted to open first-class mail in an effort to identify the sender.

[3] *Report of the Postmaster General, 1901*, 36; Wiley, "Report of Work Done [1896-99] by the Division of Chemistry . . . for the Various Executive Departments," (carbon), Miscellaneous Papers, II, Bur. of Chem. Records, RG 97, NA; Wiley, "Bureau of Chemistry, 1897-1905" (typed ms.), 89-90, Wiley Papers, box 199, Library of Congress. Jean Broderick, "Confessions of a Reformed Mail Order Quack," reminisces about events at the turn of the century. *Hygeia*, 12 (1934), 1077-80, 1144; 13 (1935), 34-37, 92-94.

mainly corrosive sublimate mixed with glycerine. Rejuvenators turned out to be petroleum jelly, or cold cream, or a mixture depending on red pepper for its zip. The flagrant fraudulency of these nostrums which Wiley analyzed for the Post Office Department may well have helped awaken him to the fact that the food and drug law for which he was fighting must contain a definition of drugs broad enough to cover patent medicines. In 1904, Wiley provided a Senate committee with data on a new batch of rejuvenators and some tuberculosis "cures" under scrutiny by postal authorities. Mormon Bishop Pills came in three colors, Wiley indicated, red, white, and blue, and Sir John Hampton's Vital Restorative in two. Sir John's first pill, containing methylene blue, would turn the urine green and frighten patients into further treatment. The second pill was licorice and saw palmetto.[4]

Wiley's analyses formed part of the evidence "satisfactory" to the Postmaster General that the nostrums under question were actually fraudulent. Since postal authorities were prohibited from opening and reading correspondence between a suspected quack and his customers, the task of securing conclusive evidence was difficult. A fraud order was too rigorous a penalty to be dispensed without due cause. When newspaper advertisements asserted categorically that a pill could cure incurable diseases, and Wiley's laboratory reported the pill to be made of inert ingredients, then action seemed justified. The pill maker was informed of the charges against him and summoned to Washington to make such defense as he might wish. If he came, he was accorded a full hearing at which both his evidence and that of the Department were presented. Then the chief legal officer for the Department, at that stage an assistant attorney general, wrote a summary of the hearing and sent it to the Postmaster General with a judgment as to what action should be taken: fraud order or dismissal of the complaint. Almost without exception the Postmaster General followed his lawyer's advice.[5]

In many mail-order ventures, advertisements in magazines

[4] *Investigations of Adulterated Foods, Etc.*, 58 Cong., 1 ses., Sen. Doc. 270 (1904), 2-4.
[5] *Report of the Postmaster General, 1902*, 39-40.

and newspapers merely hinted at the curative powers of the remedy for sale. The full gaudy gamut of promises came only with circulars mailed to all who read the ad and wrote the company pitiful letters of hopeful inquiry. Since reading this exchange of mail was taboo, postal authorities developed a technique for finding out what a quack said when he answered a poor, suffering inquirer. This technique was the test letter. Postal inspectors pretended to have cancer, tuberculosis, male weakness, venereal disease, and engaged in extensive correspondence, often under assumed names, with medicine vendors. So when a male-weakness expert came to Washington for a hearing, he might find the man who had written, "I seen your ad about that free prescription . . . ," testifying to every step in the high-pressure mail campaign touched off by such a letter.

Right at the start of its contest with quackery, the Post Office Department had been given some guidance as to ground rules. A case reached the Supreme Court, resulting in a decision that has exercised an influence over all federal regulation of medical quackery ever since.

The case arose from efforts by the Post Office Department to restrict the activities of a mental healing practitioner. In 1897 an uneducated exponent of this "science," J. H. Kelly, settled down in Nevada, Missouri, where he began practicing and teaching. The next year he incorporated his venture under the name of the American School of Magnetic Healing. Besides treating patients face to face, Kelly believed he could exert his curative powers across vast distances. Through extensive advertising, he conveyed this promise far and wide. To him and his associates, he asserted, had been committed a startling revelation whereby all human ills could be dispersed as if by magic. It was, indeed, the same power Christ had possessed 1900 years before. The human mind, Kelly held, was mainly responsible for sickness. By a proper focusing of the brain, guided from afar, men could largely control and cure their afflictions. For a price Kelly would transmit the healing regimen of his "practical scientific system"—not to be confused with Christian Science. An inquirer received from Kelly certain directions: at a specified moment of time the inquirer should rid his mind of all disturbing thoughts and compose it in a passive condition. He was then prepared to absorb influence from the mind of the healer who, at the same moment in Nevada, would exert the mysterious curative power. In actual fact, Kelly and his associated healers might never see the letters of inquiry, which were answered by female secretaries who copied form responses. Nor did the telepathic wizards necessarily concentrate at the appointed hours—they might be off vacationing in Colorado. Nonetheless the advertising was effective. By 1900 some 3,000 letters a day were arriving in Nevada for the Magnetic School, and the daily cash intake ran from $1,000 to $1,600.[6]

After a hearing in Washington, the Postmaster General directed the Nevada postmaster, J. M. McAnnulty, to refuse delivery on all mail addressed to Kelly and the School. As McAnnulty, in pursuance of the order, prepared to return all mail—stamped "Fraudulent"—to the senders, Kelly went to court. Arguing that the fraud statutes were unconstitutional, he sought an injunction to prevent McAnnulty from sending back the 25,000 letters which crowded his post office. A circuit court judge refused the injunction, saying that the constitutionality of the several laws had already been established. Kelly appealed.

The Supreme Court, although avoiding constitutional questions, sided with Kelly and against the Postmaster General. The fraud order, said Justice Peckham, rested on "a mistaken view of the law." It assumed a fact not capable of being proved, that the mail-order therapy dispensed by the Magnetic School was worthless.

Obviously, Justice Peckham argued, "the influence of the mind upon the physical condition of the body is very powerful, and . . . a hopeful mental state goes far, in many cases, not only to alleviate, but even to aid very largely in the cure of an illness from which the body may suffer." To exactly what degree this mental influence may go, no one can say.

[6] American School of Magnetic Healing and J. H. Kelly v. J. M. McAnnulty, 187 U.S. 94. Data on promotional methods derived also from Weltmer et al. [including Kelly] v. Bishop, 171 Mo. 110 (Su. Ct. of Mo. Div. 1, 1902), 17 *Southwestern Reporter* (1902), 167.

"One person may believe it of far greater efficacy than another, but surely it cannot be said that it is a fraud for one person to contend that the mind has an effect upon the body and its physical condition greater than even a vast majority of intelligent people might be willing to admit or believe." Thus Kelly's claims for his "practical scientific" therapy "cannot be proved as a fact to be fraud." "We may not believe in the efficacy of the treatment to the extent claimed" by Kelly and his supporters, "and we may have no sympathy with them in such claims, and yet their effectiveness is but matter of opinion in any court."

Justice Peckham did not rest content with making his point exclusively with respect to Magnetic Healing. He extended his argument to cover the entire field of therapy. With respect to all aspects of the healing art where medical opinions differ, he said, "there is no exact standard of absolute truth by which to approve . . . [an] assertion false and a fraud." "As the effectiveness of almost any particular method of treatment of disease is, to a more or less extent, a fruitful source of difference of opinion, even though the great majority may be of one way of thinking, the efficacy of any special method is certainly not a matter for the decision of the Postmaster General within these statutes relative to fraud."

The McAnnulty rule, coming at the very start of federal regulation of quackery, was a "roadblock" to strong control, "a source of solace and comfort to generations of nostrum vendors."[7] The decision made governmental administrators cautious. It also gave instructive lessons to quacks. They would be well advised to sell medicines for diseases still baffling orthodox physicians, to use drugs which some doctors at some time had said were worthy, to hire for their staffs physicians willing to present to a trial or hearing the medical opinion—though it might be a decidedly minority view—that the remedy under discussion was effective therapy for the advertised diseases. It was the McAnnulty doctrine which

[7] Edgar R. Carver, Jr., "The Rule in the McAnnulty Case," *FDC Law Jnl.*, 5 (1950), 494-512, an excellent discussion of the case and its continuing applicability. See also, "Proving the Falsity of Advertising: The McAnnulty Rule and Expert Evidence," *Indiana Law Jnl.*, 32 (1956-57), 350-73.

Oliver Wendell Holmes applied to let Dr. Johnson's cancer claims stay on his labels, overruling Dr. Wiley's interpretation of the 1906 law. It was the McAnnulty doctrine which molded the phrasing of the Sherley Amendment.

Justice Peckham's opinion did not, however, destroy the Postmaster General's authority to combat quackery. In Peckham's wide-ranging dicta, he suggested several limitations upon the main thrust of his central doctrine. Some medical issues had passed beyond the "empirical stage" and had entered the realm of material fact, so that the value or lack of value of a given therapy, no longer a matter of opinion, could be demonstrated scientifically. A promoter whose claims contradicted medical fact was proper prey for the Postmaster General. Even where opinions were still in conflict, Peckham intimated, fraud might occur if curative claims were absolutely unrestrained, if the promise were made "that the treatment . . . will always succeed." And there might be nostrums not assailable on the basis of their claims, the justice asserted, which could be acted against if postal authorities could prove that the "business . . . as in fact conducted" amounted to fraud.

In the Missouri state courts, it must be noted, Kelly and his associates of the Magnetic School did not fare so well as in the Supreme Court of the United States. Rebuked in a newspaper article for being "miserable charlatans," they sued for libel and won. But on appeal a Missouri supreme court justice reversed the decision. The lower judge, he said, should not have permitted the jury to decide whether or not Kelly's alleged therapy was a legitimate business, despite the long parade of former patients who testified gratefully in Kelly's behalf. "Courts are not such slaves to the forms of procedure," the high court stated, "as to surrender their own intelligence to an army of witnesses testifying to an impossibility. They are not required to give credence to a statement that would falsify well-known laws of nature, though a cloud of witnesses swear to it."[8]

The Postmaster General, restrained by the McAnnulty decision but guided by its clues, moved slowly and with great deliberation. The pace of his march against medical fraud

---

[8] Weltmer et al. v. Bishop.

can be detected by the number of analyses run for him by the Bureau of Chemistry: 21 in 1906, 13 in 1907, 5 in 1908, 15 in 1909, 20 in 1910, 21 in 1911.[9] Postal authorities assailed the most outrageous quacks, those promising sure cures for incurable diseases. Every effort was made to develop unassailable evidence in the quack's methods of promotion to demonstrate his fraudulent intent.

The great majority of Post Office cases dealt with cures for cancer, consumption, and epilepsy. Also attacked were remedies for blindness and deafness, the drug habit and the tobacco habit, lost manhood and failing womanhood. To make a fraud order stick against a concern vending a deafness cure, a postal inspector submitted thirteen symptom blanks, filled in so as to indicate various types of deafness listed as incurable in the quack's own promotional literature. In every case, the quack responded by diagnosing the deafness as due to "deep seated and chronic" catarrh, and by prescribing as the perfect treatment his own drugs and an $8 "electro-magnetic head-cap." Relying on the McAnnulty decision, the promoter went to court. Relying on a McAnnulty exception, the judge ruled against him. "What might otherwise be a legal business or profession," the judge stated, "may be so conducted as to render it a vehicle of fraud and deception." In this case, the advertising doctor, exhibiting "utter indifference" to the symptom blank, sought merely "to get . . . as much of . . . [the patient's] money as possible."[10]

Choosing its cases with care, the Post Office Department developed an excellent statistical record of success. Many mail-order promoters, hailed to a hearing, were anxious to revise their promotional methods so as to avoid the death grasp of a fraud order. In some cases this was permitted, the proprietor signing an affidavit promising to discontinue practices deemed fraudulent by postal authorities. When fraud orders were issued, they were seldom contested, and when

[9] *Reports of the Bureau of Chemistry, passim.*

[10] *Ibid. Reports of the Postmaster General* are not helpful during these years, containing few references to medical quackery as distinguished from other types of fraud. *N&Q,* I, derives a great deal of material from Post Office fraud cases. The deafness case is Branaman v. Harris, 189 Fed. 461 (1911); see also *N&Q,* I, 252-65.

contested in the courts, rarely overthrown.[11] A most discouraging fact, however, began to be evident to those within the Department charged with combatting fraud. There existed a breed of inveterate quacks who could not easily be curbed. Defeated in one venture, they launched a new one, with a new name, a new address, and a new—and often more subtle—approach. It was a somewhat risky but financially rewarding life, fleecing the sick and miserable through the mails, and called for imagination, audacity, and utter lack of scruple.

In 1904 the Postmaster General issued two fraud orders on the same day, one aimed at the Dr. Raynor Medical Company, the other at the Dr. Knapp Medical Company. In point of fact, the two companies were the same, and the moving spirit in both was a Detroit resident named Edward D. Hayes. Six years before, with help from a doctor and a chemist, Hayes had begun to play the "lost manhood" game. He had placed ads in magazines like *Mail and Breeze,* headlined "Makes 'Old Men' Boys Again," showing a grandfather type holding aloft a bouncing baby while his pretty young wife looked on. Hayes had distributed pamphlets condemning both regular physicians and "the company of quacks," and promising, "We treat and guarantee to cure absolutely the following troubles: SPERMATORRHEA (Night Emissions), VARICOCELE, LACK OF ERECTILE POWER, SMALL OR UNDEVELOPED ORGANS, HASTINESS OR PREMATURITY, URINARY TROUBLE AND KIDNEY AND BLADDER TROUBLES."[12]

The Restorative Remedies were really shotgun formulas, mostly herbal, containing drugs like damiana fabled in folklore for their rejuvenating powers. Called to Washington for a Post Office Department hearing, Hayes and his associates backed down. They signed an affidavit agreeing to abandon their enterprises and to permit the Detroit postmaster to return mail to the senders for a space of time, marked not as "Fraudulent"

[11] Carver, 494-512. That the Post Office Dept. did seek to enlarge the definition of quackery over which its controls might operate is indicated by trade reaction to the "Nature's Health Restorer" fraud order. *Druggists' Circular,* 11 (1905), 376.

[12] Fraud Order Jackets 1993 and 1995, Fraud Orders 1074 and 1076, Sep. 23, 1904, Dr. Raynor Medical Co. and Dr. Knapp Medical Co., Records of the Post Office Dept., Office of the Solicitor, RG 28, NA.

but as "Refused." But the agreement was broken: money orders were cashed and new promotional pamphlets distributed. Fraud orders followed promptly as a matter of course.

The Knapp and Raynor companies had collapsed, but very shortly Hayes was back in business. His new venture, the Interstate Remedy Company, vended the same kind of wares, but with more caution. Hayes, at least, took pains to make a great show of circumspection. On the first of many voluntary journeys to Washington, Hayes told postal authorities that it was not he, but a partner, who had cashed the money orders, and then only because of erroneous advice from the Detroit postmaster. Promotional plans for the new Interstate concern were discussed with Post Office legal officers to make sure they did not cross the border into fraud. During the next few years, Hayes dropped by the Post Office Department from time to time, just to see if there were any new rules he ought to know about. He also checked his advertising copy and direct mail pamphlets with a Chicago outfit, the Federal Guide Association, staffed by former postal inspectors who sold advice to proprietary promoters on how to avoid trouble with the law. (Hayes had taken pains to ask the assistant attorney general of the Post Office Department if the Association was run by "respectable people." So far as he knew, the legal officer had answered, it was.) And, for good measure, Hayes saw successive district attorneys in Detroit, presenting his medical literature for scrutiny.[13]

Through all this checking and rechecking, business developed nicely. During one five-day span in early 1914, the Institute cashed $1,245.80 in money orders, and only Hayes knew how much in cash and checks arrived in the 1,444 pieces of mail that was the company's daily average.

This money came mainly from men with doubts about their potency, "brought on by excesses, unnatural drains or the follies of youth." Hayes appealed to them through ads in publications ranging from the *Baptist Record* to the *Police Gazette*. "$3.50 Recipe Cures Weak Men—Free," the headline read.

[13] Fraud Order Jacket 3657, Fraud Order 7977, Apr. 17, 1914, Interstate Remedy Co., and Hearing 80, in *ibid.* See also *N&Q,* I, 266-75; II, 284-87.

This recipe was a physician's prescription, "the surest-acting combination for the cure of deficient manhood and vigor failure ever assembled." The "up-building, SPOT-TOUCHING" formula cost nothing and would be sent inquirers in a plain envelope, with all correspondence kept strictly confidential. The Interstate Company also ran advertising which promised to cure weak kidneys. Many of the ads of both kinds were signed by Dr. A. E. Robinson.

At the Interstate offices, each day's incoming mail was sorted by a large staff of clerks. Every desk bore a sign warning against the commitment of fraud. The clerks operated according to a system which, the company's lawyer said, was "almost automatic." Initial letters went into one of three piles. If the clerk interpreted the letter to describe symptoms of "lost manhood," he placed it in the "nervous" pile. There was a similar "kidney" pile. Should a letter reveal symptoms of ailments not amenable to treatment by the company's two formulas, the clerks had a third pile which Dr. Robinson would read. It seems unlikely that the doctor's labors in the company's behalf required much time.

Dr. Robinson's facsimile signature was much employed, at any rate. It came at the end of form letters sent out to all "nervous" and "kidney" patients, letters printed to resemble typewriting, with name and address typed in to enhance the illusion of personal attention. Similar letters went forth from Interstate to men who might never have seen an Interstate ad. For the company bought from brokers batches of letters written by worried males to *other* "male weakness" companies. Sometimes a promise to remedy exhausted virility might be addressed to a young boy of twelve. But accidents happen in all businesses.

True to the advertising, with the Interstate form letter went a prescription. No druggist, however, could fill the formula sent kidney sufferers. It contained two remarkable ingredients, "kydnos" and "urikol" obtainable only from the company. Happily the sufferer need not delay. For simultaneously with the letter, Interstate dispatched a fortnight's supply of medicine by express. The cost was $3.50 C.O.D., and the letter explained how the doctor was sure the sick man would want to lose no time.

The "Man Medicine" formula, mailed to the impotent, contained no trick ingredients and could be filled at any drugstore. Most men, Hayes evidently believed, would not get their prescriptions filled locally for fear news of their ailment might leak out. So the C.O.D. package, private and convenient, was a mighty safe bet. Get the package from the express office without delay, the form letter urged. "Do you think you will be better a week from now? Are you not convinced in your own mind that every week that goes by and nothing done is just seven opportunities for health wilfully squandered?"

Behind the first form letter lay a variable series of letters, to be sent according to how the sufferer behaved. If he paid $3.50 for the two-week supply, he was quickly sent enough for a month, C.O.D., costing $6. If he delayed, he was dispatched a round of increasingly frightening letters, ending with a cut in price to $1.75.

In 1913 the Post Office Department decided to check into Interstate's methods of operation. A new political administration was in office, and postal attorneys may not have known about Hayes' earlier efforts at conspicuous rectitude. Or he may have actually aroused suspicion by another visit to Washington. At any rate, postal inspectors, following their usual procedure, began to write Interstate heartrending letters.

"There is something wrong with my testicles," one test letter began, "and I don't know what to make of it. I noticed for some time that they don't hang even and that the left one hangs lower. I ain't got the nerve to ask our doctor about it so am writing to you to find out what you think about it. Please use plain envelope."

Of course, this perfectly natural condition was, to Interstate, an ailment. You have "swollen testicles," the company answered, and need Man Medicine for "quick recovery."

Another inspector asked if Interstate's prescription would "cure" him "of a weak stomach." He got a personal answer. "You say in your letter," it began, "that you are suffering from weak stomach and weak manhood. . . ."

"Ben Watkins" of Grass Lake, Michigan, was a bachelor of 23. He didn't run around much with girls, but every six or eight weeks had a "wet dream." "Now i don't feel no bad effects from them," he told Interstate, "but am kinder wondering if them dreams ain't bad for me." They were indeed, was the reply, and a special $6-package of medicine awaited Ben at the express office.

No symptoms were listed at all in the letter "Abe Rutledge" wrote. "I seen your ad about that free prescription of yours but dont know if it is the thing I need. I would of liked to ask our local doctor but kinder dont want him to know about it. I thought by writing to you I could find out if I need treatment because I don't want to eat no medicines if it ain't necessary."

Interstate sent a personal answer along with a pamphlet. If Rutledge was suffering from any of the listed troubles, the doctor said, "I am confident I can restore you to health and sexual strength." A 15-day C.O.D. treatment was being shipped by Wells Fargo Express.

Rutledge continued perversely obtuse. "I got your letter and your book," he replied, "but cant make head or tale out of it. I dont know that my sexual strength is not allright and before taking the medicine from the express office I wished you would tell me if I ought to take the treatment."

"Call at the express office at once for the treatment," the reply came back, "and commence using it." Two follow-up letters from Interstate reached Rutledge when he failed to heed this counsel.

Man Medicine was analyzed for the Post Office Department by the Bureau of Chemistry. Like Hayes' earlier Restorative Remedies, it was a mixture of "well-known tonics and laxatives," a mixture which could not rejuvenate, could not, as promised, ensure "once more the gusto, the joyful satisfaction, the pulse and throb of physical pleasure, the keen sense of man-sensation."

Once more Hayes showed up in Washington, this time summoned to show cause why a fraud order should not be issued against the Interstate Medicine Company. Into the hearing record were read the test letters and the replies, Hayes' formulas, and testimony by various physicians about the futility of treating impotency by means of such drugs. Moreover, the company kept offering the remedy when inquirers suggested no hint of an ailment, but merely normal conditions of healthy males. Diagnosis by mail on the basis of laymen's letters was simply not possible, the medical experts said. An inspector told of corresponding with 37 of Interstate's customers: two claimed they had been helped; the rest reported no benefit while taking Man Medicine for periods ranging from a month to five years.

To contradict the advertising promises of privacy, the Post Office Department revealed a letter written by Interstate to a Chicago broker handling "sucker lists." The company had 70,000 to 80,000 letters from weak-men inquirers, the letter said, "the choicest lot of Nervous Debility names to be had in the country, and have never been copied by anyone." If Interstate could get something close to a proper price, it would sell or rent.

In defending himself, Edward Hayes recounted the steps he had taken, after his earlier troubles, to stay on the right side of the law—his consultations in Washington, his conversations with district attorneys, his expensive advice from the Federal Guide Association, his reiterated injunctions to employees to function uprightly. The Interstate formulas had been devised, Hayes said, by Dr. Robinson, an M.D. from Queen's University in Toronto. Other physicians might hold a contrary opinion, but Robinson believed in his remedies, and so did Hayes.

Only once had letters written to Interstate been sold to a broker, and none was of a confidential nature. Hayes stopped the practice when told by the Federal Guide Association that the Post Office Department considered it "not very nice." The later offer to sell over 70,000 letters to the Chicago company, Hayes insisted, was not bona fide. It was a ruse to discover the going price, for while Interstate no longer sold, it often bought such merchandise.

The screening of incoming letters, Hayes admitted, was regrettably not perfect. The clerks occasionally made a mistake. No medicine should have been sent out in reply to the "weak stomach" letter, and the low-hanging testicle letter should have been given an individual, instead of a form, reply.

"You can see," Hayes' attorney amplified, "that in the multitude of letters that come in, and the number of clerks that are working on this, it is very easy for a person to get a letter that should have gone to the doctor specially, to get them into the catalogue where the debility case was and then get the regular system of follow up . . . debility letters. That is pure mistake and you can see how almost diabolically clever that [test] letter was written to trap these people, and they have simply trapped them into a mistake."

If blame there was, in short, it was on the heads of the sneaky postal inspectors.

The assistant attorney general for the Post Office Department, W. H. Lamar, did not agree. "There are facts that have developed here in connection with the actual operation of this case," he stated frankly during the hearing, "which would convince any reasonable man's mind that a fraud was being committed." Nor did Hayes' almost obsessive consultations impress Lamar. The Interstate president, Lamar told the Postmaster General, "sought advice for the purpose of enabling him so to disguise the nature of the scheme as to evade the law, or else for the purpose of being able to make a colorable showing of good faith should the business at any time be questioned."[14]

If that was Hayes' scheme, it backfired badly. On April 17, 1914, the Postmaster General issued a fraud order. But he did not stop there. By a law of 1889, using the mails to defraud had become a crime. Under this law, Hayes, his partner, and Dr. Robinson were indicted in Detroit. They pleaded guilty, and Hayes was given the maximum fine, $5,000, which the law allowed. In recommending fines instead of jail sentences, the district attorney told the judge that Hayes had agreed to turn over to the government a mailing list of half a million

[14] All of Hayes' assertions about having had the assurances of previous Post Office officials as to the propriety of his promotional methods were made orally at the hearing. When asked if he had anything in writing to substantiate his version of the conversations, Hayes said no.

names. Seven to eight tons of a "lost manhood" company's most valuable asset were converted into pulp.[15]

Hayes no longer needed the names, for he was through with prescribing for weak men. He was not done, however, with mail-order medicine. While operating Interstate, Hayes had launched an obesity cure. Marmola was to be ten times the nostrum that Man Medicine had been.[16]

One thing the Post Office Department discovered in checking on Edward Hayes' medicines was that he did not manufacture them himself. Like many mail-order operators called in for hearings, Hayes bought his wares from major ethical drug producers.

Most makers of prescription drugs, during these years, were just crossing the threshold of sophisticated science. In 1902 Parke, Davis & Company had built a research laboratory, claiming the distinction of being the first industrial concern in the country to erect a structure especially for research. The legislation of 1906, enacting the *Pharmacopeia* and *National Formulary* standards into law, forced many pharmaceutical manufacturers, who had never before had such scientific staffs, to establish laboratories for both biological and chemical assay of their products. German imports dominated the market in chemical synthetics, American concerns neglecting this scientific field. They devoted their energies chiefly to extracting the active ingredients from plants and embodying them in various pills, tablets, and elixirs. Marketing policies left much to be desired. "The advertising departments of the pharmaceutical firms . . . ," in the opinion of the director of the AMA Chemical Laboratory, "could well afford to cooperate more closely with the scientific workers before copy is sent broadcast." Even the scientific workers were viewed with some suspicion. Until past the middle of the 1920's, the American Society for Pharmacology and Experimental Therapeutics would expel a member who took permanent employment with a drug firm.[17]

[15] 25 Stat. 873 (Mar. 2, 1889); *N&Q*, II, 284-87; Kebler to A. J. Cramp, July 27, 1927, Marmola folder, Dept. of Investigation, American Medical Association.

[16] See chs. 6 and 9.

[17] Tom Mahoney, *The Merchants of Life: An Account of the American*

Whatever their other shortcomings, ethical manufacturers did one thing that deeply bothered patent medicine critics: they engaged in the surreptitious production of nostrums. Wiley and Kebler had discovered this from the flood of correspondence loosed by the passage of the Pure Food and Drugs Act. "A large majority of all the proprietary remedies," Wiley wrote late in 1906, "are made by manufacturing concerns whose names appear nowhere upon the label, and who would be, I am sure, heartily ashamed to have them there. . . . That first-class firms should lend their influence or countenance to a thing of this kind is almost incredible."[18]

Such expressions of incredulity kept recurring. "The Great Drug Laboratories of America," commented a visiting Australian, ". . . might, with ample reason, claim to be the biggest packers of quack medicines in the world. Anything from homicide to humbug, with all between, is prepared and packed to order for the nostrum-vendors." At the hearing on Congressman Richardson's abortive bill, Dr. Kebler expressed chagrin that "reputable" manufacturers were making "the most vicious frauds." "I have furthermore been informed," he added, "that some of the ethical firms actually furnish the formula, compound the medicines, supply the literature, and everything else so that these quacks can go on doing business."[19] This gloomy fact the Post Office Department kept rediscovering as it continued trying to close the mails to the most unscrupulous of the medical fakers.

The year of the victory over Interstate marked the beginning of an upsurge in Post Office activity against medical swindlers that has not slackened since. Cooperation between the Department and the Bureau of Chemistry, already close,

*Pharmaceutical Industry* (N.Y., 1959), 4, 75; Julius Stieglitz, ed., *Chemistry in Medicine* (N.Y., 1928), 397, 404-05, 414-15, 473; Paul N. Leech, "Chemistry in the Service of Pharmaceutical Medicine," *JAMA*, 85 (1925), 138-41.

[18] *Amer. Druggist*, 49 (1906), 357.

[19] *Secret Drugs, Cures, and Frauds: Report of the Royal Commission of the Parliament of the Commonwealth of Australia* (1907), I, 133; *The Pure Food and Drugs Act, Hearings . . .*, 62 Cong., 2 ses. (1912), 492. Arthur J. Cramp of the AMA did not believe that this evil had diminished by 1926. *Hygeia*, 4 (1926), 398.

was strengthened. With the arrival of Dr. Glover at the Bureau to handle Sherley Amendment matters, Lyman Kebler became a full-time liaison scientist between the two agencies. He ran the increased number of analyses which growing Post Office action required, testified at hearings and in court, and wrote numerous articles that publicized what postal authorities were doing to fight medical fraud.[20]

Protecting the public demanded close cooperation between the regulatory agencies, for each could combat quackery in ways the other could not. Where promotions were conducted mostly through the mails, Post Office action could be "more prompt and complete" than any measures the Bureau of Chemistry was permitted by law to take. The Bureau especially encountered difficulty in fighting alleged drug-habit cures that themselves contained narcotics. These were mailed direct from the proprietor to the consumer, and it was hard for food and drug inspectors to get evidence. The courts looked with disfavor on cases started with "induced shipments." So postal inspectors—whose "test letters" the courts approved—fared better in this field.[21]

The definition of fraud, under postal statutes, was broader than that of medical quackery under the 1906 Pure Food and Drugs Act. Certain promotions, therefore, which the Bureau of Chemistry was helpless to handle could be attacked by the Post Office Department. As a result of a long and hard-fought criminal case, ending in 1915, fraudulent medical devices were shown to be a proper object of postal control. The case concerned the Oxypathor, one of the "gas-pipe cures," which as a therapeutic agent "belonged in the same class as the left hind foot of a rabbit caught in a graveyard in the dark of the

[20] *Report of the Postmaster General, 1914*, 46-47; Kebler wrote a series on mail fraud for *Standard Remedies*, 6 (Feb. 1920), 21, 22; (Apr. 1920), 15, 16, 18; (Sep. 1920), 15, 16; (Oct. 1920), 15, 16; 7 (Feb. 1921), 11, 12. He also wrote "Public Health Conserved through the Enforcement of Postal Fraud Laws," *Amer. Jnl. of Public Health*, 12 (1922), 678-83, and a series for *Druggists' Circular*, reprinted in 1928 or 1929 as *The Mail-Order Medical Game*.

[21] Rexford G. Tugwell to Postmaster General, Mar. 29, 1933, Med-Rem folder, General Corres. of the Office of the Secy. of Agric., 1933, RG 16, NA; *1922 Report of the Bureau of Chemistry*, 22; *1923 Report*, 16-17; Kebler, "Public Health Conserved through the Enforcement of Postal Fraud Laws," 681.

moon." The gadget was a piece of nickel-plated tubing filled
with inert material and sealed shut. Attached to each end was
a flexible cord culminating in a garter-like band of elastic, one
for a wrist, the other for an ankle, to be worn while the cylinder
rested in a crock of water. The device purportedly permitted
the body to absorb more oxygen and hence combat almost
any ailment. Besides such crooked therapeutic devices, the
Post Office Department could take action against weight reduction drugs and certain cosmetics which the Bureau of Chemistry lacked authority to fight.[22]

During World War I, both agencies joined in battling the
rising flood of nostrums promising to cure venereal disease.
This campaign led to an effort in Congress to bar from the
mails all advertising concerned with venereal disease. To be
successful, the prohibition would have to be broad enough to
cover various euphemisms by which syphilis had recently
been disguised in order to escape postal authorities and state
advertising control bills. Everybody knew now that "blood
poisoning" in an advertisement meant venereal disease. "But
while syphilis is blood poison," as the Proprietary Association
counsel told a House committee, "it doesn't follow that all
blood poisons are syphilis." So to exclude from the mail all
venereal disguises would be to eliminate some of the oldest
and most established of family remedies. The next step would
be a law to prevent anyone from dosing himself with a proprietary remedy "unless he shall go to the doctor for a personal
examination." The bill, said another witness, had aimed at a
mountain lion but would also reach "a harmless, household
canary." The measure was not reported by the committee to
the House.[23]

What the venereal remedy quacks did in employing euphemisms was one example, of course, of what quacks always did
when regulation pressed too hard. They made some sort of
shift, especially the shrewdest enterprisers, which sought to

[22] Moses v. United States, 221 Fed. 863 (1915); *N&Q*, II, 706-13.
[23] Kebler, "Public Health Conserved through the Enforcement of the
Postal Fraud Laws," 682; *Excluding Advertisements of Cures for Venereal Diseases from the Mails: Hearings before the Committee on the
Post Office and Post Roads of the House . . . on H. R. 5123*, 66 Cong.,
1 ses. (1919).

avoid or lessen legal hazards. Another maneuver and one widely used in the late teens and twenties, was the abandonment of high-risk products, like cancer cures, in favor of wares aimed at ailments about which medical opinion was not so uniform. To judge by Post Office cases initiated between 1925 and 1930, there was a boom in remedies for reducing and for rheumatism. Postal inspectors had to work harder at their jobs, and chemical and medical analyses had to be more thorough. In earlier days, as Dr. Kebler said in 1922, schemes had been "much cruder than . . . at present."[24]

If less crude than formerly, the most disreputable remaining schemes still posed the main target for postal authorities. The burden of proving fraud was easiest against drugs and devices offering to restore "lost manhood" and against panaceas promising to cure all of mankind's ills. These categories led medical fraud cases started during the late twenties, with nostrums for tuberculosis and venereal disease also ranking high.[25] Despite constant vigilance and crash campaigns— like a 1926 effort aimed at two score Kansas City mail-order promoters[26]—the ranks of quackery were annually augmented. Numerous promoters, some naive and ignorant, others crass and clever, entered the market with products claiming to cure virtually every ailment known to man.

In its continuing contest with quackery in the mails, the Post Office Department got help from understanding court decisions. The Oxypathor case had been one instance. Equally significant was victory over a chronic offender in the "weak manhood" racket, whose Organo Tablets contained a substance extracted from the testicles of rams. This decision broadened the McAnnulty exceptions in a significant way. In that crucial case Justice Peckham had stated that no one could "lay down the limit and say beyond that there are fraud and false pre-

---

[24] Fraud and Lottery Dockets, volumes 7-9 [including 1925-1930], Office of the Assistant Attorney General for the Post Office Dept., Records of the Post Office Dept., RG 28, NA; *Report of the Postmaster General, 1928*, 66-67; Kebler, "Public Health Conserved through the Enforcement of the Postal Fraud Laws," 679.

[25] Fraud and Lottery Dockets, 1925-1930.

[26] *Printers' Ink*, 135 (June 24, 1926), 85-86, 91 [hereafter cited as *PI*]; Cramp, "Long Distance Quackery," *Hygeia*, 4 (1926), 395-98.

tenses." But in the Organo Tablets case a circuit judge did in fact draw such a line. The issue, he said, was not whether sheep's testicles were entirely worthless, about which there was some conflict of medical evidence, but whether the drug was so promoted as to constitute a fraud. Without question this "male weakness" pill had been so advertised. Thus the court blended together the panacea and the "as in fact conducted" exceptions to Peckham's main doctrine so as to cover the significant border zone wherein a remedy might not be entirely devoid of value but go forth with curative claims far beyond actual therapeutic use. This zone had become well populated with shrewd promoters, and the Organo decision aided postal authorities in driving them out.[27]

Encouraging, too, to postal authorities was evidence that the courts would keep step with advancing science. In 1916 the government had lost a Sherley Amendment case aimed at Tuberclecide. At the trial, medical opinion was evenly divided, at least quantitatively. Just as many doctors asserted the utility of creosote carbonate in treating tuberculosis as argued that the chemical had long since been discarded in proper medical practice. The judge counted noses and could not find that Tuberclecide's claims were false. Nor were they fraudulent. Granted that the nostrum's discoverer was an ignorant man. "Dr. Jenner, who discovered [smallpox] vaccine did not do it by any scientific method. He discovered it from deduction from the fact that milkmaids did not have smallpox, or, if they did have it at all, they had it only in a mild form. It did not take a graduate from any college, or a licensed physician, to make that deduction, and the same might probably be said concerning Tuberclecide."[28]

So a cruel deception continued for more than ten years, its promoter, indeed, taking a cue from the judge's words. "The greatest inventions of modern times that have benefited mankind," Charles Aycock boasted in a booklet, "have been the children of the brain of the lowly born and obscure." At a

[27] Leach, Doing Business As Organo Product Company v. Carlile, Postmaster, 258 U.S. 138 (1922); Carver, "The Rule in the McAnnulty Case," 504-505; N&Q, II, 322-26.

[28] United States v. Tuberclecide, 252 Fed. 938 (1916); N&Q, I, 165-72.

Post Office Department hearing, Aycock also sought to make a virtue of his ignorance. "I am like Jesus Christ," he said, "opening the eyes of the blind and when critics asked how it was done he said: 'I do not know, I was blind but now I see.' That is all I can say. I took it and got well. Others took it and got well. That is all I know."[29]

In 1928 a federal circuit court agreed with the Postmaster General that Tuberclecide was useless and its promotion fraudulent. More than a decade of diligent effort among scientists had as yet produced no cure for tuberculosis, the judges conceded, but some treatments earlier propounded as of value could now be discarded as futile. "Representations then made in good faith would, if now made in the light of greater scientific knowledge, and in the light of greater experience in the use of these medicines themselves, be wholly inconsistent with the theory of good faith or any honest belief in their correctness."

The Tuberclecide decision was timely. The Post Office Department—and all other agencies policing medicines vended for self-dosage—were soon to face a rigorous time of testing. For with the Great Depression came a great upsurge of questionable practices in the self-medication realm. In the meantime, the Bureau of Chemistry—and its successor, the Food, Drug, and Insecticide Administration, which in 1927 assumed responsibility for enforcing the 1906 law[30]—confronted its own version of Tuberclecide. At stake in the protracted battle over the good faith of another promoter of a tuberculosis remedy was the very integrity of the Sherley Amendment itself.

[29] Aycock v. O'Brien, 28 Fed. (2d) 817 (1928); *N&Q*, III, 108.
[30] *1928 Report of Food, Drug, and Insecticide Administration*, 1.

# 5

## B. & M.

"*This is the most important case that this [Food and Drug] Administration has ever had, and if we lose it we might just as well shut up the shop and go home.*"

—P. M. LOWELL, ACTING CHIEF, DRUG CONTROL, 1929[1]

DURING 1922 in a federal district court in Concord, New Hampshire, the United States government suffered defeat in an action to condemn "Eleven Packages of B. & M. External Remedy." Disappointed but not disheartened, officials charged with enforcing food and drug legislation set out forthwith on what was destined to be a ten-year campaign to turn the tables of justice.[2]

B. & M. labeling flaunted the boldest of claims. The list of maladies it could cure ran on and on: pneumonia, laryngitis, bronchitis, pleurisy, la grippe, asthma, hay fever, catarrh, rheumatism, lumbago, neuralgia, neuritis, peritonitis, neurasthenia, locomotor ataxia, varicose veins, blood poisoning, autointoxication, sprains, scalds, burns, cancer, and tuberculosis— above all, tuberculosis. B. & M.'s career had begun, however, more humbly.

[1] Lowell to Dr. Bowman C. Crowell, Oct. 31, 1929, Food and Drug Case 23296 (NJ 18176), Office of the Solicitor, Dept. of Agric., RG 16, NA.
[2] The early history of B. & M. and litigation concerning it is compiled from the records of F&D Case 11492 (NJ 11671), Office of the Solicitor, Dept. of Agric., RG 16, NA; Charles E. Holton, "B. & M. Case . . . Résumé of Field Investigation, 1929-1930," in F&D Case 26900 (NJ 19651), *ibid.*; *Boston Herald*, Dec. 4, 1920; Concord *Monitor*, Dec. 15, 1922; B. & M. folder, Dept. of Investigation, AMA, Chicago; *Boston Better Business Bureau Bulletin*, Aug. 27, 1932; U.S. v. Eleven Packages of B. & M. External Remedy, charge to jury, in White and Gates, *Decisions of Courts under the Federal Food and Drugs Act*, 1059-70; Ruth deForest Lamb, *American Chamber of Horrors* (N.Y., 1936), 40-44; B. & M. pamphlets in author's possession.

During the first decade of the century, a racetrack habitué named William McClellan, finding himself hard pressed for funds, marketed a liniment for horses. As to the source of his formula, McClellan later told different tales. Either it was brought from Ireland by his mother-in-law, a woman named Burns, or it was picked up from a Dr. Byrnes, who was either a doctor who played the horses or a doctor who treated them. Whatever its origin, the potent brew did not differ much from liniments long in use: its three main ingredients were turpentine, ammonia, and raw eggs. McClellan tinkered with the mixture some—the first of many modifications—adding small amounts of formaldehyde and the oils of mustard and wintergreen. The name of the liniment—destined, unlike the formula, to remain stable—derived its key letters from the Burns and McClellan initials.

Persuaded that the horse could not long hold out against the automobile, McClellan shrewdly shifted his appeal from beast to man. Pouring his excoriating concoction into small bottles, he began to peddle it around Boston for rubbing on sore muscles and aching joints. Among McClellan's customers was a court reporter plagued with rheumatic fingers. One bottle of B. & M. let him get on with his shorthand and turned his interest to the liniment. Approaching the age of 70, Frank E. Rollins was seeking a business opportunity to occupy the years of his retirement. In his youth he had worked as bookkeeper for the Ayer remedy company, so he was not unfamiliar with the promotion of proprietaries. Trying out B. & M. on others members of his family, Rollins reached the conclusion —so, at least, he was to insist unswervingly—that McClellan had far underestimated the healing capacities of his liniment. Rollins' grandniece, his sister-in-law, his daughter, all cruelly afflicted with tuberculosis, made miraculous recoveries. McClellan was pleased at the interest of the mild-mannered, round-faced, smiling court reporter, who had such good contacts in legal and religious circles. Rollins' life savings would come in handy, too. For his part, Rollins saw retirement security in the formula owned by the rough and simple racetrack man. The two got together and in 1913 incorporated as the National Remedy Company.

The situation was, as a government investigator put it, "a case of Greek meeting Greek."[3] Rollins was to win. Within a few years he had maneuvered McClellan out of his stock, and—continuing to teach a large Sunday School class the while—Rollins had amplified B. & M.'s curative compass to include the whole gamut of major human ills. He had also gone to great pains to get physicians and sanatoriums to try his remedy on tubercular patients—he had even written to Washington urging that it be used in army hospitals during the war. These efforts to reach the medical profession proved largely futile. A village doctor or two succumbed. Political influence from Rollins' court reporting days led to a test in one state hospital, but the results were not such as could be used in advertising. Much more successful was the effort to gather testimonials from laymen who had used the medicine. These Rollins reported in pamphlet and press. On them he based his rhapsodic promises.

"White Plague Conquered!!!" began one pamphlet. "The New Chemical Compound B. & M. External Remedy Has Won the Victory—Tubercular germs are entirely eradicated from the lungs, glands, or joints in four to twelve weeks . . . without any radical change in mode of life. The breadwinner need not abandon his employment. The housewife need not leave her cares to others. The student need not abandon his books. The expensive sanatorium treatment during months or years is no longer necessary. The looking forward into the grave, while dreading the approaching end, may now be only a nightmare banished forever."[4]

Such deathless prose was bound sooner or later to come to the attention of the Bureau of Chemistry. Since Rollins' interstate shipments were still on a mail-order basis, the Bureau's Boston man talked with a Post Office inspector, who took the facts to the district attorney. Rollins a menace? That could hardly be. The attorney knew him well. He would try to get the cherubic ex-court reporter to tone down his advertising. But no change occurred.

In 1919 the Bureau had some shipments of B. & M. seized

[3] Holton's Résumé.
[4] 1916 pamphlet, "B. & M. External Remedy."

in New Hampshire. While the case was awaiting trial, the Boston health commissioner took action. Asserting that Rollins' "false and misleading" advertising violated state law, the commissioner hailed B. & M.'s owner into court on an indictment of 35 counts. Rollins put two witnesses on the stand who swore that the liniment had cured them of consumption. The commissioner got their permission to have them examined by physicians on his staff and x-rayed at a city hospital. The results were sobering. Both witnesses still had tuberculosis, and one was so sick he soon would die. Another of Rollins' satisfied users, on his way to testify how he had been cured of Bright's disease, gangrene, and diabetes, collapsed while climbing the courthouse stairs and almost expired on the spot. To condemn B. & M. came distinguished physicians, including the chairman of the board governing the state's hospitals for tubercular patients, who told of the liniment's abysmal failure when it had been put to the test. When the verdict was rendered, Rollins won on 33 and lost on two counts. The judge, who was acquainted with the accused, assessed a fine of $10 and made guilt sound very much like innocence.

"I believe Mr. Rollins to be a man of the very highest type," he said from the bench, "absolutely sincere, and having the utmost faith in the efficiency of his remedy. I think the testimony shows that he was actuated by altruistic motives rather than motives of personal gain."[5]

In the Concord courtroom, a longer parade of men and women than in Boston praised B. & M. from the witness chair. Tuberculosis, pneumonia, rheumatic fever, blood poisoning, these and other ailments, they said, had been banished by the heroic liniment. A Boston minister-physician, David L. Martin, told of cures he had seen wrought. Rollins himself took the stand, beaming and benign, with a quarter-century of experience in court behind him. He made a most persuasive witness, telling of his hopes to heal mankind, his vain efforts to persuade physicians to adopt his remedy, the need, therefore, to market it himself.

The government relied on expert testimony. Concord doctors and a Harvard medical professor assured the jury that B. & M.'s

[5] Cited in 1930 pamphlet, "In the Interest of Maintaining Truth."

B. & M.

ingredients, singly or in combination, could not possibly do what Rollins' witnesses claimed. The whole thing was so medically ridiculous, it seemed pointless for government lawyers to check up on and counter the particular curative tales told by the 28 who testified. In an effort to dispel Rollins' aura of humanitarianism, the government did put McClellan on the stand. It was a mistake. Life at the track had not trained him for the ordeal of cross-examination. He contradicted himself, admitted to telling Rollins lies, revealed his own cupidity.

The judge made it clear in his charge that the Sherley Amendment required for conviction fraudulent intent as well as false claim. The jury found against the government and for the 11 packages of Rollins' medicine. Had McClellan instead of Rollins been on trial, one juror said, he would have found *him* guilty. But who could send that poor man to jail? (This, of course, was not a possibility, because conviction at the worst would have meant destruction of the seized medicine.) The juror had obviously been impressed by Rollins' demeanor and by the plea of defense attorney Melvin Johnson, that the philanthropist be given the verdict as a birthday present. He had just reached the ripe old age of 72.

With more than septuagenarian vigor, Rollins turned his court triumph into publicity. "A jury of New Hampshire men good and true," he announced in half-page advertisements, had found B. & M. to be "an efficient weapon." The conclusion was clear. "Within a few months the awfully destructive enemy, tuberculosis[,] could be put to rout in the Old Granite State."[6] The ads were supplemented by pamphlets summing up the testimony of Rollins' satisfied customers at the trial. "Vindicated"—such was the title—was distributed across the nation. B. & M. sales boomed.

The loss of this case posed a serious threat to effective control of quackery. It seemed to suggest that the burden of proof for establishing a fraudulent state of mind might be a well-nigh insuperable obstacle. Reputable doctors could all agree that the impact of turpentine and ammonia on the bare chest, excoriating as it was, could still not penetrate through

[6] *Manchester Leader*, Mar. 7, 1923, clipping, AMA folder.

[ 92 ]

to reach tuberculosis in the lungs. That was no matter. Rollins possessed no conceivable background to give him insight into the practice of medicine. That was no matter either. The experts could tell him his claims were ridiculous, as he had been advised before the trial when he visited the Bureau of Chemistry accompanied by his congressman. That was equally irrelevant. If Rollins—or any other nostrum maker—could convince a jury that he believed his remedy efficacious, the law could not interfere. This was the "joker" in the Sherley law.

What would it take to prove fraud in court? What lessons could be learned from the Concord defeat? These were significant questions for Food and Drug officials to ponder during the decade of the twenties.

Despite the spreading wave of B. & M., the patent medicine scene was vastly improved in one significant respect compared with the days preceding 1906. The giants of the proprietary industry found it good business to live within the law. Ever larger, as combinations continued in the favorable economic climate, the major concerns had never before been so respectable or so proud of respectability. "Many of us remember the days," said Frank Blair, perennial president of the Proprietary Association, in 1928, "when the business was laughed at. Today it is a most substantial, firmly established, constantly growing industry." Doctors of the present day were not like "barber surgeons and crude empirics" of a former age, asserted a Proprietary Association stalwart, and no more did major medicine makers resemble "street fakirs of the past." The disrepute in which proprietary manufacturers had once been held by the financial community had largely dissipated. Ownership of many major proprietaries had passed from family hands into corporations with stocks traded on all the exchanges and owned by investors around the globe. Overseas sales had expanded too to the point that American proprietors were the largest exporters of packaged medicines in the world. The Department of Commerce itself urged them to be even more "aggressive."[7]

[7] George H. Simmons, in Foreword, *N&Q*, III, [iii]; *Standard Remedies*, 14 (Mar. 1927), 31; 15 (June 1928), 11-12; William H. Gove,

In this aura of respectability, the president of a trade association representing smaller remedy makers shared. "I am sure," said H. E. Woodward of the United Medicine Manufacturers of America, "there is not a man nor a member of our association, nor, indeed, scarcely a package medicine manufacturer in the country, who does not regard his business as entirely honest and legitimate in every way and himself as a self-respecting citizen serving humanity in general quite as fully as does the manufacturer of cotton thread or washing machines."[8]

Perhaps the insistent assertion of respectability might indicate secret doubts. *Standard Remedies* at least recognized "a need for concerted action by package remedy makers to remove the reproach which the average man unconsciously fastens upon the term 'patent medicine.'" It was nonetheless a token of how accustomed major proprietors had become to the fact of governmental regulation that in 1920 a drug journal could give the Proprietary Association major credit for having secured the enactment of the 1906 law.[9]

Believing in that law, the big concerns sought to avoid trouble, expense, and bad publicity by keeping their labeling within the law's limits. The Proprietary Association, screening applications for membership, offering advice on labels, suggesting some restraints on advertising, played the major role. Blair was sure that the industry's enhanced respectability was due almost entirely to the Association's efforts. To keep aware of officialdom's thinking about regulatory problems became, for manufacturers, a necessary task. Lawyers for trade associations and for individual proprietors moved to Washington and paid frequent calls at the Bureau of Chemistry offices. "The Proprietary Association," asserted the editor of *Standard*

---

President, Lydia E. Pinkham Medicine Co., to *Chicago Tribune*, Aug. 29, 1916, Pinkham folder, AMA; M. C. Bergin, *Markets for Prepared Medicines* (U.S. Bur. of Foreign and Domestic Commerce, Dept. of Commerce, Trade Promotion Series, No. 48: Wash., 1927). *Standard Remedies* during the decade was filled with information about export markets.

[8] *N.Y. Times*, Sep. 13, 1927.

[9] *Standard Remedies*, 6 (Aug. 1920), 5; *Drugdom*, cited in *ibid.*, (Nov. 1920), 18.

*Remedies,* "if it had no other claim upon its members, would more than justify itself by its bureau contacts."[10]

Bureau officials, for their part, desired the largest measure of compliance with the law that could be attained. They realized that voluntary cooperation from the regulated industries, if it could be secured and maintained, was quicker and less expensive than compliance wrung from recalcitrant offenders through legal action. Wiley had so asserted in his early annual reports, and his successors were to reiterate frequently that their purpose was primarily educational. "The food and drugs act," said the acting chief in 1922, "is corrective rather than punitive." Legal action would come only as a last resort, when suggestions and warnings had not been heeded. At the start of the twenties, proprietary attorneys could not get Bureau officials to pass on label claims before labels were glued to the bottles. But long experience in listening to nuances of conversations let the lawyers shrewdly guess at how far their clients might go and still be safe. Informal procedures expanded as the decade went by. Bureau officials became willing to discuss formulas and criticize labels before proprietors took their wares into the marketplace: in 1928-1929, 15,000 such letters of inquiry were received in a single year. An ever-expanding list of diseases and symptoms was made known to the trade: the mere mention on a label of appendicitis, Bright's disease, cancer, diabetes, and so on through the alphabet to venereal disease, brought the threat of quick seizure without mercy. Public warnings predicted campaigns soon to start against specific labeling abuses, providing the wise proprietor with time to set his house in order. Other helpful counsel was given in press releases, speeches, conversations. Except for references to the dread diseases, label violations discovered by Food and Drug inspectors were called to the manufacturer's attention, so that he might, if he chose, voluntarily undertake the needed change.[11]

[10] *Standard Remedies,* 8 (May 1922), 12; 11 (May 1925), 12; 15 (June 1928), 11-12; 19 (June 1932), 5.

[11] *1907 Report of the Bureau of Chemistry,* 3-4; *1908 Report,* 13; *1922 Report,* 25; *1925 Report,* 20; *1926 Report,* 20; *1928 Report,* 4-5; *Standard Remedies,* 8 (Oct. 1922), 16, 18, 24; (Nov. 1922), 8, 10, 12; 14 (May 1927), 46, 48; *F&D Rev.,* 9 (May 1925), 13-17; 10 (Sep.

A Bureau drug officer, addressing the Proprietary Association in 1927, could express pleasure that the trade's earlier "suspicion" of bureaucrats had disappeared. And in the journal that spoke for the Association, there was, during the twenties, more of exultation than of anguish. Bureau government might not be perfect, but it was not too onerous either. The names of Association members appeared in the Notices of Judgment, by which actions under the law were publicized, hardly at all.[12]

To be sure, there were the inevitable tensions between the regulated and the regulator. Manufacturers chafed under certain rulings decreed from Washington, two being especially upsetting during the decade. Piqued at proprietors who toned down the phraseology on their labels, only to make bold claims in advertising, Bureau officials developed a new interpretative device. When a medicine label bore some such vague and elastic phrase as "stomach troubles," the therapeutic meaning which the manufacturer really intended to convey was determined by reading his advertising. Seizures were made on such a basis. This procedure, many proprietors believed, unduly stretched the law.[13]

Even worse were multiple seizures. The threat that the government might initiate legal actions against a proprietor's

---

1926), 19-22; 13 (Dec. 1929), 416; Paul Dunbar, cited in Harvey W. Wiley, *The History of a Crime against the Food Law* (Wash., 1929), 375-76. The list of diseases and symptoms that could not be mentioned on labels had evolved by 1930 into the following (FDA Decimal file 530-.11 for 1930): appendicitis, Bright's disease, cancer, diabetes, diphtheria, female pills (amenorrhea, dysmenorrhea, ovarian and uterine diseases, menstrual disorders, vaginal diseases—venereal), flu and synonyms, heart disease, high blood pressure or hypertension, kidney pills (other than "diuretic to the kidneys"), la grippe and synonyms, "lost manhood" restorers, malaria (except for remedies containing quinine or cinchona alkaloids in a sufficient dosage), pneumonia, pyorrhea, rheumatism (if this appeared in the name of the product), scrofula, tuberculosis, venereal diseases (except for recognized treatments).

[12] Alexander G. Murray, acting chief of the Drug Control Laboratory, *Standard Remedies*, 14 (May 1927), 46; *ibid.*, 11 (May 1925), 12.

[13] *Ibid.*, 8 (Apr. 1922), 5; Waldon Fawcett, "The Government's Position on Control of Collateral Advertising," *ibid.* (Sep. 1922), 20, 22, 24; Bur. of Chem. mimeographed "Information on Drugs," cited in *ibid.*, 12 (May 1926), 94-96.

product at a dozen sites at once, according to *Standard Reme-dies*, provided the "one great abuse" that had arisen from the enforcement of the 1906 law. The practice was "monstrous." It let the government "paralyze and destroy a business, no matter how reputable, no matter how old, no matter how great the investment, no matter how meritorious the prepara-tion."[14]

Bureau officials admitted the effectiveness of multiple sei-zures. That, indeed, was the indispensable value of this legal weapon. It provided the most certain method of quickly stop-ping the grossest frauds. And it was so used, being resorted to rarely and when the public threat was great. The attack by industry struck bureaucrats as ingenuous and unfair. "The fan-cied threat of multiple seizure," said Walter Campbell, chief of the agency, "seems to have been set up as a straw man for the purpose of inspiring terror in the drug manufacturing industry and a zeal for a modification of the Federal food and drugs act which would practically amount to nullification as far as patent medicines are concerned." Such ripper bills, which would have outlawed the multiple seizure weapon, were constantly before Congress. They failed to pass, and so did other bills of contrary intent, which would have strengthened regulation by expanding controls to cover nostrum advertis-ing.[15]

Campbell's tiff with industry came at the end of 1929, when the public climate was beginning to change. For most of the prosperity decade, despite occasional strains, major proprie-tors and bureaucrats did business together politely. Campbell was key man in enforcement, as he had been, indeed, from the day that the law had gone into effect. Wiley had brought the young lawyer to Washington from the Kentucky Agricul-

[14] *Standard Remedies*, 10 (June 1924), 12; 13 (Nov. 1926), 13; 14 (May 1927), 22.

[15] Charles W. Crawford to Florence Kirlin, Apr. 9, 1935, "Correspond-ence on Legislation," FDA Records, Office of Commissioner, Legisla-tion, 1927-40, Bills-Regulations, box 12, RG 88, NA; Campbell, Press Notices, I, Nov. 8, 1929, Office of Information, Dept. of Agric. On vari-ous bills intended either to weaken or strengthen the law, see *Standard Remedies*, 10 (Mar. 1924), 11; 12 (May 1926), 20-21; (June 1926), 21; 16 (June 1929), 11; 18 (Mar. 1931), 4-6; 19 (Jan. 1932), 7-8; *F&D Rev.*, 10 (Nov. 1926), 8-10; 13 (Feb. 1929), 86-87.

tural Experiment Station. His state boss had written a glowing recommendation: "He is the best inspector . . . we have yet had . . . [,] familiar with chemical terms, and . . . very easy with figures. . . . He is a thorough gentleman, he has a big fund of commonsense." The chief chemist had been equally impressed. When Wiley resigned, Campbell stayed on to help Alsberg set up and adopt the "project" system, a method of priorities by which the Bureau's limited resources could be concentrated on those abuses that seemed most threatening. Serving briefly as acting chief when Alsberg left, Campbell refused the full title since he believed a chemist should hold the post. He saw a conflict between the research and regulatory functions of the Bureau, believing that each could operate with greater success if administratively separate. This step was taken in 1927. The Food, Drug, and Insecticide Administration (three years later the "Insecticide" was deleted) was created with Campbell as chief. Into the new Administration came the old Bureau's Drug Control Laboratory, created in 1923, with the surveillance of proprietaries as part of its task.[16]

Dr. Wiley misread the abolition of the Bureau as a blow to law enforcement, one more proof of the cumulative "crime" that had destroyed the law he had worked so hard to secure. He had himself sought compliance through education, but during the 1920's he thought his successors were carrying the process much too far. The pressure groups which ousted him, he felt, were calling the tune. Other critics, equally bitter, although not for reasons so personal, agreed with Wiley. They were convinced the consumer was being sacrificed to the forces of Big Business which had captured America, and namby-pamby enforcement of this particular law was but one case in point. "The control of foods and drugs in America," so the authors of one book saw it, had been "characterized by inex-

[16] R. M. Allen to Wiley, May 24, 1904, Bur. of Chem., Letters Received, RG 96, NA; Gustavus A. Weber, *The Food, Drug and Insecticide Administration* (Inst. for Govt. Research, Service Monograph No. 1950: Baltimore, 1928), 23-24, 33, 43-45, 62-63; Campbell, "The Project Plan Fundamental in Regulating Commerce in Food and Drugs," *F&D Rev.*, 5 (Nov. 1921), 1-2; *1928 Report of Food, Drug, and Insecticide Administration*, 1; *1930 Report of Food and Drug Administration*, 1; *F&D Rev.*, 7 (Jan. 1923), 4. Chief of the Bureau of Chemistry during the mid-20's was C. A. Browne.

cusable official indifference and negligence." There had been shocking "administrative incompetence, shiftiness, and a preference for backstairs methods," as well as "a progressive weakening of official activity and concern for the public health through the pressure of concealed commercial forces in close touch with food and drug administrators."[17]

This criticism was much too harsh, but, truth to tell, the national political climate during the golden glow of prosperity made it impossible to be a crusader and a bureaucrat. Wiley's successors, so many of them—like Campbell—chosen by him, were really not interested in being crusaders in any case, certainly not crusaders of the Wiley stamp. They agreed with Dr. Alsberg in having "no desire to be known as a great personage, a fighting character or a man who has killed a dragon." What they sought for was personal anonymity in an esteemed agency. Campbell and his subordinates believed that "publicity for the service, rather than for any individual" was "the rational course to be followed for a business-like execution of the job." Without a Wiley, with his flair for personal publicity, they were quick to admit, it was virtually impossible to get the agency on the front page and into public attention. This could mean lack of the kind of fervent support that led to adequate appropriations and remedial amendments. It could even mean a threat of retrogression. The ripper bills did not evoke a ripple of public interest. "We have no publicity value," an administrator wrote. "Not since Wiley resigned have we had a headliner."[18]

It was fortunate for Food and Drug officials—and for the American public—that the plan of compliance through education worked as well as it did. They were not equipped to tackle the enforcement problem in any other way. Business was

[17] Wiley, *The History of a Crime*, 372-76; Arthur Kallet and F. J. Schlink, *100,000,000 Guinea Pigs* (N.Y., 1933), 195-96. A judicious assessment of the risks inherent in close fraternizing between regulator and regulated is presented in E. Pendleton Herring, "The Balance of Social Forces in the Administration of the Pure Food and Drug Act," *Social Forces*, 13 (1935), 358-66.

[18] *Minneapolis Journal*, Oct. 12, 1913; Crawford to David F. Cavers, Aug. 1, 1933, "Correspondence on Legislation"; *1926 Report of Bureau of Chemistry*, 19; T. Swann Harding, *The Popular Practice of Fraud* (N.Y., 1935), 273.

in the saddle economically, politically, and mythically. In the prevailing mythology of prosperity, the businessman was not the suspicious character he had been in the decade when the food and drug law was enacted. Now a figure of popular veneration, he was engaged in ushering in a millennium of material comfort. No bureaucrat could treat such a noble figure too roughly. Whereas Henry Wallace, Sr., while Secretary of Agriculture, had been sympathetic with the agency, his successors were, in the phrase of one administrator, "men typical of the last half of the 'Roaring Twenties.'" Appropriations were meager and staff was small. While the regulated industries kept expanding, the resources of the Bureau did not. At the end of the decade, the agency, taking into account inflation, was worse off than it had been in 1910. One estimate put the total annual appropriation at only one-third of one per cent of the retail sales of proprietary drugs alone. The fewer than a hundred inspectors could barely scan the field. To gain compliance by voluntary action not only took less precious time than going to court, it was much swifter. Court dockets were crowded with prohibition cases. Many district attorneys were reluctant to undertake food and drug cases, because the issues were so complicated and the fines so small.[19]

The sanctity of business did not, even in the twenties, cloak the unmitigated fraud. Nobody liked the most unscrupulous of medical quacks, except themselves and their as-yet-undeceived patients. The large-scale manufacturers of packaged remedies wanted quacks eliminated both as competitors and discreditors, for they injured the good name of the trade. Eternal vigilance was necessary against nostrum vendors either completely ignorant or utterly unscrupulous. One operator might be put out of business, but another was right at hand to

[19] James Harvey Young, "The Myth of Prosperity in the 1920's," *Emory University Qtly.*, 13 (June 1957), 99-111; Crawford to Cavers, Oct. 6, 1934, "Correspondence on Legislation"; Kallet and Schlink, 254; Lauffer T. Hayes and Frank J. Ruff, "The Administration of the Federal Food and Drugs Act," *Law and Contemporary Problems*, 1 (Dec. 1933), 24-25, 30. In the group of Notices of Judgment numbered 5,001-10,000 (issued Jan. 1918-Mar. 1922), 1,765 Notices related to drug products and preparations; the number fell off to 691 in the 10,001-15,000 group (Mar. 1922-June 1927). Munch, "Notices of Judgment—Nos. 5001-15,000," *FDC Law Jnl.*, 11 (1956), 201.

take his place—if not the first fellow with a new product. Walter Campbell was as aware as his collaborators in the Post Office Department of the hardy perennials. "Not infrequently," he wrote, "firms are encountered which repeatedly violate the law, paying the fines imposed . . . , but apparently regarding these penalties as in the nature of a license fee for doing an illegitimate business."[20]

The wartime contest against "cures" for venereal disease continued through the early postwar years, the Bureau also campaigning against such allied products as "lost manhood" remedies and abortifacients. The next project placed special emphasis on nostrums claiming to cure serious ailments, especially kidney disease. Then, after a nation-wide survey, came an attack upon purported radioactive drugs, some dangerous because they contained radioactive material, others deceptive because they did not.[21]

Projects combining much pressure for voluntary improvement in labeling with some legal action sought to reduce excessive claims being made for cod liver oil preparations, for pyorrhea-curing toothpastes, and especially for so-called antiseptics. After a wide survey of the market, nearly half the soaps, douches, mouthwashes, and gargles analyzed were found to be "wholly ineffective" as germicides. Some even contained live bacteria. Virtually all the rest of the products exaggerated their germ-killing powers. Indeed, the survey revealed, few manufacturers had really ever tested the germicidal qualities of what they sold as antiseptics. The FDA, combining press releases and seizures, warred on this front for several years.[22]

The routine enforcement of a prosperity decade could not meet the needs of a nation in depression. With competition sharpening in a declining market, promotional practices deteriorated in honesty and taste. The tempo of criticism in-

[20] *1931 Report of Food and Drug Administration*, 4.

[21] *1921, 1925, 1926 Reports of Bureau of Chemistry*; Press Notices, 1, July 13, 1926, Office of Information, Dept. of Agric.

[22] *1928, 1929, 1931*, and *1933 Reports of Food and Drug Administration*; Press Notices, 1, June 18, 1928, Aug. 12, 1929, Office of Information, Dept. of Agric.; *F&D Rev.*, 10 (Sep. 1926), 11-14; (Dec. 1926), 3-7; 11 (June 1927), 22-23; (Aug. 1927), 27; 15 (1931), 86.

creased. Business seemed not so sacrosanct as in the good years now gone by. A particular spur to public interest in drug matters was a Congressional investigation, undertaken because of scare stories about imported ergot. The long hearing made clear that the Food and Drug Administration did not have staff and funds to do an adequate job. The FDA itself, welcoming this revival of public concern, sought to enlarge it. Through press releases, radio programs, an openhanded welcome to writers, the agency sought to inculcate in consumers a read-the-label habit. At the same time the FDA made pointedly clear what the law would not permit it to do.[23]

The new temper of the times emboldened regulatory officials to more vigorous enforcement. Congress, despite the depression, enlarged appropriations, and Campbell and his aides made good use of them. J. J. Durrett, who had taken charge of drug work in 1928, believed in tight controls over questionable practices. A Southerner with a Harvard medical degree, he pursued the anti-"antiseptic" campaign with added intensity and began a new one against malaria medicines short on quinine. Conversations between Durrett and proprietors became more formal, even chilly, than similar conversations in the pre-depression years. When the Proprietary Association's general representative came by to make the complaint that the proprietary branch of the drug industry received more rigorous attention from the FDA than did manufacturers of prescription drugs, the results of the interview must have been dismaying. "I told Mr. Kemp," Durrett wrote in a memorandum, "that I was very glad that he had called, that it had caused us to review our activities and we were inclined on first results to believe that his group was receiving by far the most lenient treatment and that we might have to revise our activities accordingly."[24]

[23] *N&Q*, iii, xii; Ralph W. Hower, *The History of an Advertising Agency: N. W. Ayer & Son at Work, 1869-1949* (Revised ed.: Cambridge, Mass., 1949), 147-50; Harding, 4, 186, 201-202; *PI*, 169 (Oct. 11, 1934), 63-64; *1930, 1931,* and *1932 Reports of Food and Drug Administration; F&D Rev.,* 13 (Dec. 1929), 429.

[24] *1929* through *1932 Reports of Food and Drug Administration; Standard Remedies,* 15 (June 1928), 40; 16 (Jan. 1929), 7-8; Press Notice, i, Jan. 3, 1929, Office of Information, Dept. of Agric.; Durrett

Dr. Durrett was particularly incensed at the way even the mightiest proprietors jumped on the epidemic bandwagon when a wave of influenza swept the country in late 1928 and 1929. The FDA acted quickly. It sent letters to hundreds of manufacturers and issued a trade notice warning against the temptation to label salves, gargles, and aspirins as preventives or treatments of influenza, la grippe, pneumonia, and related diseases. Proprietors laggard in complying were assailed by seizures, some 300 products suffering this fate during 1929. The Post Office Department helped out. Since the most direct appeal to the public came through advertising— some newspapers solicited ads against the flu from remedy makers—the FDA also besought the Federal Trade Commission for aid. "Out of that joint effort," Durrett told the Proprietary Association, "had come probably what is a permanent working agreement between these regulatory governmental agencies."[25]

The combination of Durrett and depression brought cries of protest from the drug industry. The doctor was personally arrogant, trade journals charged, and his medical views were wrong. A "therapeutic nihilist," he and the FDA were "working toward a bureaucratic prohibition of drugs." Carloads of antiseptics, chest rubs, antipyretics, and analgesics had been seized during the influenza epidemic merely because manufacturers sought to tell the people how physicians treated the disease. "The drug industry is long-suffering," an editorial complained. "It apparently is afflicted with some sort of inferiority complex. It has been law-ridden for ages, and it seemingly knows not how to get rid of its 'old Man of the Sea.'" The law itself was all right. But the regulations under it, aimed at curtailing the use of medicines, were something quite different. "When will the drug trade . . . shake off its

memorandum of interview with Ervin F. Kemp and Alexander G. Murray, Apr. 29, 1930, FDA Decimal file 530-.11 for 1930.

[25] *F&D Rev.*, 13 (July 1929), 231-38; Trade Notices, 1, Jan. 16, 1929, Office of Information, Dept. of Agric.; R. W. Dunlap, Acting Secy., to Sen. Otis F. Glenn, Dec. 5, 1929, FDA Decimal file, 530-.11 for 1929; *1929, 1930,* and *1931 Reports of Food and Drug Administration*; Lamb, 134-40, 316-17.

fear of over-zealous officials, become truly unified in its common cause and fight as it could fight, for its rights?"²⁶

A fight was not far off. In the meantime, the FDA, in a spirit of new hopefulness, turned its attention to some unfinished business. Short, round, amiable Frank E. Rollins, the retired court reporter, was still flooding the country with his mixture of turpentine, ammonia, and raw eggs. A case prepared more carefully than for the New Hampshire trial, FDA officials reasoned, might rid the market of this tuberculosis "cure." In December 1928 and January 1929 agents seized shipments of B. & M. from Maine to California, charging adulteration and misbranding. At the same time the most elaborate preparations were begun to build an air-tight case. Experts on tuberculosis were lined up to testify about the consensus of medical opinion. Other doctors began clinical trials, rubbing B. & M. on tubercular patients to observe how it affected them. Dr. Charles E. Holton of the FDA's Boston station was ordered to track down what he could discover about every testimonial-giver ever used by Rollins in B. & M. advertising.²⁷

Three years went by before the issues were tried before a jury. The government's enforcement officials were not the only parties to learn a lesson in New Hampshire. Rollins and his urbane lawyer, Melvin Johnson, realized that something more

²⁶ *Oil, Paint and Drug Reporter,* May 13, 1929, and *Druggists' Circular,* June 1929, cited in *Standard Remedies,* 16 (June 1929), 5-6 and 44-46; *Drug and Cosmetic Industry,* Nov. 1933, "Clippings on Food and Drug Legislation," Scrapbooks, FDA Records, RG 88, NA.

²⁷ Information on the 1928-1932 campaign against B. & M. is from records of F&D Cases 23295 and 23296 (NJ 18176), Office of the Solicitor, Dept. of Agric., RG 16, NA; F&D Case 26900 (NJ 19651), *ibid.*; records of Interstate Office Seizure Case 5067 (NJ 19651), RG 88, NA; correspondence in Medical Remedies folder, General Corres. of the Secy. of Agric., 1929, 1931, and 1932, RG 16, NA; Records of the District Courts of the U.S., Nos. 4666 and 4667, RG 21, Federal Record Center, Region 3, General Services Adm.; interview with Simon Sobeloff, July 13, 1956; United States v. 17 Bottles, Large Size, and 65 Bottles, Small Size, of an Article of Drugs Labeled in Part "B. & M.," 55 Fed. (2d) 264 (DC. Md; 1932), reprinted in White and Gates, 1287-1322; *Baltimore Sun,* June 28–July 20, 1932; B. & M. folder, AMA; *1931* and *1932 Reports of Food and Drug Administration; JAMA,* 99 (1932), 578-82; *Standard Remedies,* 18 (Nov. 1931), 3-5. Very useful is the 94-page mimeographed "Summary of the Trial, U.S. of America vs. Certain Bottles of B. & M., F. E. Rollins Company, Claimant," a copy of which is filed with Seizure Case 5067.

than an appearance of amiable innocence might be desirable. So, as testimonials continued to pile up, Rollins handed over inquiries and symptom-forms to the minister-physician, Dr. Martin, to handle. Rollins also hired a pharmacist, Benson Fenwick, to perform experiments, both laboratory and clinical, that could be cited in B. & M. pamphlets, copy for which both Martin and Fenwick approved. More than that, attorney Johnson went to New York to the Pease Laboratories, a private research center much patronized by manufacturers as a source of medical studies to be cited in advertising. Johnson put B. & M. into Dr. Herbert D. Pease's hands for tests. Science as well as empiricism could be a weapon in the fight against the government.

So too could legal maneuvering. Johnson wrote the Secretary of Agriculture reasserting the good faith of B. & M.'s maker, as newly attested by the thousands of research dollars he was expending. Let the government but state what claims might legally be made, Johnson declared, and Rollins would adopt them. At the same time Johnson sought an injunction against the Secretary to stop further seizures of B. & M. until a test case could be tried. The letter did no good, but the suit did. An appeal court decreed that the injunction must be issued, crippling the FDA's use of multiple seizures in its effort to suppress nostrums.

On the eve of the trial in Baltimore, Rollins and Johnson backed out. Fenwick had erred in making a test, they said, and the label was wrong in stating the potency of B. & M. compared with carbolic acid. The government was welcome to destroy the bottles seized.

B. & M. was soon on the market again with labeling approved by Dr. Pease. He himself, indeed, had penned most of the text that went to the printer, and the new pamphlet showed the fruits of his research in picture, table, and text. "Tabulations of Results," the heading on one exhibit read, "Showing the Number of Surviving Germs in (a) Circulating Infected Horse Serum and (b) Circulating Infected Beef Broth after Flowing from Animal Membranes with Undiluted B. & M. on the Opposite Side of the Same."

What relevance, FDA officials wondered, reading the new

circular, did Dr. Pease's experiments have to Mr. Rollins' claims? And what about the reappearance of the same old glowing testimonials, about which Dr. Holton had been finding some interesting, indeed, shocking, facts?

So the government seized more B. & M., and this time the company did not concede. The case came to trial in Baltimore during a scorching heat wave in late June 1932. Melvin Johnson, as he had done since 1920, headed Rollins' defense. Dignified, able, authorized to practice up to the Supreme Court of the United States, university law professor, college trustee, chairman of a medical school board of visitors, Johnson had even been elected president of the B. & M. company. This fact embarrassed him, he said, and it had happened in his absence. Fighting the case for the government was a young district attorney named Simon Sobeloff. Funds had been set aside to employ special counsel, but the depression made it seem advisable to save the money. The year 1932 was one in which all federal employees sacrificed one month's pay, and Sobeloff's month was that of the B. & M. trial. Keen, quick, witty, indefatigable, Sobeloff outpointed the more experienced Johnson.

The B. & M. presentation at the trial aimed at persuading the jury that no one had been guilty of fraud. It could not be the saintly Rollins, who, through thick and thin, continued to believe in the efficacy of his remedy, even to the point that only grudgingly would he modify his claims at the insistent urging of his medical advisers. And why should he not have faith in B. & M.? In some empirical way, mysterious and unknown to science, the medicine wrought cures. There were all the early tales, so often recited in the pamphlets, that could be told again. More recent successes could be demonstrated by healthy people in the witness chair. Gibbs L. Baker, a Washington attorney, had been told by a doctor to go to a sanatorium. He had refused and had used B. & M. Now he was well. Russell Ricker of Philadelphia, who laid hardwood floors, had contracted tuberculosis. Life in the country, working in the mornings, resting in the afternoons—and B. & M.—had cured him. John Frank Havens of Morehead, Kentucky, full of despair, had left the sanatorium to die. But B. & M. had worked a miracle, and he had resumed his trade of butchering. There were many more to bless Rollins for their health and happiness.

Rollins himself bespoke his own faith. He told how doctors, most of them now dead, had used B. & M. with great success. One, on the staff of Harvard, would not now testify, he said, for fear of retribution from the medical profession. Rollins told of paying Fenwick, who had died the year before, more than $80,000 to conduct his valuable experiments, and he had paid Dr. Pease $15,000 more. He did not understand all that they told him, but he followed their advice.

Was B. & M. a general germicide? It could, Rollins believed, cure any germ disease in the body, except, perhaps, in the brain. The skull was too thick. How did it work? Rubbed on the body, Rollins said, B. & M. "penetrates to where the germs are, if enough is used to reach that far, and combines with the poisons of the germs, destroying the soreness. We can find the poisons on the outside that we know are inside and the discharge from the sores is the same as the sputum shows by an examination. The skin eruption will be exactly over the infection if the infection is local. But where the infection is all through the blood stream, the eruption will be generalized."[28]

One doctor did come to Baltimore to speak for B. & M., the same Dr. Martin who had testified in Concord. He recited how he had used the remedy at Camp Oglethorpe during the war, and how it had kept 24 men from succumbing to the flu. Since then he had prescribed B. & M. with outstanding success for dozens of ailments, including numerous cases of blood poisoning. Rollins himself had had a bad case of ulcers and had heroically kept applying the liniment. The medicine cured him, drawing the ulcers right up through the skin. How did it work? "We render an antitoxin in the system," Dr. Martin explained, "which gives Nature a chance to heal and throw off whatever germ is attacking the place."[29]

Attorney Johnson, who had his own separate version of how B. & M. worked, pointed to Martin to show that medical thought was not united with respect to his client's remedy.

[28] Cited in "Summary of Trial," 27.
[29] *Ibid.*, 38.

The consensus of medical opinion, in any case, was not necessarily right. By the consensus of medical opinion George
Washington had been bled to death.

Such skepticism did not deter Soboloff from seeking to persuade the jury that reputable modern medicine was of one
mind regarding the utility of B. & M. Twenty-two doctors, of
various medical specialties, spoke for the government side.
Night after night until two in the morning they met in Sobeloff's office working on the case. One by one, Soboloff called
them to testify. There was Eugene Maximilian Karl Geiling,
Johns Hopkins' brilliant pharmacologist, who walked to the
stand with a suitcase in each hand. Why, the judge asked, did
he have the suitcases? "I have brought my authorities," replied
Geiling in his Dutch accent.[30] No medicine or combination of
medicines, the authorities all agreed, could kill the tuberculosis germ in the human body. Certainly not the ingredients of
B. & M. The harsh liniment could indeed blister the skin, but it
could not penetrate into the body. Its use was mischievous in
tuberculosis, because the discomfort of irritated skin prevented
rest and the sharp ammonia fumes stimulated coughing. Rollins' theory of germs coming out through blisters in the skin
was absolute nonsense. "To me it appears as so stupid," Dr.
Geiling said, "just as if I . . . was to ask you gentlemen, 'Close
your eyes and you will see a green angel.' "[31]

In this judgment the other physicians concurred. From
leading medical schools and sanatoriums throughout the nation, America's distinguished doctors came to call Rollins'
claims ridiculous.

Soboloff did not stop this time, as had the attorney at Concord, with presenting the judgment of medical experts. Dr.
Victor F. Cullen, superintendent of a state tubercular hospital
in Maryland, told of using B. & M. on 22 patients. Not one
had been helped, and some had lost rest from the blistering
and coughing. The same disheartening results were reported
by a Vanderbilt University professor who had tried out B. & M.
on 25 patients in Tennessee. A veterinary from the Bureau of

[30] Soboloff interview.
[31] "Summary of Trial," 7.

Animal Husbandry said he had duplicated one of Fenwick's guinea pig tests, reported in B. & M. literature, and found that the remedy did not prevent tuberculosis in the little animals. A technician who had helped Fenwick do his original experiment testified that the same had been true then. A Johns Hopkins physiologist asserted that Dr. Pease's animal membrane test in no way simulated conditions in the human body.

Still other doctors were heard in Baltimore. They told of treating the men and women whom Rollins had cited in his pamphlets. In many instances, patients had never suffered from the illnesses from which, according to their testimonials, they had been delivered by B. & M. In other cases, patients had died from tuberculosis, so doctors testified and death certificates revealed, and Rollins had gone on using their letters thanking B. & M. for curing them. There was poor Mrs. Edith Merchant of Ashland, New Hampshire. At the Boston trial she had lauded B. & M. Then a doctor had examined her and told her she was still afflicted. Mrs. Merchant's praise remained in Rollins' booklets, as did her promise to write inquirers about her case. This she persevered in doing, even on her deathbed. Rollins furnished her a desk, stationery, stamps, and, out of sympathy for her suffering and impoverishment, $1,143.10. Her letters, he once wrote her, were an important part of his advertising. When Mrs. Merchant died at last, her son sent the news to Rollins. The amiable proprietor replied, saying that it was important to his company to learn the cause of death. People attacking B. & M., he noted, would probably say that it was tuberculosis. Was it, perhaps, cancer of the rectum? "Yes, Mr. Rollins," the son replied, "you have it right. It was cancer of the rectum. The cause of mother's death."[32]

Soboloff introduced the death certificate which Dr. Holton had tracked down. Mrs. Merchant had died, it showed, from pulmonary and intestinal tuberculosis.

Mrs. Merchant's was not the only example of conflict between testimonial and death certificate presented in court. Indeed, there were more than 60. Holton had gone around, Rollins complained, stealing epitaphs from tombstones. "Well, that may be extreme," Sobeloff replied, "but do you blame the Department for looking for your customers in graveyards if you send them there?"[33]

The government sought also to impeach the testimony of living witnesses. When the Kentucky butcher, John Frank Havens, stepped down, Sobeloff called Dr. Paul Turner to the stand. Havens had been less than candid, Dr. Turner said. He had failed to state that after fleeing from the sanatorium to pursue self-treatment with B. & M., he had paid a return visit to the hospital. Dr. Turner had examined him and found that he was still sick. Havens had been given the gloomy report and warned that it was illegal for him to work, as he was doing, in a restaurant.

Dr. Turner's appearance with Havens' hospital records startled the defense. "I did not know until yesterday," one of Rollins' lawyers told the judge, "that Havens was going to testify." "Evidently the district attorney did," the judge replied.[34] Sobeloff did not inform them how a woman in Washington, gossiping over the fence, had told her neighbor she was going to have guests from Kentucky, the man to appear in a food and drug case in Baltimore. The neighbor's husband worked for the FDA. The B. & M. case, the Administration had earlier informed its branch offices, must take precedence over all other matters, and any leads sent down must be developed instantly. The backyard gossip had led promptly to Dr. Turner.

Havens could not have been too surprised when an examination by a Johns Hopkins physician brought out the sad truth that tuberculosis still held him in its grip. Other B. & M. witnesses did not have the same forewarning. The Washington lawyer and the Philadelphia carpenter learned to their dismay, as a doctor showed their x-ray plates to the jury, that B. & M. had failed them too. A French Canadian who had put his trust in Rollins' remedy found out in open court that he was in the last stages of consumption and soon would die. He broke down and wept. The jury was much moved.

Nor did B. & M.'s scientists stand up well. The dead Fenwick was shown to have lost his job as hospital pharmacist be-

[33] *Ibid.*, 54.       [34] Sobeloff interview.

cause of a liquor scandal. His research for Rollins, government witnesses said, was worthless. Under Sobeloff's relentless cross-examination, Dr. Martin revealed how remote were his views from those of modern medicine. He took Rollins' pay and prescribed B. & M. for the gravest maladies after looking at mailed-in symptom-sheets filled out by laymen. When asked what he knew about the tetanus bacillus, Martin replied: "Well, I don't know that they have isolated the particular germ. I was taught it was streptococcus."[35] Dr. Pease, head of the large New York laboratories, sat through the presentation of the government's case. Later he said he had not been hired to testify, but during the trial Johnson desired to put him on the stand. Pease was not to be found. Even a court subpoena could not stir him up. "I have no excuse to offer you," Johnson told the jury, ". . . for his not being here, except that he walked out on us." And the urbane attorney, pointing out that Rollins had paid Pease $15,000, pleaded with the jury to have sympathy for a saintly man whose scientist had "welched."[36]

This appeal did not impress the twelve good men and true. They had heard Judge Calvin Chesnut charge them: "If . . . you find that the statements made by" Rollins and his allies "were made with knowledge of their falsity, or recklessly made without reasonable grounds for making them, in defiance of known authoritative information which was reasonably available to them and the failure on their part to make said reasonable inquiry, then you may find that they were acting in bad faith and fraudulently."[37] The jury returned in an hour and 35 minutes to report that the makers of B. & M. had violated the Sherley Amendment and the seized bottles of the blistering liniment should be condemned.

After more than ten years of time and at a cost of more than $75,000, the Food and Drug Administration had cleaned up the labeling of a horse liniment sold as a tuberculosis cure.[38] Immediately Walter Campbell sent out an order to

[35] "Summary of Trial," 44.
[36] Lamb, 53.
[37] White and Gates, 1306.
[38] Crawford memorandum, Jan. 24, 1938, "Statements in Connection with F.D.C. Act Legislation," Office of the Commissioner, FDA Records, RG 88, NA.

seize misbranded B. & M. wherever it could be found. A criminal suit was launched against the corporation, to which, in time, its officers pleaded guilty. At $100 for each of twenty counts, the fine amounted to $2,000.[39]

The B. & M. verdict furnished a much-needed tonic for FDA morale. The agency had recently lost major misbranding cases against Chi-Ches-ters Pills for female disorders and a bottled concoction called Lee's Save the Baby.[40] The B. & M. victory saved the agency's officials from despair; they did not need to shut up shop; they could remain in business. Nonetheless, the unbelievable effort it had taken to win the B. & M. case was one more spadeful piled atop a growing mountain of proof that Dr. Wiley's law was out of date and in need of drastic overhauling.

While the B. & M. trial was taking place in Baltimore, out in Chicago the Democrats were holding a quadrennial convention. Before many months had passed, a new regime and a new spirit were installed in Washington. With the New Deal came a new fight for a new law.

[39] F&D Case 30186 (NJ 22177), Office of the Solicitor, Dept. of Agric., RG 16, NA.
[40] White and Gates, 1240-61.

# 6

## "TRUTH IN ADVERTISING"

---

*"Thou shalt have no other gods in advertising but Truth."*

—THE TEN COMMANDMENTS OF ADVERTISING, ASSOCIATED ADVERTISING CLUBS OF AMERICA, 1911[1]

---

WHILE Frank Rollins fought with the Food and Drug Administration over the fate of B. & M., a court contest equally decisive sought to determine the anti-nostrum powers of another federal agency. One contestant in this struggle was Edward Hayes, erstwhile promoter of male-weakness remedies, now vending Marmola, an obesity cure. Hayes' court opponent was the Federal Trade Commission.

Like food and drug legislation, the Federal Trade Commission statute was a product of the Progressive period. Enacted in 1914 under President Woodrow Wilson's leadership, the law sought to make safeguards against business monopoly more effective. A five-man independent body, granted extensive authority to investigate, publicize, and prohibit all "unfair methods of competition," the FTC, in the eyes of its proponents, should hew to a strict and impartial line of vigorous antitrust activity. Definitions of what was "unfair" were left deliberately vague, so that the Commission would not be hamstrung by new techniques tending toward monopoly which wily entrepreneurs might be expected to devise. Although the task of getting organized took time, and wartime problems diverted the Commission from its main task, Wilson's appointees viewed big business with the skepticism characteristic of the Progressive mood.[2]

[1] Cited in H. J. Kenner, *The Fight for Truth in Advertising* (N.Y., 1936), 23.

[2] G. Cullom Davis, "The Transformation of the Federal Trade Com-

With the postwar Republican ascendancy, this mood changed. No longer enemies, business and government became friends and collaborators. On the Federal Trade Commission, the shift came sharply in 1925: President Coolidge's appointment of William E. Humphrey reversed the voting balance. A Republican party regular from Washington state, Humphrey was close to lumber interests which had been given unflattering publicity through an investigation by the FTC. Avowing "a profound distrust of the reformer," Humphrey termed the pre-1925 Commission "an instrument of oppression and disturbance and injury instead of a help to business." All this was destined to change under Humphrey's committed and effective leadership. Sweeping investigations of industrial malpractice were curtailed. Procedures became more informal, with greater emphasis on voluntary reform if grievances were indeed discovered. This meant a reduction of unfavorable publicity. All in all, Humphrey's new approach was "friendlier, more trusting, and more co-operative toward business." In the main, when regulation was needed, business could regulate itself, and government would smile benignly, using its authority only against incorrigibles.[3]

One of the practices, among the incorrigibles, most damaging to respectable businessmen was false advertising. Hardly had the Federal Trade Commission been set in operation when, in November 1915, a delegation from the Associated Advertising Clubs of the World appeared before it. The statutory phrase "unfair methods of competition," the delegation urged, should be so interpreted by the Commission as to include false and fraudulent advertising.[4] Such a definition would join government efforts to those of an already active private crusade.

"Out of the foulness of the nostrums and quackery which

mission, 1914-1929," *Mississippi Valley Historical Rev.*, 49 (1962), 437-55; Milton Handler, "The Jurisdiction of the Federal Trade Commission over False Advertising," *Columbia Law Rev.*, 31 (1931), 527-60.

[3] Davis, 445-55; Pendleton Herring, "Politics, Personalities, and the Federal Trade Commission," *Amer. Political Science Rev.*, 29 (1935), 21-26; Myron W. Watkins, "An Appraisal of the Work of the Federal Trade Commission," *Columbia Law Rev.*, 32 (1932), 272-89.

[4] Kenner, 65; "Untrue Advertising," *Yale Law Jnl.*, 36 (1926-27), 1161-62.

flourished in the 1890's and the first years of the new century," wrote one of the most articulate of these crusaders, "the desire took root to clean out the Augean stables of what some critics called a defiled and subsidized press." It became increasingly clear to advertising men, amid the harsh rigor of the muck-raking attack, that advertising's grossest examples made all advertising suspect in the consumer's mind. In 1907 the Associated Advertising Clubs of America, founded two years before, acknowledged that the "value of advertisements depends largely upon the credence placed in them by the public," and hoped to regain public confidence by outlawing "pernicious practices" through state laws. Four years later *Printers' Ink*, long a spokesman for decent advertising, proposed a Model Statute, enacted in subsequent years by many states, although seldom well enforced. In 1911 also, the crusade for self-regulation reached a new peak of evangelistic fervor. In Boston, once the citadel of Puritan culture, members of the AACA pledged themselves to obey "The Ten Commandments of Advertising," the first being "Thou shalt have no other gods in advertising but Truth."[5]

To survey the observance of this new decalogue, a National Vigilance Committee was set up, and local Better Business Bureaus were created in many cities. Such scrutiny was necessary, for, in advertising, the sins of one might well become the sins of all. There was a tendency, wrote the Vigilance Committee's first chairman in 1913, for misrepresentation by a few to impel the honest advertiser "to adopt in some degree the policy of misrepresentation followed by his competitors." Efforts were made in 1913 at Baltimore and in 1914 at Toronto—where "the World" replaced "America" in the Association's name—to tighten up controls, by persuading each branch of the advertising industry, as well as the media, to set up codes detailing what practices were wrong and to police them. Trade association membership depended to some degree on abiding by the standards. A "National Commission" of

[5] Kenner, 7-24; Alfred M. Lee, *The Daily Newspaper in America* (N.Y., 1937), 329; Handler, "False and Misleading Advertising," *Yale Law Jnl.*, 39 (1929-30), 32; "The Regulation of Advertising," *Columbia Law Rev.*, 56 (1956), 1057-1065.

referees chosen by each branch adjudicated the knottiest problems. "The scheme," its chairman remembered, "worked extraordinarily well in the first few years when it was followed." Then it "got submerged by the conditions accompanying the war" and "disintegrated from lack of continuity."[6]

The dilemma of self-regulation was reflected by attitudes in the proprietary industry. The Proprietary Association in 1915 endorsed the *Printers' Ink* Model Statute and wrote advertising taboos into its own code. Yet in that same year the Association's journal, explaining that publishers' costs were rising because of the European war, could exult: "Advertisements that a short time ago were rejected with disdain are now accepted with alacrity if not cheerfulness."[7]

The National Vigilance Committee, equipped with a paid permanent staff in 1915, persevered in its labors, including Nicotol, a tobacco-habit treatment, and Addiline, a tuberculosis cure, among its notable opponents.[8] In 1915, also, representatives from the parent body, the Associated Advertising Clubs of the World, besought the new Federal Trade Commission to combat false advertising as a method of competition legally "unfair."

The Commission was not averse to using this "left-handed control"—as a later commissioner termed it—over advertising. Indeed, its first two formal cases dealt with advertising abuses, and, even during the years when Wilson's appointees were dominant, this type of case was statistically ascendant. Some 2,000 of the first 3,000 cease and desist orders issued by the Commission sought to restrain false and misleading advertising. Among them were a relatively few cases involving patent medicines. With the nostrums, as with other products, the object of action was to protect competitors more than to protect the public. In 1918, for example, in the first drug case receiving formal attention, a company was ordered to stop

---

[6] Roland Cole, "Review of the Ten-Year Fight against Fraudulent Advertising," *PI*, 114 (Feb. 24, 1921), 17-20, 25-26; (Mar. 3, 1921), 121, 125-26, 129-30; William H. Ingersoll [chairman for three years of the Ntl. Commission], "Where We Go from Here," *PI*, 175 (June 4, 1936), 73-76. Ingersoll cites Harry D. Robbins, first chairman of the Ntl. Vigilance Comm.

[7] Cole, 122; *Standard Remedies*, 1 (Feb. 1915), 27.

[8] Cole, 125, 129.

calling its ointment "Mentholanum," and to cease from using a label imitative of the already flourishing Mentholatum brand. Other early cases concerned unfair promotion of electric belts, aspirin, Bacilli-Kill, and soaps with therapeutic claims.[9]

A marked increase in the attack on false advertising characterized the Humphrey-dominated Commission during the years of Republican ascendancy. To do this while neglecting fundamental monopolistic trends was, for Progressive-minded critics, to swat at a gnat while swallowing a camel. Yet, in his much more limited crusade, Humphrey was unquestionably sincere. As with the self-regulators, his hatred of the lunatic fringe in advertising arose from his desire to promote and protect business. A little "puffing" in advertising, exaggeration of the facts which consumers would recognize as such, was perfectly all right. But exaggeration beyond the border of truth, where it misled the consumer, hurt competitors and tarnished the reputation of all advertising. It must be stopped.

Americans "are annually robbed of hundreds of millions of dollars through these fake advertisements," Humphrey said in a 1926 address. He did not mean those "that may be in the twilight zone or near the border line, but only those that are brazenly and shamelessly fraudulent: . . . 'antifat' remedies, medicines [for incurable diseases], soaps, belts," fake industrial schools. "All of these prey upon the weak and the unfortunate, the ignorant and the credulous. There is no viler class of criminal known among men" than the perpetrators of such schemes. But equally guilty, in Humphrey's judgment, was the publisher in whose journal such advertisements appeared. He shared in the promoter's "ill gotten gains." "These disreputable publications," the commissioner asserted, "are the most power-

---

[9] Commissioner Albert A. Carretta, "Extravagant Advertising Claims," speech before Pa. Council of the Painting and Decorating Contractors of Amer., Jan. 29, 1953, Speech File, FTC Library; James W. Cassedy, "Progress of Federal Law against False Advertisement of Food, Drugs, and Cosmetics," *FDC Law Qtly.*, 4 (1949), 357; Otis Pease, *The Responsibilities of American Advertising: Private Control and Public Influence, 1920-1940* (New Haven, 1958), 90; FTC v. Block & Co., 1 *FTC Decisions* 154 (1918); FTC v. The Electric Appliance Co. of Burlington, Kansas, 2 FTC 335 (1920); FTC v. Albany Chemical Company, 3 FTC 369 (1921); FTC v. M. G. Slocum, 4 FTC 155 (1921); FTC v. Williams Soap Co., 6 FTC 107 (1923).

ful instruments for unfair practices and fraud that we have to combat in the conduct of the nation's business."[10]

The number of offending publications, happily, was small. "The newspaper columns of the country," said Humphrey, "are most commendably free from such advertisements. Most of the magazines exercise great care in the selection of their advertisements, and deserve great credit for having done more than perhaps any other agency in bringing about truth in advertising." The vast majority of American publications need have no fear "of any possible hardship" from regulatory action by the Federal Trade Commission.

And action there had to be. The courts seemed helpless to reach "this gigantic evil." Efforts by the Post Office Department had proved "ineffectual." FTC action up to this time had "not brought encouraging results. We have tried to reach the originators of these schemes. We have accomplished something, but comparatively little. They are usually fleet and cunning crooks that engage in this business. When located, they fold their tents and silently vanish, and commence business again in some new locality, under some new name."

The new FTC approach, Humphrey reported, would be to bring a joint action against both advertiser and publisher. One such case was already under way. "I have persuaded the Federal Trade Commission to commence a war," said Humphrey, "that, if I have my way about it, will be a war of extermination." "We want not only to protect the public from these fakers and crooks, but we want also to protect the honest publisher from their unfair and dishonest competition."

Humphrey's bellwether case combined an obesity cream, Reducine, and *True Romances* magazine. The advertisements told potential buyers that upon applying the cream to the body "a harmless chemical reaction takes place during which the excess fat is literally dissolved away, leaving the figure slim and properly rounded, giving the lithe grace to the body every man and woman desires." By careful application, even spot reducing was possible, and the results were permanent. Such claims, the FTC concluded, were utterly false, as the

[10] "Publishers and False Advertising," speech before Ntl. Petroleum Assoc., Sep. 17, 1926, FTC Speech File.

manufacturer must know. The publisher of *True Romances*, by accepting and publishing such advertisements, had "purposely and knowingly become a party to, and part of, said false and fraudulent plan." Then came the Commission's order: maker and publisher must "cease and desist" from making the claims complained of in any Reducine advertising appearing in the magazine.[11]

If the Reducine case was intended as a first shot, no war of extermination followed it. No long series of orders issued from the Commission linking disreputable advertisers and their advertising media. Indeed, the battle strategy changed. The Commission decided to delay its firing at magazines until the self-regulators had had a chance.

The agencies of self-regulation, disrupted by wartime conditions, drew strength from the favorable business climate of the twenties. A better-financed National Vigilance Committee sought, in the words of its motto, "to create maximum public confidence in advertising by making all advertising trustworthy." Truth-in-Advertising had paid off particularly, the Committee believed, in a drastic reduction in the amount of advertising of cures for dread diseases. But, like Humphrey, the Committee recognized there still was work to do. "FINISH THE JOB," read the headline on a bulletin issued in 1925: "Organized Advertising and Publishing *vs*. Exploitation of Disease Victims."[12]

In that same year the National Vigilance Committee was transmuted into a stronger agency, the National Better Business Bureau. Publicity exposing the disreputable fringe in advertising expanded. And the NBBB resumed the effort of a decade earlier to promote industry-wide cooperation with respect to advertising practices. Sponsoring "fair trade practices" conferences, the Bureau sought to secure concurrence from competitors in various industries on codes regulating advertising behavior.[13]

In using the mechanism of the fair trade conference, the

[11] In the Matter of McGowan Laboratories, Inc., and Womanhood Publishing Corporation, 11 FTC 125 (1927).

[12] "Finish the Job," Ntl. Vigilance Comm. Bull. [May 1925], NBBB files, New York.

[13] Pease, 49-50; Kenner, 183-87; numerous bulletins in NBBB files.

NBBB was borrowing a page from the Federal Trade Commission's own book. From the beginning, the FTC had used this device occasionally as a hopefully quick and inexpensive method of bringing questionable trade practices within an industry into line. Commissioner Humphrey's pro-business orientation caused him greatly to expand the method. A new division within the Commission was created to spur the effort, and the yearly number of trade practice conferences more than quintupled. An industry was enabled "to make its own rules of business conduct . . . in cooperation with the commission"; these rules might be approved by the FTC and given the force of law.[14]

In a sort of conjunction or intertwining, the trade practice conference techniques of both the FTC and the NBBB came together in 1928 to set rules for periodical advertising. It was the Commission that called the meeting. Some magazine publishers were skeptical, fearing FTC censorship and too ready initiative as in the Reducine–*True Romances* case. Preliminary consultation ironed out this problem. The FTC would not act against a publisher, even when advertising was unquestionably fraudulent, until self-regulation had had its chance. Self-regulation meant the NBBB. The unanimous resolution adopted at the New York conference, Commissioner Humphrey presiding, recognized the NBBB as "the most competent agency of assistance to the business of advertising in preventing fraud in advertising." Since the Bureau was willing, the resolution continued, the conference requested the Bureau to investigate advertising, calling any that it deemed fraudulent to the attention of the advertiser. Then the Bureau could advise all periodical publishers of the fraud and, if it saw fit, could report the matter to any governmental agency.[15]

Several months later, after consultation with both the FTC and leaders in the publishing industry, the NBBB announced its plan of procedure. This included a one-by-one survey of various classifications of periodical advertising, the results to go to publishers, permitting them to "censor" as they saw

[14] *FTC Annual Report, 1926*, 47-50; Davis, 449-50.
[15] *FTC Annual Report, 1929*, 47-48; *PI*, 145 (Oct. 11, 1928), 26-52 *passim*; Pease, 77.

fit. "If satisfactory adjustments cannot be obtained from publishers on advertising of a fraudulent character," the NBBB
announced, "a formal complaint will be presented to the Federal Trade Commission." Of all the advertising classifications
which the Bureau intended to survey, only jewelry and puzzles
fell outside the drug and cosmetic field. And all the cosmetics
had therapeutic overtones. Leading the list were "Fat Reducing" products.[16]

In the wake of the trade practice conference, the tempo of
anti-quackery action quickened on the part of both self- and
governmental regulators. From the NBBB poured a series of
critical bulletins, aimed at individual nostrums and at classes
of specious wares: obesity remedies, "health foods," radioactive
waters, and the like. From the FTC came more cease and desist
orders restraining nostrum advertising. In even greater numbers the FTC accepted stipulations from erring advertisers,
informal agreements to abandon shady practices, with no
names made public.[17]

This combined campaign against disreputable advertising,
so promisingly launched, encountered confusing trouble on
two scores. A significant court decision restricted the Federal
Trade Commission's authority to police. And the Great Depression, shattering most patterns developed during the decade of prosperity, increased the need for the policing of adver-

[16] *NBBB Commercial Dept. Bull.*, No. 20, Mar. 6, 1929, NBBB files.
Besides fat-reducing remedies, the bulletin listed these categories of
medicinal drugs: glands, asthma, piles, female weakness, bladder, fits,
stomach troubles, colds, goiter, dropsy; and these kinds of "external
health and beauty appliances": facial skin cures, bone straighteners, hair
dyes, fat reducing, bust developers, baldness, rupture, deafness, hair
removers, piles, eyelash growers, panaceas, leg sores, rheumatism, corns
and bunions, optical. Tobacco cures were also cited. Bull. No. 139,
Aug. 15, 1929, listed NBBB's "Tentative Censorship Regulations" to
govern publishers in assessing copy. These too gave prominent emphasis to proprietary medicines.
[17] *NBBB Bulletin* files; *FTC Annual Reports* and *Decisions. NBBB
Commercial Dept. Bull.* No. 50, May 3, 1929, reports that the FTC had
taken action against 300 advertisers and publishers during the preceding
fortnight, many in the medical field; a specific list of FTC complaints
is included in Bull. 71, May 24, 1929. The *FTC Decisions* reveals a
great increase in stipulations concerning proprietary drugs. The stipulation was introduced as part of Humphrey's plan to achieve results
by cooperating with business. *FTC Annual Report, 1926*, 7-8; Davis,
448-49.

tising as many hard-pressed businessmen, hitherto cautious, scrambled for a share of the shrinking market by employing promotional methods they had formerly held in disdain.

The critical court decision concerned Marmola.[18] Back in 1907, at about the same time he was launching Man Medicine, Edward Hayes set up another company to vend his weight-reducing remedy. The formula, given to Hayes by a business partner, owed its key ingredient to reputable medical research. A decade or so earlier, physicians had discovered that they could speed up body metabolism and reduce weight for some patients by dosing them with the dried thyroid glands of various animals. By 1907 alert doctors had learned the dangers inherent in such therapy and were using the glandular substance with great caution.[19] Some physicians, indeed, had abandoned thyroid completely and turned to safer remedies and regimens. Nostrum promoters, however, considered thyroid a great find. For one thing, it really worked. Many fat people who dosed themselves heavily with desiccated thyroid actually lost weight. Also, some of the large pharmaceutical houses were glad to sell the substance and to give scientific advice about dosage instructions and labeling claims. Obesity, moreover, was not considered a disease, so "cures" for that condition were not subject to the 1906 Pure Food and Drugs Act. Hayes was by no means the only entrepreneur to market a fat-reducing formula.

Besides desiccated thyroid, Marmola contained laxatives and several other ingredients, relatively inert. But the formula did not remain fixed from year to year. In 1911 the amount of thyroid was cut because of its rising price. During the war, the laxative phenolphthalein, a German import, got scarce, so it was dropped and the amount of cascara—an American herbal laxative—was upped. In 1922 the thyroid in each Marmola tablet was reduced again, to half a grain, on the advice of the

[18] The basic sources for the discussion of Marmola are the FTC files, In the Matter of Raladam Company, Docket 1496, RG 122, NA; 12 FTC 363; material in the Marmola folders, AMA Dept. of Investigation; and the court decisions.

[19] David Hunt and Atherton Seidel, "Commercial Thyroid Preparations," *JAMA*, 51 (1908), 1385-89.

pharmaceutical manufacturer who compounded the tablets for Hayes.[20]

If the formula varied, the main theme of Marmola advertising persevered without change. "Take Off the Fat Where It Shows," urged the headline on an early ad, under the picture of a huge-busted woman. "Famous Beauties Never Get Fat," assured another advertisement: grand ladies might indulge in a "lifelong loaf," drink liquor "not illiberally," and abandon "table restraint," all without risk of obesity—if they used Marmola. "Beneath Your Fat a Graceful Figure Dwells," cajoled another message.[21]

The moderate market of the days of the Gibson girl became, in the twenties, a golden opportunity. Style decreed that men must be lithe and athletic, women slim to the point of emaciation. "There seems, indeed, to have come upon the women of America," wrote the editor of the *Journal of the American Medical Association*, "a veritable craze for reduction which has passed the bounds of normality and driven women and young girls to a type of self-mutilation impossible to explain on any other basis than the faddism of the mob." "Fabulous sums are spent for . . . anti-fat frauds," said Commissioner Humphrey, "since the female skeleton has become the fashion of this country." The first general NBBB bulletin dealt with this racket. Marmola told flaming youth and the would-be young about "The Pleasant Way to Banish Excess Fat" and presented the testimony of movie actress Constance Talmadge: "The demand for slender figures is so universal that movie stars must have them. Not only beauty, but good health and vitality argue against excess fat." The argument was persuasive. Marmola's sales climbed to the sum of $600,000 a year.[22]

[20] FTC Docket 1496.

[21] *N&Q*, I, 388; *JAMA*, 70 (1918), 1163; [*Chicago Examiner*] clipping, Marmola folder, AMA.

[22] Morris Fishbein, *The New Medical Follies* (N.Y., 1927), 91; Humphrey, "Fraudulent Advertising," speech over NBC network, May 22, 1930, FTC Speech File; "Obesity Remedies," *NBBB Commercial Bull.* No. 65, May 16, 1929; Talmadge ad in *Photoplay*, Jan. 1929 clipping, Marmola folder, AMA; sales from FTC Docket 1496.

Business was just too good to run risks that could be avoided. When his old nemesis, the Post Office Department, called upon Hayes to show cause why a fraud order should not be issued against the Marmola Company, Hayes sent a lawyer to talk things over. The upshot was an affidavit signed early in 1927, in which Hayes swore that the company had "absolutely abandoned" its business and would "not resume it at any time in [the] future." Nor did it. But Hayes immediately launched the Raladam Company—the name was composed by the girls in the office—which did no mail-order business, dealing only with wholesale and retail druggists and shipping Marmola only by express.[23]

When an attack came from another quarter the next year, Hayes had to stand and fight. The Federal Trade Commission challenged the Raladam Company's advertising. "People used to think that excess fat all came from over-eating or under-exercise," some ads had said, whereas "fat people, it was found, generally suffered from an under-active thyroid." These statements, the FTC complained, were wrong. So was the advice Marmola advertising offered to consumers. It was not a "scientific way" to reduce, the complaint alleged, to "simply take . . . four tablets daily [of Marmola, each containing half a grain of desiccated thyroid], until weight comes down to normal."[24]

According to FTC procedure, hearings were held before an examiner. Dr. Kebler of the Food and Drug Administration testified that, at the most, only 5 per cent of the overweight owed their obesity to an under-active thyroid. Thus for 95 per cent of fat people, the use of desiccated thyroid, even carefully administered, would do no good. For many people, with various ailments, *any* extra thyroid was highly dangerous. For anybody, even the most healthy, too much thyroid posed a threat. The Marmola dosage, said Dr. Kebler, was "very unwise." Another witness, Dr. William E. Clark of the Georgetown Medical School, painted a grim picture of the potential results of Marmola dosage for many people if continued over a period of time. "Rapid pulse" could develop, as well as "headache, nervousness, tremor, often bad diarrhea, weight loss, sweating, and often a toxic state." Prescribing the same

[23] Fraud and Lottery Docket Book 8, 131, Office of the Solicitor, Post Office Dept. Records, RG 28, NA; FTC Docket 1496.
[24] *Ibid.*

amount of thyroid for each patient, a Northwestern University medical professor thought, was criminal. In addition to the thyroid danger, he said, Marmola posed a threat of creating the laxative habit—after the war phenolphthalein had been restored.

Other medical professors were similarly appalled at Marmola's hazards. But Hayes found six physicians—some of them medical professors and all members of their local medical societies—who took his side. Taken as directed, they asserted, Marmola was both effective and safe. The pharmacopeial dose of dried thyroid was, after all, a whole grain. And the Marmola label warned self-dosers to consult their doctors upon encountering "unusual conditions." Thyroid worked for their patients, the doctors said, when they prescribed it for obesity. One of them testified that he gave from 6 to 40 grains a day. The average person, Hayes' medical witnesses insisted, could take Marmola safely for 60 to 90 days without medical supervision and attain the desired results.

Dr. Arthur Cramp, head of the American Medical Association's Bureau of Investigation and himself a witness against Marmola, was stunned to find established physicians arrayed for pay in favor of the thyroid remedy. "Here, then, is a sweet spectacle," Cramp wrote in a *Journal* editorial, "the American Medical Association attempting to protect the public against quack remedies, while individual members testify in behalf of exploiters of quack remedies!" Cramp published their names for all their professional colleagues to see. A spokesman for the proprietary industry thought the editorial an "outrageous attempt to influence testimony."[25]

It was Cramp's side of the argument which seemed the more persuasive to the hearing examiner and, later, to the full Commission. In April 1929 an order was issued demanding that the Raladam Company stop advertising Marmola as a scientific, accurate, and harmless method for treating obesity. If Marmola was to be promoted for reducing weight, the order

[25] "Lending Aid and Comfort to Quackery," *JAMA*, 91 (1928), 1377-78. Cramp acknowledged authorship in letter to F. J. Schlink, Apr. 3, 1931, Marmola folder, AMA; the Chicago Medical Soc., Cramp wrote, censured two of the physicians and took no action against three others who expressed contrition for having been inveigled into testifying for Marmola. *Standard Remedies*, 15 (1928), 708.

said, the company must include a statement that the remedy could not be taken with safety to physical health except upon the advice of a competent physician.[26]

Hayes did not bow to the order and tone down Marmola advertising. Instead, taking the appropriate steps under the law, he petitioned a circuit court to vacate the order. The Federal Trade Commission fought this petition and countered with an appeal to the same court, asking for an injunction that would forbid the Raladam Company from carrying on with its false advertising.

When the three judges had weighed the matter, they gave their judgment to Marmola, canceling out the Commission's order. Physicians had testified on both sides about Marmola's value. Words like "scientific" and "safety" were so flexible that they could properly be used in different ways by doctors of contrary views. Marmola's role lay not in the realm of fact but —shades of the McAnnulty decision—in the realm of opinion. "The specific question . . . ," said the court, "is whether this amount of thyroid taken in this way is so inherently and characteristically dangerous to the patient as to make that danger a fact, as distinguished from a reasonable scope of conflicting opinion." The answer must be negative on the basis of the FTC's own order, for the Commission would permit a citizen to take Marmola—if he got a doctor to supervise.[27]

Despite the court's excursion into medical opinion, however, the real reason for the reversal had nothing at all to do with therapy. More basic, said the judges, was a "broader question of the jurisdiction of the Commission." The law forbade methods of competition that were unfair. If the Commission failed to demonstrate that competitors had been hurt, it had no case. That lack was obvious in the action against Marmola. The Commission had sought to show injury to the public, but had paid no explicit heed to any competitors. Might they be discovered by indirection? Possibly the medical profession, the court posited. "It cannot be seriously contended," the judges went on, destroying their own hypothesis, "that the act was intended to protect any profession against encroachment—

[26] 12 FTC 363.
[27] Raladam Co. v. Federal Trade Commission, 42 Fed. (2d) 430 (1930).

[ 126 ]

the aid of the Commission might be as logically given to physicians and surgeons as against chiropractors, or to lawyers as against incompetent will draftsmen." How, then, about competing nostrums "commercially exploited . . . for obesity?" Could they be considered competitors deserving protection? "It is fairly to be inferred," the court stated, "not only that these are on the same *index expurgatorius* as Marmola, but that they are relatively disreputable. Again, it cannot be seriously contended that the machinery of the Commission was intended to give governmental aid to the protection of this kind of trade and commerce."

So, while the Commission appealed the decision to the Supreme Court, Marmola advertising reached a new level of audacity. "Obesity Frauds," a headline ran. "Time was when there was a great cry against obesity frauds," the text continued. "Methods either harmful or useless. That cry has led many to fear a method that is right and scientific. But now frauds are few. All things wrong or harmful are short-lived. Marmola prescription tablets have been sold for 24 years— millions of boxes of them—during all this furore of folly. . . . You can trust a help so time-tested, so endorsed."[28]

The Supreme Court gave this time-tested weight-reducer a verbal blow—but also handed Marmola the victory. "If the necessity of protecting the public against dangerously misleading advertisements of a remedy sold in interstate commerce were all that is necessary to give the Commission jurisdiction," wrote Justice Sutherland, "the [FTC] order could not successfully be assailed. But this is not all." Competition must be demonstrated, and this task the Commission had failed to undertake.[29]

The Raladam decision was "a staggering set-back," which "greatly limited" the Commission's "sphere of usefulness" in controlling advertising abuses. To be sure, the Commission could and did prove injury to honest competition in many actions against bogus medicines. But the Supreme Court's needlessly rigid interpretation of the law proved a real barrier and a psychological deterrent.[30] The decision also came at a

[28] Unidentified ad [late 1930], AMA Marmola folder.
[29] Federal Trade Commission v. Raladam Company, 283 U.S. 643 (1931).
[30] Carretta, FTC Speech File; Handler, "The Jurisdiction of the Fed-

most inappropriate time, a time when defenses against dishonest advertising could ill afford weakening, but rather needed shoring up. The integrity of advertising behavior, under the impact of the depression, was skidding fast.

"So far as advertising goes," wrote an executive in this line of business during 1932, "we are fallen on evil days." Truth in advertising was being dragged down by declining demand. In desperation manufacturers employed whatever claims they thought might possibly persuade. Few advertising media had the financial strength to turn down copy offered them. Better Business Bureaus were confronted, said the NBBB general manager, "with the most trying advertising transgressions on the part of advertisers who are normally regarded as honest advertisers." Nor were the smaller companies the only sinners. "More and more," noted the NBBB official, "our work involves negotiations with the largest advertisers in the country."[31]

What chance had self-regulation to keep American advertising decent when makers of cigarettes, soap, deodorants, yeast, and sanitary napkins adopted promotional pitches very like those of the most unscrupulous medical quacks, and when advertisers somewhat more scrupulous walked close to the border of rectitude, presenting their wares with an ever-more-sophisticated psychology that might have the ring but not the content of truth?[32]

The depression not only made advertising more ruthless. It made advertising's critics more bitter. The menace of quackery had not been forgotten during the golden glow of prosperity. But in the disenchantment accompanying the depression, a new tide of muckraking swept over even the most respectable of medicine proprietors—indeed, threatened to engulf the institution of advertising itself.

---

eral Trade Commission over False Advertising," 527 [referring to the Circuit Court decision]. The Supreme Court relaxed its taboo on FTC regulation of noncompetitive practices in 1934 in FTC v. R. F. Kappel and Bros., 291 U.S. 304.

[31] H. A. Batten, "An Advertising Man Looks at Advertising," *Atlantic Monthly*, 150 (1932), 53; Hower, *The History of an Advertising Agency, N. W. Ayer & Son at Work, 1869-1949*, 148-49; Pease, 60-61; Edward L. Greene, "Advertising Generally," *NBBB Bull.*, Sep. 7, 1932.

[32] Hower 148, 609 note 6; Pease 167-97.

# THE NEW MUCKRAKERS

*"Thou* shalt *covet thy neighbor's car and his radio and his silverware and his refrigerator and everything that is his."*

—THE TEN COMMANDMENTS OF ADVERTISING, *Ballyhoo*[1]

THE American Medical Association's continuous, relentless, excoriating critique of quackery formed a bridge between the patent medicine muckraking of the Progressive period and the "guinea pig" exposure of the Great Depression. In charge of this important task for the AMA was a shy and dedicated man.

Arthur J. Cramp had joined the AMA staff as an editorial assistant during the same year that the Pure Food and Drugs Act had been passed by Congress. Then a man of 34, he had shortly before received his M.D. degree from the Wisconsin College of Physicians and Surgeons. Born in England, Cramp came to America in his late teens and taught science in Milwaukee high schools. A sense of personal mission sent him to medical school. His daughter ill, Cramp had called a man to treat her who turned out to be a quack. The young girl died. Thus was born in Cramp an implacable hatred of quackery and a desire to train himself to know the true from the false in the realm of medical care. Practicing medicine proved not congenial to Cramp's personality, and he welcomed the offer of a position on the *Journal* staff. It provided him the opportunity to devote his entire career to fighting medical quackery.[2]

---

[1] Cited in E. S. Turner, *The Shocking History of Advertising!* (N.Y., 1953), 243. *Ballyhoo* was a magazine which spoofed advertising during the depression.

[2] Obituary, *JAMA*, 147 (1951), 1773; interviews with Dr. W. W. Bauer, May 2, 1961, and Aug. 15, 1962.

When Cramp came, the AMA was already deeply involved in combatting fake "ethical specialties" promoted to physicians. In 1905 the Council on Pharmacy and Chemistry had been set up to determine which proprietary products were worthy of being granted permission to advertise in the *Journal* and which were not. The next year, mainly to run analyses for this project, a Chemical Laboratory was set up. The results of these investigations, good and bad, were printed in the *Journal* and issued as pamphlets. Into Dr. Cramp's careful editorial hand fell the task of preparing this material for the press. Soon, as the bulk of work grew, this became his key task. The Propaganda Department was created with Cramp as director.[3]

The line had never been hard and fast between "pharmaceutical humbugs" promoted to physicians and proprietaries peddled to the general public. In being concerned with one, the AMA could not avoid the other. The Association was, after all, the major national organization possessing the expert skills needed to differentiate valid from specious medication. It was inevitable that Cramp's department broaden the audience for its propaganda to include laymen being fleeced by quacks.

Public interest in patent medicines at this time was already high. Cramp fanned the flames by reprinting as a small book Samuel Hopkins Adams' recent *Collier's* series on "The Great American Fraud." By 1913 a fourth edition was exhausted and a fifth in press. The Propaganda Department issued other best-selling documents. From exposés written for the *Journal*, Cramp assembled blue-backed pamphlets on various quackish themes—like "Cancer Fakes" and "Medical Institutes"—and dispensed them cheaply far and wide. The pamphlets in their turn were pulled together into green-bound books. Working with remarkable diligence, Cramp issued the first in 1911, a 500-page volume, *Nostrums and Quackery*, which gave case histories of scores of nostrums, throwing light, as Cramp said,

[3] Austin Smith, "The Council on Pharmacy and Chemistry," in Morris Fishbein, *A History of the American Medical Association, 1847 to 1947* (Phila., 1957), 866-77; Bliss O. Halling, "The Bureau of Investigation," in *ibid.*, 1034. Burrow, *AMA*, contains three excellent chapters treating the anti-quackery work of the AMA.

"into the innermost recesses—the holy of holies of quackery." Within a year, the printing was sold out, and a second edition issued, larger by 200 pages than the first. In 1921 Cramp assembled his new material into a second volume, over 800 closely printed pages long. The work was, indeed, as Cramp believed, "a veritable 'Who's Who in Quackdom.' "[4]

In the variety of his appeals to those who needed knowledge, Cramp sought to emulate his adversaries. He devised posters for exhibit at fairs and schools, with bold headings proclaiming "TESTIMONIALS ARE WORTHLESS" or naming "QUACK EPILEPSY CURES." He worked out several series of lantern slides for loan to any interested party, some merely pictorial to accompany lectures, others including slides with explanatory text. Whenever he could possibly spare the time, Cramp himself went forth from Chicago to deliver lectures. With his carefully prepared and lucid manuscripts, his crisp delivery, his irony and bitter wit, the doctor made a telling presentation. But Cramp preferred the written to the spoken word, and expressed his anti-quackery convictions more effectively in writing. He wrote incessantly, not only for the *Journal*, but for many medical and lay magazines.[5]

Cramp's correspondence was enormous. Doctors wrote in asking about nostrums which they found their patients using. Scarcely an investigation was launched by a regulatory agency but that an inquiry went to Cramp to see what information the AMA already had on hand. As early as 1910 Cramp's office contained over 12,000 cards in a "Fake File," listing

[4] "Report of the Propaganda Department for 1913," Reports of the Bureau of Investigation folder, AMA; *N&Q*, I, 8, and ad in back; *N&Q*, II, 3-6.

[5] *Material Prepared and Issued by the Bureau of Investigation of the American Medical Association* (Chicago, n.d.) includes facsimiles of posters and lists of pamphlets and lantern slides. Cramp mentions his speeches in various annual reports, Bureau of Investigation folder, and his style can be detected from addresses that were published. A few of his articles include "Modern Advertising and the Nostrum," *Amer. Jnl. of Public Health*, 8 (1918), 756-58; "The Nostrum and the Public Health," *New England Jnl. of Med.*, 201 (1929), 1297-1300; "The Fight on Crooked Advertisers of Toilet Goods," *PI*, 138 (Mar. 24, 1927), 25-36 *passim*; "Therapeutic Thaumaturgy," *Amer. Mercury*, 3 (1924), 423-30; "Patent Office Magic—Medical," *ibid.*, 8 (1926), 187-94; "The Work of the Bureau of Investigation," *Law and Contemporary Problems*, 1 (Dec. 1933), 51-54.

products, firms, and names of promoters. His "Testimonial File" held the names of over 13,000 American and 3,000 foreign doctors who had given testimonials for proprietary drugs. Foreign health officials also, on tour or by mail, concerned about American proprietaries exported to their shores, availed themselves of the department's resources. From Australia, India, most of the countries of Europe, came appeals for information.[6]

The Propaganda Department proved a mainstay for "Truth in Advertising" campaigners. Newspaper advertising managers, officials of local Better Business Bureaus, members of the national Vigilance Committee not only bought Cramp's pamphlets and borrowed his slides but posed thousands of individual questions about particular patent medicines. So too did authors writing textbooks in college economics and in elementary general science. As prohibition spread, the Anti-Saloon League and Woman's Christian Temperance Union inquired about nostrums of high alcoholic content. When the war came, Cramp gave the army counsel on remedies purporting to cure venereal disease. And as the years passed, an increasing number of common citizens, concerned about their own health problems, wrote seeking assurances about therapeutic claims made in nostrum advertising.[7]

To answer an inquiry, Cramp often needed to do no more than consult his folders or send a reprint of a *Journal* article. But sometimes a question prompted a thorough investigation, including consultation with anti-quackery specialists in government, the buying and analysis of the product under consideration, and a lengthy interchange of letters with the proprietor himself. Cramp could be ingenious. The Professor Scholder Institute, Inc., in New York City, a cure-for-baldness concern more bold than most, claimed—after they were dead and unable to contradict—that Theodore Roosevelt and Harry Houdini had both been satisfied customers. Scholder advertising besought the balding to write in, enclosing a few specimens of hair, so that the professor might make a microscopic analysis,

[6] AMA files, especially annual reports for 1910 and 1913 in Reports of Bureau of Investigation folder.
[7] Annual reports, 1910-1934.

[ 132 ]

diagnose the particular trouble, and prepare an individual prescription to counteract the gloomy trend. Central to the cure, of course, was a secret formula learned by the professor in Galicia from a Dominican friar. Under an assumed name, Cramp submitted some hairs plucked from the fur cuff of a secretary's platinum fox fur coat. "A microscopic examination," Scholder replied, "discloses that the roots are in a seriously undernourished condition. You are in grave danger of continuous and increasing loss of your hair, but it can still be saved by prompt treatment." The professor would be glad to undertake the case, and promised to "positively restore your hair and scalp to normal, healthy condition."[8]

Much cheered, Cramp wrote a second letter under a second name, enclosing this time hairs from the collar of another coat, this one made of fur known to the trade as wolf (Siberian or Japanese dog). Scholder's answer was word for word the same. In the spirit of the game, Cramp tried again and again and again. He sent in short lengths of hair, with roots removed, from a girl whose long, luxurious tresses had never been bobbed. And in two other envelopes he mailed to the professor short strands of twine, some dyed black and some dyed brown. In all cases Scholder's analysis was identical, "the roots are in a seriously undernourished condition," and his promise of a cure equally sure.

Data in hand, Cramp sat down and laughed Professor Scholder out of business. It was not a jolly laugh, Cramp's account of hoaxing a hoaxer, for indignation lay just beneath the humor. "Seriously, though," the doctor wrote, "one wonders just how far it is possible to go in humbugging the bald and still keep out of jail." There was humor, indignation, and still something more in Cramp's piece on Scholder—an air of incredulity. On his desk Cramp kept a copy of *Alice in Wonderland*. Before writing up a case, he always took the book and read a chapter. It put him in the mood, he said, for the job he had to do.[9]

Cramp required the mood of fantasy, perhaps, because his

[8] Prof. Scholder Institute folder, Dept. of Investigation, AMA; Cramp, "Some Bald Facts," *Hygeia*, 5 (1927), 497-99.

[9] *Ibid.*; Dr. W. W. Bauer to author, Aug. 20, 1962.

temperament was so alien to the qualities almost mandatory for a successful career in pursuing quackery. About him there was nothing at all sly, boastful, callous, coarse, or mean. Cramp was slight in build, with ruddy cheeks, clear blue eyes, a clipped mustache, and an imperial. A fastidious man, he was always impeccably and conservatively dressed. His tastes in food and drink were discriminating, his hobbies quiet: photography and ornithology. Dignified, even austere, by nature, he made friends slowly and always retained a sense of reserve. A dedicated man, Cramp was both modest and sensitive. Linked by an editor once with two outstanding medical scientists, Sir William Osler and Carl Von Noorden, Cramp wrote a letter of protest. To find himself classed with "such giants of the profession," he said, made him "feel like a damn fool" and subjected him "to the ridicule of the profession."[10]

Cramp's work was his life, and in it he was a perfectionist. He pursued quackery, wrote George Simmons, the *Journal* editor, who supervised Cramp's efforts, "with necessary caution, with courage, and with honesty of purpose."[11] Thorough preparation, a fine sense of style, a recognition of the absurd, and moral conviction, these traits made Cramp's writing vivid, eloquent, and effective.

Dr. Cramp and the American Medical Association fought not only the most unscrupulous of quacks. They opposed virtually all proprietary preparations with secret formulas advertised to laymen for self-dosage. That the formula for a general consumption medicine should be nobody's business but the manufacturer's, Cramp wrote, was "mid-Victorian nonsense." Secrecy permitted the promoter to fool the public by making his impossible claims. "In the case of general merchandise," Cramp admitted, "there may be some excuse for these attempts to create in the minds of the public a desire for certain things it would not, otherwise, want. Some economic argument may conceivably be built up in defense of the proposition that the public should be impelled, through plausible and persuasive advertising, to purchase more pianos, more motor-

---

[10] *Ibid.*; Bauer interviews; interview with Dr. Walter Alvarez, Aug. 13, 1962; interview with Juelma Williams, Aug. 14, 1962; Cramp to Campbell Bradshaw, Apr. 17, 1919 [regarding item in Feb. 1919 *Mich. Food and Drug Monthly*], Warner Safe Cure Co. folder, AMA.
[11] Foreword to *N&Q*, III.

cars, more hats or more clothes than it really can afford or has use for. No such excuse can be put forward in the case of medicaments. No man has a moral right so to advertise as to make well persons think they are sick and sick persons think they are very sick. Such advertising is an offense against the public health."[12]

The public, moreover, could detect if a motor-car did not run or a hat did not fit. But "the healing power of nature" entered into the evaluation of nostrums in a critical way. Spontaneous cures occurred in an "enormous percentage" of dispositions. A patient was not qualified to judge whether he got well because of a proprietor's product or in spite of it. This point was what invalidated the claim that extensive sales over many years proved the efficacy of a patent medicine. It also negated the relevance of any testimonial, however sincere the testator.[13]

Cramp had to keep defending the medical profession's integrity in its opposition to nostrums. "Why," an official of the Lydia Pinkham company queried the public rhetorically on one occasion, "should you be persuaded or compelled to give . . . [packaged household remedies] up . . . and call a physician for every little ailment for which you do not need him . . . ?" The answer was that "some illiberal physicians, jealously desirous of a complete monopoly" were "taking advantage of the present mania for muck-raking and pseudo-reform to serve their own selfish purposes." Such charges of greed Cramp continually refuted. If financial profit were the physician's motive, Cramp said, patent medicines would receive the medical profession's blessing. Nostrums ruined health and created business for the doctor.[14]

Physicians were not entirely against self-dosage. Cramp made clear that he did not expect the ordinary citizen to run to his doctor with every little ailment. For a limited sphere of minor health problems, home remedies were perfectly natu-

[12] *Ibid.*, ix; "Modern Advertising and the Nostrum Evil," *Amer. Jnl. of Public Health*, 8 (1918), 756-58.
[13] *Ibid.*; PI, 149 (Nov. 7, 1929), 74; "The Part Played by the Testimonial," *Hygeia*, 1 (1923), 170-74.
[14] W. H. Gove in *Charities and the Commons*, 18 (Apr. 13, 1907), 85; Cramp, "The Nostrum and the Public Health," *JAMA*, 72 (1919), 1530-33.

ral and proper. Legitimate medicines of this type should, Cramp believed, meet certain standards: they must contain no dangerous or habit-forming drugs, must not be recommended for diseases too serious for self-treatment, and must be truthfully advertised, so the buyer would not be tempted to exaggerate an ailment and dose himself unnecessarily. Remedies meeting these specifications were to be found among the simpler products on every druggist's shelf—nonsecret recipes listed in the *Pharmacopeia* or *National Formulary* and hence standardized in strength by force of law. "When the public is properly informed," Cramp wrote, "so that it knows what preparations to call for in order to treat its simpler ailments, advertising of secret remedies will be entirely unnecessary."[15]

Whether the key role in so educating the public lay with a scientific society like the AMA or with an agency of government like the Public Health Service, Cramp was not quite sure. In the 1920's the AMA did determine that it had a larger obligation to furnish laymen with health information than it had up to that time fulfilled. The result was a new popular journal, christened *Hygeia,* which began publication in April 1923. Its editor was Morris Fishbein, an articulate physician who had come to the AMA in 1913 to assist Simmons in editing the *Journal* and who took over its editorship when Simmons retired in 1924. Unlike Cramp, Fishbein was a primary figure in the AMA's power structure, and he was just as ardent a foe of quackery as Cramp himself. Dr. Fishbein encouraged Cramp, whose department was now called the Bureau of Investigation, to employ *Hygeia* as a new and more effective avenue for reaching public awareness with his anti-quackery messages. During the first year Cramp wrote a four-part series, lavishly illustrated, analyzing the nostrum evil. Hardly an issue went by thereafter without a new and trenchant attack from his pen on some facet of patent medicine promotion.[16]

The organ of the major proprietary manufacturers gave *Hygeia* a sarcastic greeting. "Beside such a magazine as 'Physi-

[15] Cramp, "The Nostrum and the Public Health," *New England Jnl. of Med.,* 201 (1929), 1299-1300.
[16] *Ibid.;* Fishbein, *A History of the American Medical Association,*

cal Culture,'" jibed *Standard Remedies,* "this publication is as lively as the U.S. Crop Report for 1893." The AMA's new publishing venture would "fall flat as a tapeworm."[17] The prediction proved as inaccurate as the appraisal.

Bernarr Macfadden's *Physical Culture* was one of Morris Fishbein's targets, condemned for both its reading and advertising columns. Fishbein aimed at a score of others, using his quick and clever pen to ridicule such widely assorted "medical follies" as chiropractic, antivivisectionism, rejuvenation, and muscle-building. One target he willingly shared with Cramp and numerous other foes of quackery: the Electronic Reactions of Albert Abrams.[18]

Abrams "easily ranked," in Cramp's phrase, "as the dean of twentieth century charlatans."[19] Claiming to have received a medical degree from Heidelberg at a very early age, Abrams became in the 1890's a professor of pathology at the Cooper Medical College in San Francisco. Performing legitimate research and publishing scientific articles, Abrams also wrote precious literary essays on medical topics. Among his themes was the hazard of quackery. "The physician," Abrams wrote on one occasion, "is only allowed to think he knows it all, but

---

280-81, 343, 349, 1184-85. Cramp's series in the first volume (1923) of *Hygeia, A Journal of Individual and Community Health,* was "What Is a 'Patent Medicine' and Why?," 43-45; "What Protection Does the National Food and Drugs Act Give?," 104-107; "The Part Played by the Testimonial," 170-74; and "Secrecy and Mystery—the Essentials," 243-48. The Propaganda Dept. became the Bureau of Investigation in 1924; *Hygeia* was rechristened *Today's Health* in 1950.

[17] *Standard Remedies,* 9 (Apr. 1923), 3.

[18] Fishbein's lively articles were assembled into two books, *The Medical Follies* (N.Y., 1925) and *The New Medical Follies* (N.Y., 1927). Material from these books with new essays was published as *Fads and Quackery in Healing* (N.Y., 1932).

[19] *N&Q,* III, 112. The account of Abrams is based on *ibid.,* 112-14; Albert Abrams folders, AMA Dept. of Investigation; "Albert Abrams, A.M., M.D., LL.D., F.R.M.S.," AMA reprint of *JAMA* material on Abrams of various dates; Cramp, "The Electronic Reactions of Abrams," *Hygeia,* 2 (1924), 658-59; Fishbein, *The Medical Follies,* 99-118; Martin Gardner, *In the Name of Science* (N.Y., 1952), 205-208; interviews with Dr. Walter Alvarez, May 19, 1961, and Aug. 13, 1962; the 12-part *Scientific American* series between 129 (Oct. 1923), 130, and 131 (Sep. 1924), 158-60, 220-22; Ernest W. Page, "Portrait of a Quack," *Hygeia,* 17 (1939), 53-55, 92, 95; Nathan Flaxman, "A Cardiology Anomaly, Albert Abrams (1863-1924)," *Bull. Hist. Med.,* 27 (1953), 252-68.

the quack, ungoverned by conscience, is permitted to know he knows it all; and with a fertile mental field for humbuggery, truth can never successfully compete with untruth."[20]

What some people cannot lick, they join. When Abrams joined the ranks of quackery is hard to say, and perhaps he never knew he had. While a medical school professor, he seems not to have been perfectly scrupulous. His course in physical diagnosis was a thin and shoddy affair, but he let students know he also gave an evening course on his own, much meatier in subject matter, for which he charged $200 a head. This and similar tawdry actions eventually cost him his professorship. Abrams' first clear deviation in print from medical orthodoxy came in 1909 and 1910 when he published books on a new theory of healing called spondylotherapy. He could diagnose disease, he said, and cure it too, by a steady, rapid percussing or hammering of the spine. A review in the AMA *Journal* was critical, but Abrams twisted the wording to make it favorable and used it in his advertising. He began to give lectures, both in San Francisco and on tour, explaining his new theories for a fee to cranks and quacks and gullible M.D.'s.

Several years later, "apparently having percussed the back to the fullest extent of what it would yield monetarily," as Dr. Fishbein put it, "Dr. Albert Abrams turned the patient over and began to percuss the abdomen."[21] His new system, however, was much more complex than spondylotherapy, and it was gadget-oriented. Electricity had always provided a tremendous storehouse of power for quackery. Now America was beginning to thrill at the wonder of radio. "The spirit of the age is radio," Abrams wrote, "and we can use radio in diagnosis."[22] Abrams developed a series of machines, linked together, that permitted him to harness the marvelous new force. Into the first contraption, the dynamizer, he put a piece of paper containing a few drops of the ailing person's blood, removed no matter when nor where, but only while the patient

[20] Cited in Gardner, 205.
[21] Fishbein, *The Medical Follies*, 101.
[22] Cited inside front cover, *Jnl. of Electronic Medicine*, Jan. 1925, Abrams folder, AMA.

was facing west. From the dynamizer a wire ran to the rheostatic dynamizer, from that to the vibratory rate rheostat, from that to the measuring rheostat. And from that a wire also extended, ending in an electrode. The use of this Rube Goldberg sequence for diagnosis required the participation of a healthy third party whom Abrams called the "subject." When the moment for diagnosis came, Abrams, operating in dim light, stripped the subject to the waist, faced him westward, and affixed the electrode to his forehead. Then the doctor tapped the subject's abdomen, determining by the various areas of resonance and dullness what diseases plagued the patient, however distant, whose dried blood lay quietly four machines back up the line. Such was the method of determining what their discoverer was pleased to call the "Electronic Reactions of Abrams."

ERA was superbly sensitive. Not only would Abrams' chain of devices detect syphilis, tuberculosis, and cancer, but the precise location of these diseases within the body. The sex of the patient could be determined, and, if female, whether or not pregnant. More remarkable still, even religion could be detected. In the September 1922 issue of his journal, *Physico-Clinical Medicine,* Abrams printed a chart showing abdominal areas of dullness for Catholic, Seventh Day Adventist, Theosophist, Jew, Protestant, and Methodist—the last two quite some distance apart. But wonder of wonders! Abrams discovered that a patient's autograph served the diagnostic purpose as well as did dried blood. This permitted excursions into the past. Pepys, Dr. Johnson, Longfellow, and Poe, Abrams reported, all had had syphilis, and for Poe there was also a "reaction of dipsomania."[23]

ERA was harnessed not only for detection but also for cure. This involved one more machine, the oscilloclast, capable of producing vibrations in consonance with the vibratory rates of all known diseases. Applied to a sufferer, and set by its operator to produce the proper rate, the machine stepped up the force of vibrations somehow so as to shatter and destroy the ailment. Abrams sold his diagnostic devices, but would

[23] "Albert Abrams, A.M., M.D., LL.D., F.R.M.S.," 2-3.

only lease the oscilloclast. The fee was fancy, and the lessee agreed by contract never to open the apparatus, which was hermetically sealed.

In fact, the insides were a weird jumble of ohmmeters, rheostats, condensers, and other parts, wired together without any sense at all. "They are the kind of device," said the physicist Robert Millikan, "a ten-year-old boy would build to fool an eight-year-old."[24] One of Cramp's West Coast friends, the physician Walter Alvarez, tracked down the electrician who was making the oscilloclasts. Shamefacedly he admitted the feeling that he was "prostituting" himself. But the pay was irresistible.[25] Abrams must be coining money, the electrician said, at the rate of many thousands a week.

No question about it, money was flowing in. Practitioners from all over the nation had assembled at Abrams' San Francisco laboratories to sit at the master's feet, and he went forth on propaganda tours. A beachhead had been established in England with the recruitment of a past president of the British Medical Association to ardent discipleship. In a paternity case, the judge had accepted Abrams' report, based on electronic vibrations in the blood, that pinned on a protesting man the fatherhood of a baby.[26] But widespread national interest in Abrams and his claims awaited a 1922 article by Upton Sinclair, who made ERA one of a long succession of fads to which he gave his outspoken allegiance. "His name," wrote the editor of *Scientific American*, "carried a brilliant and convincing story to the masses, who quite overlooked the fact that Sinclair's name meant no more in medical research than Jack Dempsey's would mean on a thesis dealing with the fourth dimension, or Babe Ruth's on the mathematical theory of invariance."[27]

Cramp and Fishbein had followed Abrams' dubious pathways from the start. The upsurge of public interest following Sinclair's avowal of support made Abrams for a time the main task of Cramp's department.[28] Reluctantly, for he ad-

[24] Cited in Fishbein and William Engle, "Medical Hucksters, The Black Magic Box," *Amer. Weekly*, Feb. 1, 1948, 16-17.
[25] Alvarez to Cramp, Nov. 13, 1922, Abrams folder, AMA.
[26] *San Francisco Examiner*, Feb. 13, 1921, clipping, *ibid*.
[27] 131 (1924), 96.
[28] 1922 annual report, "The Propaganda Department," Reports of Bureau of Investigation folder, AMA.

mired the outspoken reformer in many ways, Cramp engaged
Sinclair in a public debate in print over Abrams' validity. "Mr.
Sinclair says that he has spent time in Dr. Abrams' clinic,"
Cramp wrote, "and is wonderfully impressed with Dr.
Abrams' achievements. So is the small boy impressed with the
marvelous facility with which the magician extracts the white
rabbit from the silk hat. Mr. Sinclair is convinced 'that Albert
Abrams has discovered the great secret of the diagnosis and
cure of all the major diseases.' The small boy is equally convinced that the prestidigitator has solved the mystery of producing snow white bunnies from airy nothings." More in
sorrow than in anger, Cramp concluded that Sinclair's "naïveté
may be childlike, but it is not scientific," and hoped that in
time the author would abandon ERA as he had given up earlier panaceas that had once caught his fancy.[29]

Besides his own writing, Cramp furnished raw data for
other critics taking aim at Abrams, among them Paul DeKruif
and H. L. Mencken. "I met this wizard casually in San Francisco," Mencken wrote to Dr. Fishbein, "the usual pince nez
and torpedo beard . . . [and] something quackish in his
scheme." Cramp suggested the name of Dr. Alvarez as a member of the blue-ribbon panel created by *Scientific American* to
assess Abrams and gave much help to the committee's chairman, Austin Lescarboura, the magazine's editor and an expert
in electricity and radio. The twelve long articles which resulted, one a month for a whole year, seemed to Cramp like
giving Abrams more exposure than was his due, but Cramp
concurred heartily with the concluding judgments. ERA had
no objective existence, the committee found, occurring only in
the minds of Abrams' practitioners. "At best," the scheme "is
an illusion. At worst, it is a colossal fraud." Recent trends in
electricity and radio had "given rise to all sorts of occultism
in medicine . . . , a renaissance of the black magic of medieval
times." ERA was just the most dramatic example.[30]

While this series was in midstream, Dr. Abrams, a man of
60, died of pneumonia, leaving an estate valued at $2,000,000.

[29] The original Cramp-Sinclair correspondence is in one of the Abrams
folders, AMA. It is cited in "Albert Abrams, A.M., M.D., LL.D.,
F.R.M.S.," 6-8.
[30] DeKruif, "Albert Abrams, Wonder of the West," *Hearst's International*, 43 (Jan. 1923), 76; Mencken, *Prejudices: Sixth Series* (N.Y.,

He left also hundreds of machines around the land, in the hands of practitioners able to diagnose syphilis not only in the blood of human patients, but also (unknowingly) in the blood of guinea pigs, chickens, and sheep. And he left a hard corps of disciples, dedicated to his name and system, organized as the American Association for Medico-Physical Research.[31]

Albert Abrams was but one of hundreds of medical messiahs whose message of hope Arthur Cramp brought into question, always with Morris Fishbein's unflagging support. During Cramp's tenure as director of the Bureau of Investigation, despite numerous threats, only two libel suits were actually brought to trial, and only one was lost. In 1914 articles in the *Journal* called Wine of Cardui, made by the Chattanooga Medicine Company, "a vicious fraud." Its alcoholic content high, the *Journal* charged, the remedy contained no ingredient capable of lifting up a fallen womb. The article also contained disparaging comments about the brothers who made Wine of Cardui, one of them, John A. Patten, a leading layman nationally in the Methodist Church. The company countered with two suits, a personal suit by Patten for $200,000, which lapsed during the course of trial when Patten died, and a partnership suit for $100,000. After 13 tempestuous weeks of testimony, the jury gave a verdict against the AMA. Damages, however, were not $100,000, but just a single cent, and the Chattanooga Medicine Company had to pay its own court costs. Despite the defeat and the staggering $125,000 in expenses incidental to the trial, the AMA was satisfied. "Technically guilty; morally justified!" the *Journal* reported the verdict. "To the Association a moral triumph; to the 'Patent medicine' interests a Pyrrhic victory."[32]

---

1927), 98; Mencken to Fishbein, Oct. 6, 1921 (copy), Abrams folder, AMA; Alvarez to Cramp, Feb. 7, 1924, *ibid.*; Cramp, "The Electronic Reactions of Abrams," *Hygeia,* 2 (1924), 658-59; *Scientific American,* 131 (1924), 158-60, 220-22.

[31] *Ibid.*, 130 (1924), 159; *JAMA,* 79 (1922), 2247; *N&Q,* iii, 112. Two years after the master's death, a follower boasted in the group's journal: "Hiccough Germ Tracked to Its Lair . . .," *Jnl. of Electronic Med.*, Jan. 1926, AMA file.

[32] Cramp, "The Work of the Bureau of Investigation," *Law and Contemporary Problems,* 1 (Dec. 1933), 54; Fishbein, "Libel Suits against

Through the 1920's and into the thirties, Cramp continued to set his clever traps for nostrum promoters and to reach for *Alice* when it came time to write up the fantastic results. Pamphlets mailed out based on Cramp's investigations passed the 2,000,000 mark. By 1930 more than enough data were on hand to warrant a third volume of *Nostrums and Quackery*, but the depression did not permit the AMA to get it out. In 1934, while attending the Association convention, Cramp suffered a heart attack, retiring to Florida the next year. There, far away from the scene of his former labors, he finished editing his manuscript. The third green-bound volume was published in 1936.[33]

Cramp, in his swan song, acknowledged that the situation with respect to self-medication, largely because of federal action, was improved as compared with the time when he had arrived at the AMA. But a "Utopian period" was not close at hand. "In the field of medicine human credulity learns little from experience." And in some ways, especially relating to advertising, things were, if less blatant, more tricky than before. "In this line of 'patent medicines' as in other lines," Cramp wrote, "the direct falsehood has given place to the falsehood by implication."[34]

As long before as 1920, Cramp had detected a significant transition through which most advertising was passing. The emphasis was not so much on "offering copy," which presented a product quite straightforwardly for a reader to buy or not as he had need of it, but upon "selling copy," the creation of desires where no craving had existed. Patent medicine pioneers had long sold the fear of suffering and death, the hope of well-being and health. During the early 20th century, all advertising was learning "scientifically" what the nostrum promoter had learned empirically, that the most effec-

the American Medical Association," *FDC Law Qtly.*, 2 (1947), 180-82; Fishbein, *A History of the American Medical Association*, 495-98; Burrow, 124-25. AMA, *The Wine of Cardui Suit* (n.p., 1916), reprints most of the testimony in behalf of the AMA.

[33] Cramp, "The Work of the Bureau of Investigation," 53-54; "Report of the Bureau of Investigation for 1931," AMA; *N&Q*, III, v; interview with Juelma Williams; *JAMA*, 147 (1951), 1773. Cramp died in 1951.
[34] *N&Q*, III, vii, xii, 21.

tive appeal was to the emotions. At the very same time that the advertising self-regulators were striving to stamp out the worst abuses in patent medicine advertising, they were themselves eagerly adopting nostrum advertising's basic approaches. In the same years that advertising agents were urging truth-in-advertising statutes, they were beginning to find answers to questions posed for them by professors of psychology. "How many advertisers," inquired Walter Dill Scott of Northwestern University in 1904, "describe a piano so vividly that the reader can *hear* it? How many food products are so described that the reader can *taste* the food? How many advertisements describe a perfume so that the reader can *smell* it? How many describe an undergarment so that the reader can *feel* the pleasant contact with his body?"[35]

For Albert Lasker, hard-driving and audacious advertising agent, the new day dawned with vivid force. As part of his appeal to the public in behalf of Palmolive soap, Lasker had been using the slogan, "Keep That School Girl Complexion." One day he saw an ad worked out for a competing soap by J. Walter Thompson, a rival agency. Woodbury was urged for "The Skin You Love to Touch." In an instant Lasker grasped the real thrust of this ad and was both envious and indignant. "You see what Thompson has done," he told his staff. "They have gone us one better and put *sex* into soap advertising." Lasker snorted, "Sex ... SEX!"[36]

Sex was not the only basic emotion to be sold to Americans in the new day. The trend toward stressing primary appeals accelerated and gained respectability during the war, when advertising agents were recruited by the government itself to promote patriotism. George Creel, who did the recruiting, once said that prior to this time most advertising men were viewed with much suspicion, classed with check-suited salesmen and sideshow barkers. They emerged from their wartime

[35] Cramp, "Truth in Advertising Drug Products," *Amer. Jnl. of Public Health*, 10 (1920), 781, 784; Walter D. Scott, "The Psychology of Advertising," *Atlantic Monthly*, 93 (1904), 34; Frank Presbrey, *The History and Development of Advertising* (Garden City, 1929), 441-43.

[36] John Gunther, *Taken at the Flood: The Story of Albert D. Lasker* (N.Y., 1960), 74-75.

duties ready to play in the twenties roles of the highest prestige.[37]

Many reasons underlay the "awesome persistence" with which advertising expanded after the war: the needs of emancipated woman, tax policy, the birth of brand-new industries, a disillusionment with the great internationalist crusade leading to a delight in materialistic pleasures. Fundamental were the pro-business orientation of the nation's politics and the needs of the economy. American industry became too productive for the ready and easy absorption of its wares. "The American citizen's first importance to his country is no longer that of a citizen," editorialized Middletown's favorite paper, "but that of a consumer. Consumption is a new necessity." Advertising was called on to make people buy more goods. In doing so, advertising men perfected their technique of approaching potential customers by aiming at their basic emotions. Indeed, during these years, advertising created a business civilization's concept of Utopia, "an Arcady of material prosperity and social ease (and of questionable moral worth)." Liberating "a middle-class people from the tyranny of Puritanism, parsimoniousness, and material asceticism," the advertising of the twenties presented an ideal vision of the healthy, happy American family, securely at home, avoiding pitfalls which would hamper romantic love, and enjoying a superabundant leisure crammed with material pleasures.[38]

The appeal in advertising, then, was largely to buy those things which fit one into this grand scheme. Not soap and perfume were sold—not explicitly, at any rate—but youth, beauty, sex, romance. Not automobiles, but manly dominance and social prestige. Not a bathroom as "a mere utility," but "a spacious shrine of cleanliness and health."[39]

"Appeal to reason in your advertising," a practitioner of the craft told his fellows assembled in convention, "and you ap-

[37] Pease, *The Responsibilities of American Advertising*, 17.
[38] *Ibid.*, 11-15, 20-44; Robert S. and Helen M. Lynd, *Middletown* (N.Y., 1929), 88; Leo Spitzer, "American Advertising Explained as Popular Art," in *Essays on English and American Literature* (Princeton, 1962), 265n.
[39] Turner, 213.

peal to about 4 per cent of the human race." The percentage of non-rational in the total span of advertising was not quite so high as 96. A 1924 survey showed—advertising men sought to make their profession as scientific as statistics would permit —that 72 per cent of the advertising in general magazines took aim at the emotions. "We advertising men must be practical as well as truthful," wrote an agency president. "Advertising will not pay unless it is directed at the grade of intelligence of the reading public. To tell the naked truth might make no appeal. It may be necessary to fool people for their own good. Doctors, and even preachers, know that and practise it. Average intelligence is surprisingly low. It is so much more effectively guided by its subconscious impulses and instincts than by its reason."[40]

To be sure, few, if any, Americans believed that the dream world presented in advertising was a strictly literal place, already achieved in the twenties, or even just around the corner. Even the 96 per cent, if pushed, would grant it was a "never-never land." "Puffing"—legitimate exaggeration—was taken for granted by consumer as well as by court of law. "No sane woman," asserted the president of the American Association of Advertising Agencies, "is going to believe seriously that soap can restore youthful charm." Yet the illusion was cheering, and soap helped keep the woman clean. "The American people like advertising," he went on. "They like to buy from it. It suits their temperament. It is cordial and optimistic. It gives them a value that goes beyond use. It appeals to the instincts and desires of the human heart in suggesting benefits which arouse and keep them alive. It helps us all to carry on."[41]

Such a mystique was especially apt for advertising automobiles and cigarettes, cosmetics and toothpaste. And it worked superbly with proprietary medicines. For health was a fundamental emotional concern, and one easily linked to other

[40] *Ibid.*, 214; Neil H. Borden, *The Economic Effects of Advertising* (Chicago, 1942), 661-64; John Benson, "Pseudo Scientific Arguments in Advertising," *Advertising and Selling*, 8 (Feb. 23, 1927), 85.

[41] Spitzer, 264-65; Borden, 760; James A. Horton, FTC chief examiner, "Regulation and Cooperation," in Amer. Drug Mnfrs. Assoc., *Twenty-Ninth Annual Meeting* (Baltimore, 1940), 108; Benson cited in Lee, *The Daily Newspaper in America*, 336-37.

moods men lived by. Americans surpassed citizens of all other
nations, foreign observers stated, in their concern for health
and physical vigor. This helped explain nostrums and gadgets
designed to "charge the body with the bubbling joy of wing-
foot manhood." For major proprietors with much at stake,
confronting the FDA, the FTC, the AMA, and the NBBB, the
old days were happily gone. The old-fashioned cure-all was
dead, noted an expert in the marketing of proprietary remedies, and the listing in advertising of a long string of ailments
now had a "ludicrous" and "unreasonable" sound. Good markets existed for articles like vitamins, minerals, foods, soft
drinks—even coffee roasters—carefully advertised to link
them with health. Before the war a cottage cheese called
Sanatogen had soared forth on a spectacular career, and
Nuxated Iron had elicited high praise from Jack Dempsey
and Ty Cobb. The twenties were replete with such products.
Pseudo-scientific arguments, statistics, and testimonials
abounded. Only in fundamentalist Sunday School papers,
observed one commentator, did God still wear a long white
beard; in American advertising he wore a pince-nez and an
imperial and brandished a test tube. So often was the science
of the advertisements distorted and partisan, that even advertising men began to worry. "After all," one of them queried,
"is science not a dangerous jade for advertising to flirt with?"[42]

Some proprietors abandoned the old diseases and created
new ones, ailments that might bring pain to their victim, but
also might threaten him in other ways as well. Listerine had
first been marketed in the late 19th century as a proprietary
promoted to physicians and was named after Sir Joseph Lister,
antiseptic surgery's pioneer. Touted as "the best antiseptic for
both internal and external use," it was recommended for treating gonorrhea and for "filling the cavity, during ovariotomy."
In 1921 the ebullient Gerald Lambert, son of the founder,

[42] Borden, 431-34; George H. Knoles, *The Jazz Age Revisited: British
Criticism of American Civilization during the 1920's* (Stanford, 1955),
33; *Standard Remedies*, 6 (Sep. 1920), 23, and 18 (Sep. 1931), 3;
1916 AMA pamphlet, "Sanatogen: Cottage Cheese—The New Elixir of
Life"; *N&Q*, I, 470-78, II, 535-43, 560-62; Benson, "Pseudo Scientific
Arguments in Medicine," 28, 84-85; James Rorty, *Our Master's Voice:
Advertising* (N.Y., 1934), 231; the final quotation is from Benson, 84.

decided to vend his product direct to the public in a massive way. Within a few years, the company's sales had spurted phenomenally, and net earnings had multiplied 40-fold. Much of Listerine's success must be credited to "halitosis." This coined word frightened the continent, not because bad breath was a fatal malady but because it was a social disaster. Listerine advertising raised worrisome doubts in each reader's mind with telling slogans like "Even your best friends won't tell you," and "Often a bridesmaid but never a bride."[43]

With the advent of the depression, Listerine's attack on America's complacency became harder hitting still. While sponsoring radio broadcasts of the Metropolitan Opera, the company recaptured an echo of its earliest days: "Wet feet? Cold hands? Fatigued? Gargle with Listerine to ward off colds and sore throat. Safe antiseptic reduces number of germs as much as 99 per cent." In another ad came the warning, "3 out of 4 times it begins as a common cold: PNEUMONIA." But there were other threats besides that of personal illness. "Protect Baby, Mother," urged one appeal. "Don't transmit your cold . . . rinse hands with Listerine before any contact with children." In similar vein: "After their prayers are said, send those youngsters of yours into the bathroom for a good night gargle with Listerine." Economic security was also fair game. "Jobs are still scarce, so we say to you: If you have one, hold onto it. Keep well; fight colds as never before. Use Listerine." Nor was the threat to romance forgotten. "You 5,000,000 women who want to get married: How's Your Breath Today?"[44]

Halitosis pioneered a whole host of plagues against which proprietary products promised to protect Americans in prosperity and in depression. Assembling the maladies all in one

[43] Lambert's Lithiated Hydrangea and Listerine, pamphlet of late 1880's, Toner Collection, Rare Book Div., Library of Congress; Gerald B. Lambert, "Lessons from Listerine's Success," *PI*, 141 (Nov. 10, 1927), 3-8, 200, 203; *Printers' Ink: Fifty Years, 1888-1938* (N.Y., 1938), 362; *Standard Remedies*, 15 (Apr. 1928), 60.

[44] Listerine ads from *Sat. Eve. Post, Ladies' Home Jnl., Farmer's Wife, Physical Culture, Liberty*, and *Hearst's International-Cosmopolitan* for the mid-1930's, from file of Advertisements of medicinal preparations and devices, 1933-37, FDA Records, RG 88, NA.

place, as *Printers' Ink* was bold enough to do in 1934, the list was staggering, a massive threat to health, happiness, and social acceptance. Among the hazards were acid indigestion, athlete's foot, body odor, calendar fear, coffee nerves, dry skin blight, folliculitis, intestinal fatigue, paralyzed pores, sandpaper hands, scalp crust, sneaker smell, and underarm offense.[45]

Depression pressures not only lowered the taste of big-time proprietary advertising. The economic disaster also brought many new small-scale proprietors into the already keener competitive fray. Bankrupts from other lines of business, believing the medicine game easy and lucrative, and, after the repeal of prohibition, unemployed bootleggers, put their therapeutic wares upon the market. Many old and extinct nostrums, as well as outmoded versions of thriving proprietaries, got into trade channels when salvaging houses bought bankrupt stores and sought to unload the goods acquired. Some of the patent medicines sold in this way antedated 1906.[46]

The depression aggravated still another problem of central significance to the ethics of proprietary advertising: the role of radio. One of the boom industries of the twenties, radio's early policy forbade direct advertising over the airwaves, but it was soon to come. In 1924 major medicine proprietors were being told that "direct radio advertising talks at a rate of $100 for 10 minutes is not exactly cheap advertising." The cost rose, but so did the value received, as chain broadcasting, beginning that same year and culminating in NBC (1926) and CBS (1927), assembled for advertisers a national listening audience. In the year the crash came, radio was "moving definitely toward recognition as a major advertising medium."[47]

By then a sordid pioneer of radio promotion had for six years been demonstrating how effective this method of advertising could be. Out in Milford, Kansas, Dr. John R. Brinkley had in 1923 set up KFKB—"Kansas First, Kansas Best"—

[45] "Plagues," *PI*, 169 (Oct. 11, 1934), 63-64.
[46] Denver Station Annual Report, 1933, and Eastern District Annual Report, 1934, Decimal file .053, FDA Records.
[47] Hower, *The History of an Advertising Agency*, 132-38; *Standard Remedies*, 10 (Dec. 1924), 17; *Printers' Ink: Fifty Years*, 379.

one of the nation's most powerful stations. In between country music, fundamentalist sermons, and market reports, Brinkley talked into a gold-plated microphone about rejuvenation. Fusing public fascination with glands, a by-product of developments in regular medicine, with folklore traditions about the billy goat, Brinkley actually transplanted the sliced gonads of goats into the scrotums of inadequate males—even permitting each patient to choose, from a herd in the doctor's back yard, his own animal. In mesmeric fashion, Brinkley, facing his microphone, would drone on for elderly men to hear throughout the Midwest, "Don't let your doctor two-dollar you to death . . . come to Dr. Brinkley . . . take advantage of our Compound Operation . . . I can cure you the same as I did Ezra Hopkins of Possum Point, Missouri."[48]

The Federal Radio Commission, set up in 1927, proved three years later that it could quash outrageous quackery such as Brinkley's by failing to renew his license (though for a time the intent of this action was thwarted while Brinkley telephoned his broadcasts to a radio station in Mexico ten times as powerful as any in the United States). Concurrently, however, even the most reputable radio stations, in the view of one critic, were tolerating advertising pitches "far more deceptive and dishonest" than the best periodicals would admit to their pages. Even before the depression *Hygeia* had voiced a similar lament. "Barred from the newspapers by sincere and honest editorial supervision, the patent medicine mongers, the promoters of strange notions concerning the cause and cure of disease, the leaders of extraordinary cults of healing and of faith, find an outlet on radio, not yet subject to intelligent control." The depression made things worse. Radio, "too young to have developed an ethical conscience," took advertising away from periodicals and presented so much disgusting pseudo-medical copy that the chorus of criticism swelled. One of many protesters, using radio to condemn radio proprietary advertising, was director of the New York Tuberculosis and Health Association, Harry L. Hopkins.[49]

---

[48] Gerald Carson, *The Roguish World of Doctor Brinkley* (N.Y., 1960), is a sound and lively biography.

[49] *Ibid.*, 145-48, 176-77, 180-87; T. Swann Harding, *The Popular*

The depression brought an avalanche of criticism of varying kinds and degrees aimed at a business civilization whose recent promises of unending prosperity now seemed to lie in ashes. Especially vulnerable was advertising, which had presented the most glowing version of the New Era's vision of Utopia. The faults of advertising, not unobserved during prosperity, now, during disillusionment, seemed and, indeed, *were* worse.

Within the industry new pangs of conscience stirred renewed efforts at self-regulation. "Advertising needs a thorough purging," admitted one agency official who was especially disturbed by the tactics of the medicine makers. "Now I maintain," he wrote, "that the man who climbs to wealth by exploiting the fears and foibles of his fellow men, and destroying their peace of mind, is little better than the creature who fattens on the dreadful produce of the battlefield." A committee of the Affiliated Better Business Bureaus drafted a new code. The Association of National Advertisers and the American Association of Advertising Agencies cooperatively developed a list of ethical principles and established a "Supreme Court" to assume jurisdiction when a violator refused to accept the NBBB's recommendation that an offensive practice be curtailed. Radio networks tightened advertising censorship. Trade associations in many industries formulated more rigorous taboos. The Proprietary Association created an advertising advisory committee to compile a new code and hired a marketing professor from the University of Wisconsin to scrutinize proposed copy.[50]

Conscience alone does not explain these rekindled efforts by the advertising fraternity at reform from within. To a significant degree they were provoked from outside by the harshest

---

*Practice of Fraud* (N.Y., 1935), 186; "Station WCFL," *Hygeia*, 5 (1927), 645-46; "Quackery in Medicine," *ibid.*, 8 (1930), 514; *FTC Annual Report, 1934,* 102; "Quackery Adopts Radio," *Hygeia*, 8 (1930), 384-85.

[50] H. A. Batten, "Wanted: A Pillory," *Advertising and Selling,* 19 (Aug. 4, 1932), 14, 41; Lee, 333; *Hygeia*, 13 (1935), 764; *Standard Remedies*, 21 (June 1934), 12-13; (Aug. 1934), 3-5, 12; (Sep. 1934), 3-6, 13; *N.Y. Herald-Tribune*, Aug. 17, 1934; *PI*, 168 (Aug. 16, 1934), 24-28. For criticism of these efforts see Pease, 74-75, and Lamb, *American Chamber of Horrors*, 141.

criticism to which advertising had ever been subjected. Even during the fat years, some social scientists, like most creative writers, were not enamoured of the materialistic dream world conjured up for consumers in national advertising. In *The Tragedy of Waste*, published in 1925, the economist Stuart Chase argued that American productive energies were too largely devoted to creating not wealth but "illth," goods and service not useful for satisfying basic human wants, but harmful, or at least unnecessary. Among them he included not only such things as vice and crime, adulterated goods, and harmful drugs, but also super-luxuries and fashions. Standing as "a sort of godfather" to all forms of illth was advertising. "National advertising for the education of the consumer," Chase wrote, "if conducted by some impartial and scientific body might conceivably provide a great channel for eliminating wastes in consumption. But nine-tenths and more of advertising is largely competitive wrangling as to the relative merits of two undistinguished and often indistinguishable compounds —soaps, tooth powders, motor cars, tires, snappy suits, breakfast foods, patent medicines, and cigarettes."[51]

Business and government, in making their purchases, set precise specifications of quality and required suppliers to meet them. Not so the consumer, said Chase, in *Your Money's Worth*, which he wrote in collaboration with F. J. Schlink, a mechanical engineer. Confronted with advertising, the American consumer was "utterly unorganized, with no defense except a waning quality of common sense"; he pursued "his blundering way; a moth about a candle." What was needed was organization, so that consumers could be equipped with accurate information about the quality of products based on scientific testing. Was such organization possible? Chase and Schlink answered, "Perhaps."[52]

In 1929 Schlink offered a more positive answer, when, with Arthur Kallet, he organized Consumers' Research. After testing, products were described and compared in bulletins issued to paying members, so they could know what they were buying—brand names were given—and thus "defend them-

[51] Chase, *The Tragedy of Waste* (N.Y., 1925), 30-31, 113.
[52] Chase and Schlink, *Your Money's Worth* (N.Y., 1927), 41, 256.

selves against the aggressions of advertising and salesman-ship." By mid-1934, 48,000 would-be literate consumers had joined the group. Chase's critique, delivered during prosperity, sounded more persuasive in the depression. More and more vigorous propaganda was needed. Kallet and Schlink wrote *100,000,000 Guinea Pigs*, a mixture of technological analysis and fiery tract, that sped through 27 printings in a year. Other volumes of similar import quickly followed—*Skin Deep; Eat, Drink and Be Wary; Facts and Frauds in Woman's Hygiene; Paying through the Teeth; Our Master's Voice: Advertising.* The hazards to health in foods, drugs, and cosmetics were made vividly real in these exciting pages. And the irrationality of a helter-skelter, wasteful, unplanned economic system was asserted with equal vigor.[53]

The debate over advertising was keen and bitter between intellectuals in the business camp, who believed in its social utility, and intellectuals in the consumer's movement, who decried its value. Chase's attack was amplified in scope and fervor. Not only was advertising a sterile wrangling over products almost identical. Even worse, the kind of appeals it used degraded American life, exalting material and destroy-ing ethical values, and leading the citizenry by the nose to a drab culture of dead-level conformity. Consumers were cheated, the press was subverted, and the rationality upon which democracy depended was threatened by advertising's avowed stress upon subconscious drives and emotional ap-peals. Self-regulation by the "Goose Girls" of the advertising profession had failed, the critics said, and new gestures in that direction were just another effort to hoodwink the public.[54]

The "guinea pig" muckrakers found proprietary products

[53] A copy of the 28th printing of *100,000,000 Guinea Pigs* is dated Feb. 4, 1935, and gives the 1st printing date as Jan. 12, 1933; data on growth of Consumers' Research in M. C. Phillips, *Skin Deep: The Truth about Beauty Aids—Safe and Harmful* (N.Y., 1934), vii-viii; F. J. Schlink, *Eat, Drink and Be Wary* (N.Y., 1935); Rachel Lynn Palmer and Sarah K. Greenberg, *Facts and Frauds in Woman's Hygiene* (N.Y., 1936); Bissell B. Palmer, *Paying through the Teeth* (N.Y., 1935). There were many other similar books, and the *Nation* and *New Republic* pub-lished like material.

[54] Pease summarizes and analyzes the debate, 87-114, 138-66. The "Goose Girls" phrase is in Rorty, 179.

affecting the health a fertile field for dramatic exposure. Most of the basic facts they presented, to be sure, were quite like those of other critics, the American Medical Association, the regulatory agencies, the National Better Business Bureau. Indeed, most of the basic facts came from the pamphlets and releases of these organizations. Nonetheless, "guinea pig" muckraking had a noticeable difference. Kallet and Schlink and others of their school wrote up the facts so as to take greatest advantage of their shock value. They tended too to regard all sinners as of nearly equal culpability, condemning the big borderline advertiser exploiting body odor or bad breath with a rigor resembling that used to castigate the small operator vending a lethal radium water. Of course, one was worse than the other as a hazard to health, but neither would perform the function held out in advertising promises. Measured by the yardstick of utility to consumers, both fell equally short. Thus the "guinea pig" muckrakers saw proprietary promotion as a particularly glaring example of the bootlessness of advertising.

"Almost *no* advertising intended to influence the general public," Kallet and Schlink asserted, "is honest in the sense that a decent scientist understands honesty." Nor was anything better to be expected so long as "the profit motive continues to dominate all manufacture and distribution." Codes of ethics were mere eyewash. Should an advertising agency try to abide by them, it soon would lose its clients and go bankrupt.[55]

"In the eyes of the law," then, "we are all guinea pigs, and any scoundrel who takes it into his head to enter the drug or food business can experiment on us." The poisons fed to the American public might be expected to shorten normal life expectancy by several decades. For food and drug manufacturers engaged in killing. Their crime required a new name; perhaps an accurate one would be "statistical homicide." "But whatever we call it, they are responsible for the death of very large numbers of persons—death through premature old age, disease of stomach, bowels, and kidneys, which weakened organs cannot resist, and death because good medicine or

[55] Kallet and Schlink, *100,000,000 Guinea Pigs*, 178, 181-83.

medical care was needed, and a patent medicine for pneumonia or tuberculosis or cancer was taken instead."[56]

Were proprietary medicines safe? "The answer is No—an emphatic No." The consumer should abstain completely from using them. For, in taking nostrums, the ailing person was having, not a doctor, but an advertising copywriter prescribe for his pains. "With a laboratory in his mind and a medical dictionary in his hand, the copy-writer is ideally equipped to help the medicine and food manufacturers hoodwink and poison the public." Big agencies were as bad as small, big periodicals as bad as small, big manufacturers as bad as small.[57]

Listerine and similar so-called antiseptics, wrote Kallet and Schlink, were "of trifling worth for the galaxy of purposes" listed in their advertising. The proprietors worried the public mind with "groundless fears." They exaggerated the germ-killing potency of their wares. They did not tell of hazardous germs which were not killed. And they failed to advise that the massacre of bacteria in a test tube was no proof that a proprietary would kill germs in mouth, teeth, gums, or tonsils. Listerine's merits as an antiseptic, said the founders of Consumers' Research, citing the AMA, were "infinitesimal," and, by appropriating his name, Listerine debased "the fame of the great scientific investigator who first established the idea of antisepsis." No antiseptic should be advertised, Kallet and Schlink believed, "without a forthright and standard statement of germicidal power based on a standard test made by a designated testing agency, official and not for profit."[58]

Other grim examples crowded the pages of *100,000,000 Guinea Pigs*, and though these were taken mainly from AMA records and cases before regulatory agencies, this debt did not mean that Kallet and Schlink refrained from turning their critical spotlight in those directions. While complimenting Arthur Cramp for "the able direction" of his bureau, Kallet and Schlink rebuked the AMA for the unreliability of its *Journal* advertising. They criticized the Post Office Department for

[56] *Ibid.*, 6, 10, 16.
[57] *Ibid.*, 15, 62, 170, 176-78, 180, 183, 297.
[58] *Ibid.*, 63-64, 100-14, 194.

settling so many cases without criminal action and characterized the FTC as "unhappily dying of inanition." The strongest
castigations, however, were reserved for the Food and Drug
Administration.[59]

Behind the nostrum vendor, according to the "guinea pig"
muckrakers, lay "an incompetent and indifferent and quite
cold-blooded Government régime," characterized by "shiftiness, and a preference for backstairs methods." Granted
that the basic law was "feeble and ineffective" as written and
that it had been further weakened by court interpretation.
Granted that funds for enforcement were incredibly inadequate: the Food and Drug Administration had only 65 inspectors to police 110,000 different products, manpower hardly
sufficient to check on Philadelphia alone. There were, indeed,
more inspectors than this pitiful handful in the Department
of Agriculture's program to control hog cholera and in the
effort to enforce plant quarantine along the Mexican border.
Granted all this, Food and Drug officials deserved much
blame. In the first place, charged Kallet and Schlink, officials
had failed to urge new laws to plug the loopholes, to repair
the "niggardliness" of appropriations for protecting the public
health.[60]

FDA administrators were dull, unimaginative, and smug,
their critics charged, but their major failing lay in bending
the law to favor not the consumer but the manufacturer. This
policy underlay their preference for seizure to criminal actions
—only one offender had ever received a jail sentence under
the law—their announcement of warnings to proprietary manufacturers before launching an enforcement program, their
secret negotiations with manufacturers, their avoidance of
using publicity as a weapon against quackery. FDA Chief,
Walter Campbell, deserved the severest condemnation for
his "naïve interpretation" of his job. "Could anyone be kinder
than Mr. Campbell," Kallet and Schlink inquired, "to the
quacks and crooks who are purveying cures and treatments
for Bright's disease, cancer, pneumonia, and tuberculosis?"[61]

[59] *Ibid.*, 159, 190-93, 213.
[60] *Ibid.*, 4, 195, 206, 212, 232, 255-56.
[61] *Ibid.*, 7, 119-20, 129-30, 133, 204, 214, 240, 251.

Neither Campbell nor his boss, the Secretary of Agriculture, in the judgment of the authors of *100,000,000 Guinea Pigs*, had the right to decide "that in pursuance of the general ideas and social policies of Messrs. Harding, Coolidge, and Hoover, they may turn the statute from its original punitive purpose protecting the public interest, to the guiding and educational one of bringing the manufacturers into a harmonious understanding with the changed and attenuated purposes of the Federal officials."[62]

Thus Messrs. Kallet and Schlink cast regulated and regulators into the same den of iniquity. Such condemnation Food and Drug officials felt to be outrageously unfair, just as they were persuaded—and so were many others—that numerous factual statements made by Consumers' Research were careless and inaccurate. Yet the beleaguered bureaucrats welcomed whatever pressure Kallet, Schlink & Co. might generate that would help secure a remedial law.

"I have been pursuing for years a policy calculated to correct these defects by seeking amendatory legislation," wrote Campbell to Simon Sobeloff, his ally in the B. & M. trial. "If this muck-raking publication [*100,000,000 Guinea Pigs*] furthers these ends it will not have been published in vain."[63]

[62] *Ibid.*, 215.
[63] [1933] letter, Accession job 446-548, FDA Records, RG 88, NA. Examples of critical reviews are those by T. Swann Harding in the *Sat. Rev. of Literature*, 9 (1932-33), 402, and by James A. Tobey in the *Amer. Jnl. of Public Health*, 23 (1933), 530-31.

# 8

## THE NEW DEAL AND THE
## NEW LAWS

---

*"Every slimy serpent of a vile manufacturer of
patent medicine is right now working his wiggling way
around this Capitol. I have heard heretofore about the
effort dear old Dr. Wiley made to secure the passage
of the original law 28 years ago. Historically I was familiar with it, but now from experience I am familiar
with it. I know the devious ways of those who are seeking to defeat the effort of the Congress to give protection to the health and lives of our people."*

—ROYAL S. COPELAND IN THE SENATE, 1935[1]

---

A FEW DAYS after the inauguration of Franklin D. Roosevelt, the Chief of the Food and Drug Administration, Walter
Campbell, walked across the street to pay a call on a new
Assistant Secretary of Agriculture, Rexford G. Tugwell. Tugwell had raised a point about a letter prepared for his signature in Campbell's office, and the Chief felt a personal explanation was in order. The matter settled, the two men went on to
a general conversation about the way in which existing food

[1] *Cong. Record*, 74 Cong., 1 ses., 5138 (1935). Charles Wesley Dunn,
in *Federal Food, Drug, and Cosmetic Act: A Statement of Its Legislative Record* (N.Y., 1938), has reprinted all the pertinent portions of the
*Congressional Record* relating to the efforts from 1933 into 1938 to secure the law. The work also contains other material, especially the portions of Congressional hearings citing testimony of FDA and FTC
spokesmen. For leads on material used in this chapter, the author wishes
to express appreciation to graduate students who prepared course
papers on various aspects of the law's background: David L. Coker,
Norman B. Ferris, William J. Harkins, Shirley Hinton, Charles O. Jack-
son, Robert L. Keele, Jr., Bartlett C. Jones, Anne Lide, Choice McCoin,
R. L. McConnell, Joseph C. Ray, Jr., Jane Stubbs, and Edwin H. Trainer.

and drug legislation failed to provide proper safeguards for the consumer.[2]

That same afternoon Campbell was again summoned to Tugwell's office. "Mr. Campbell," the Assistant Secretary said, "since I saw you this morning I have talked with the President. I repeated our conversation to him, and he has authorized a revision of the Food and Drugs Act." Thus began a five-year battle.

Inadequacies in Dr. Wiley's 1906 law had been recognized from the start. Wiley and his successors—despite what the "guinea pig" muckrakers said—had not been negligent in pointing out the scope which supplementary legislation should have.[3] From time to time bills had been presented to the Congress to rectify this or that omission. Only a few had passed.[4] No broad-gauge measure had been given serious consideration. Not since the Sherley Act of 1912 had Congress dealt with the drug provisions of the law. During the golden glow of prosperity particularly, the political climate had not been conducive to reform. Now there was a dramatic change.

The situation "goes so far beyond the boundaries of what we dreamed to be a possibility six months ago," wrote Charles W. Crawford, in charge of enforcement for the FDA, in August 1933, "that it does not seem possible. Perhaps I have not oriented myself to the tempo of the 'new deal.' "[5]

After the Campbell-Tugwell conversation, things moved fast, perhaps too fast. In order to get a bill to present to the emergency session of Congress, the drafting process had been hurried. FDA officials and Department of Agriculture lawyers, aided by young law school professors secured by Tugwell, had quickly concluded that their goals could not be satisfied by

[2] Ruth deForest Lamb, *American Chamber of Horrors*, 278-79.

[3] Wiley expressed his views in testifying before a House Committee in 1912. *The Pure Food and Drugs Act: Hearings before the Committee on Interstate and Foreign Commerce, House of Representatives* (62 Cong., 2 ses.). Carl Alsberg, Chief of the Bureau of Chemistry, described "serious limitations" of the law in his *1917 Report of Bureau of Chemistry.*

[4] The several amendments that had been passed since 1906 are summarized in *1931 Report of Food and Drug Administration.*

[5] Crawford to David F. Cavers, Aug. 8, 1933, "Correspondence on Legislation," Office of the Commissioner, Records of the Food and Drug Administration, RG 88, NA.

mere amendments to Dr. Wiley's law. Some of the 1906 language might be retained, but an entirely new bill was necessary. The draft was not yet in final form when preliminary conferences were held with representatives of the drug, food, and publishing industries. Tugwell and his cohorts saw an advantage in seeking ideas from the business community without revealing a specific text upon which criticism could focus. The businessmen, hoping to see such a text, were unnerved to discover that they were being asked to make suggestions about a new law without knowing exactly what government officials had in mind. The mystery of the unpresented bill struck them as ominous, especially since Rexford Tugwell was known to be its sponsor.[6]

Of all that new breed of "brain trusters" whom Roosevelt had brought to Washington, none was more suspect to the ranks of business than the handsome young Tugwell. This Columbia University economics professor was frank to say that he believed in a planned economy. He had spent two months in Russia—in company with Stuart Chase. In a book published in May 1933, Tugwell had stated, "It is doubtful whether nine-tenths of our sales effort and expense serves any good social purpose." He was soon to assert that "property rights and financial rights will be subordinated to human rights." These frightening phrases appeared in the middle of extended discussions of political economy also frightening because of the abstruse, academic, sophisticated nature of Tugwell's thought. In manner also Tugwell upset businessmen: his "gallant confidence" struck them as haughty and imperious. The reaction came quickly. This outspoken theorist was soon presented, in a nightmare dreamed by a business-oriented educator, as a key villain, playing the role of Stalin to Roosevelt's Kerensky.[7]

[6] David F. Cavers, "The Food, Drug, and Cosmetic Act of 1938: Its Legislative History and Its Substantive Provisions," *Law and Contemporary Problems*, 6 (Winter 1939), 7-8; the FDA prepared summary statements concerning the conferences with industry which are reproduced in Dunn, 1033-47; Bernard Sternsher, *Rexford Tugwell and the New Deal* (New Brunswick, N.J., 1964), 248; *N.Y. Journal of Commerce*, Apr. 11 and 28, 1933, "Clippings on Food and Drug Legislation," Scrapbook, FDA Records, RG 88, NA.

[7] Rexford G. Tugwell, *The Industrial Discipline* (N.Y., 1933), 180;

When the proposed new food and drug law was at last revealed, its greatest handicap to acceptance in business circles and to some degree in Congress was not its particular provisions, worrisome as many of them were, but the name by which it was known, the "Tugwell bill." Indeed, opponents of particular provisions sought to gain allies by deliberately brandishing Tugwell's frightening name.[8] This was in a measure unfair, for the Assistant Secretary had nothing to do with the exact terms of the draft bill. But such are the realities of politics. Wiley had been a bureaucratic wild man to opponents of legislation during the first decade of the century. During the thirties Tugwell was cast in a similar role.

There are other similarities between the two crusades. Both were protracted, requiring half a decade of intensive effort. Both ended with laws much modified from earlier drafts. So all-pervasive are foods, drugs, and cosmetics, and so complex the details of regulation, that there was both necessity and room for the politician's art of compromise. By 1938, as by 1906, there had come to be somewhat too much of compromise for the general welfare. Both Theodore and Franklin Roosevelt favored food and drug reform, but in a moderate rather than an energetic way, and neither was prompt to give the issue top priority. In both decades, industries to be regulated lobbied with greater effectiveness than did consumers. Women's organizations both times were the most important and steadfast of consumers' champions. To those who took part in both struggles, there was a feeling of familiarity about the second fight. They had been that way before. The opponents of reform used many of the same basic arguments, even the same angry adjectives.[9] In the end, the achievement of

---

Elliott Roosevelt, ed., *F.D.R.: His Personal Letters* (N.Y., 1950), I, 372-73; Sternsher, 228-30; *Current Biography 1941* (N.Y., 1941), 874-76; Cavers, 6. The late John J. McCann of FDA told the author that, at a small informal meeting held by Tugwell and FDA officials to discuss what form the new law should take, Stuart Chase was present.

[8] Sternsher, 244.

[9] Charles H. LaWall, "Fads and Frauds in Foods and Drugs," *Amer. Jnl. of Pharmacy*, 109 (1937), 115-23; Dr. A. T. McCormack, *Foods, Drugs, and Cosmetics: Hearings before a Subcommittee of the Committee on Interstate and Foreign Commerce, House of Representatives . . . on H.R. 6906 . . . and S.5* (74 Cong., 1 ses., 1935), 103-104.

legislation depended upon upsurges of public pressure felt in Congress, generated in each case by a dramatic threat to the public health. Instead of the fear of impure meat, there was, in 1937, the "Elixir Sulfanilamide" disaster.

The events preceding 1906 and 1938 had also their differences. The 1933 bill was presented more dramatically, with less of a gradual conditioning of industry to the general idea than was true at the turn of the century, and thus struck the business community with greater immediate shock. During the second campaign the public did not develop the degree of interest and concern that characterized the Wiley crusade. One reason is that the 1906 law had done much good, especially respecting food. There was widespread popular feeling, indeed, mistaken but sincerely held, that the first law had solved almost all the problems. A supplementary crusade, perhaps, cannot elicit the fire and zeal of the initial one. Another reason for the lesser impact in the thirties of food and drug efforts upon public awareness was the total political and economic environment. The United States was struggling to lift herself from the worst economic disaster in her history by relief, recovery, and reform measures of unprecedented novelty. Competition for headlines and front-page space was keener than during the more prosperous days of the Square Deal.

Muckraking was different also. In Wiley's day, popular magazines had carried stark tales of food and nostrum evils into half the homes of the land. This did not happen in the thirties. The development of national advertising had made the slick, wide-circulation magazines more cautious. And since food, drug, and cosmetic advertising was a field over which the proposed new law sought to extend control, some of the same journals that fought hard for reform in 1906 were initially hostile in 1933. Partly for the same reason, perhaps, newspapers gave very little space to the continuing efforts in Congress to enact a new law. Medicine proprietors sought to frighten publishers, as they had done at the turn of the century, about how advertising revenue would tumble if the law should pass.[10] A St. Louis editor wrote Tugwell that opponents of the bill had generated the hottest "heat" he had felt in a

[10] An example is reproduced in Lamb, 307.

quarter of a century.[11] It is hard to say how much of a club this proved to be in the thirties. Editors, like the broader public, were just more interested in other issues. Insofar as food and drug matters did concern them, they might favor some aspects of a new bill but be leary of bureaucratic control over advertising.

The "guinea pig" muckrakers of the thirties reached their public through books and slender-circulation magazines. Thus the number of people aroused was a smaller proportion of the public than that which had reacted to the exposés of Mark Sullivan, Upton Sinclair, and Samuel Hopkins Adams. These old muckrakers had worked hand-in-glove with Wiley to secure the 1906 law. The new muckrakers stood in a different relationship to Walter Campbell and his aides, not collaborators but critics. Using the same harsh adjectives they employed for adulterators and quacks, the Consumers' Research spokesmen belabored Food and Drug officials for indifference to the public welfare. Kallet and Schlink thought the FDA draft of a bill not rigorous enough to be acceptable, whereas Campbell and Crawford considered Consumers' Research proposals too extreme to be practicable. The more the FDA yielded to political realities in the hope of getting some kind of a law, the more Consumers' Research rebuked the inconstancy of bureaucrats.

Tugwell and Campbell had hoped that a food and drug law might be swept through Congress during the New Deal's first hundred days. This did not happen. Recovery was the prime national concern, and other measures held priority. The President did not label this particular reform a "must"; indeed, the bill's proponents did not make public the fact that Roosevelt had specifically authorized their effort. Even had the President spoken out firmly, the bill might well have failed. Every state, every Congressional district, had manufacturers, wholesalers, and retailers concerned with foods and drugs. "The connections between businesses engaged in doubtful conduct and local politicians," as Tugwell later said, "turned out to be very direct in many places." There was even difficulty in securing a Congressional sponsor for the bill. The

[11] Sternsher, 234.

Food and Drug Administration was a unit in the Department of Agriculture, but the chairmen of the Committees on Agriculture in both the Senate and the House expressed their inability to consider the measure. Finally Royal S. Copeland came forward and volunteered for the assignment.[12]

Copeland was not the ardent reformer's picture of a reforming Senator. A Tammany Democrat, his economic views were not noted for their liberalism. Copeland did not look like a crusader. A debonair man, he bore himself jauntily and was widely known for the fresh red carnation worn in his buttonhole each morning. Courteous in debate, he gave the impression of being much more anxious to compromise than to stand resolute. His physician's training had been homeopathic. He had written a health column for the Hearst papers, which soon would bitterly oppose his bill. All this made Copeland suspect among the more extreme crusaders. Yet there is no question that the dapper Senator was deeply devoted to the cause of food and drug reform. While serving as health commissioner of New York City, he had encountered evils which the 1906 law could not prevent. Coming to the Senate, he had introduced bills aimed at plugging some of these loopholes. Now he accepted the draft measure from Campbell and, as the emergency session of Congress drew to a close, introduced the bill. Copeland had not yet read it through.[13]

When four months later Copeland did read the bill, he found that it would expand drastically the government's control over proprietary remedies. The 1906 law had provided a few "Thou shalt nots" regarding remedy labeling. The draft measure added to the prohibitions and included sweeping "Thou shalts." No longer would the government have to prove the fraudulent state of mind of a proprietor, as it had so expensively done in the B. & M. case: a drug was misbranded, according to the Tugwell bill, if its labeling made

[12] *Ibid.*, 230; Tugwell, *The Democratic Roosevelt* (Garden City, N.Y., 1957), 464-66; Cavers, 4, 8. Lamb, 287, says there was no expectation that the bill would pass during the emergency session.

[13] *Wash. Post*, June 18, 1938, FDA Scrapbook; Cavers, 10; Tugwell, *The Democratic Roosevelt*, 466; Sternsher, 249; Campbell to Cavers, June 14, 1933, "Correspondence on Legislation"; Copeland in Senate, May 16, 1934, *Cong. Record*, 73 Cong., 2 ses., 8957.

any therapeutic claim, even by ambiguity or inference, that was "contrary to the general agreement of medical opinion." The misbranding ban fell too on labels which gave the names of diseases for which the remedies were palliatives instead of cures, unless the labels clearly stated that the drugs were not cures. No longer would the names of only eleven drugs appear on labels; the draft bill required that all proprietary medicine labels list the common names and quantities of all medicinal ingredients. Medicines containing certain narcotic and hypnotic drugs must caution the consumer: "Warning—May be habit forming." And the list of dangerous drugs was longer than in the old law, for many new products—like the barbiturates—had developed or come into wider use since 1906. Germicides and antiseptics, if they would escape misbranding, must bear an accurate label statement telling under what precise conditions they would actually kill micro-organisms.[14]

Whole categories of proprietary products which Dr. Wiley's law had not touched were covered in the Tugwell bill. Taboo were those remedies, like radium-containing liquids, which were desperately risky to take even though the labels, by avoiding therapeutic claims, told no untruth. A drug was adulterated, the draft bill stated, if it was dangerous to health when used according to directions on the label. Banished also were mechanical devices, like "electric" belts and Rube Goldberg machines with flashing lights, sold with claims to cure whatever ailed the customer. The definition of "drugs" was broad enough to encompass "devices intended for use in the cure, mitigation, treatment, or prevention of disease." Restricted too were remedies and gadgets that, strictly speaking, had nothing to do with illness, like weight-reducers, bust-expanders, and nose-straighteners, for the draft bill brought them under its control.

False advertising would also be illegal if the Tugwell bill should pass. The promotion of drugs, as well as of foods and the newly included cosmetics, must adhere, in general, to the same strict standards that were to apply to labeling. With respect to certain ailments, indeed, for which self-treatment was considered dangerous or futile, no remedies at all

[14] *Ibid.*; Dunn cites the text of S. 1944, the "Tugwell bill," 37-50.

could be advertised to the lay public. The list was long, including appendicitis, blood poisoning, carbuncles, sexual impotence, sinus infections, and venereal disease. And the FDA could add to or subtract from it as the state of medical knowledge warranted.

Makers of proprietary drugs were also subject to general provisions of the bill. Their factories would be inspected by FDA agents. A permit system meant that their interstate shipments might be restrained; conflicts with the government could lead to widespread unfavorable publicity; and, should they be proved guilty of violating the law, proprietors would suffer penalties much stiffer than under Dr. Wiley's law. There was even a real threat of prison for the first offense.

Such, then, were the rigorous provisions of the Tugwell bill, no longer suspected items for fearful guessing, but now a matter of record for all to see. The target was in plain view, and firing began at once. It reached a peak at subcommittee hearings which Copeland held in December 1933.[15] The proprietary manufacturers, asserted the *New Republic* in that month, became "the first group of industrialists openly to declare war on the Roosevelt administration."[16]

There was no need for a new law, they insisted. The old one served the purpose of controlling quackery well enough. What troubles there were resulted from "misdirected inforcement." To destroy the Wiley act would produce widespread confusion, wiping out a quarter of a century of legal precedents and disrupting the harmony between federal law and state laws enacted in imitation of it. Granted a few rascally charlatans still operated. The way to attack them was not to enact such a drastic new "un-American" bill. "To catch a rat in the garret," need Professor Tugwell "burn down the entire house?" "If a criminal is believed to be in a house with 9 other men who may be innocent of any wrongdoing," do we "surround the house with police and shoot down every man in it to make sure that the criminal will not escape?" The Tugwell bill posed just such a grave threat. ". . . I have never in my life,"

[15] *Food, Drugs, and Cosmetics: Hearings before a Subcommittee of the Committee on Commerce, United States Senate, . . . on S. 1944* (73 Cong., 2 ses., 1933).
[16] 77 (1933), 119.

asserted the general counsel of the Proprietary Association at the hearings, "read a bill or heard of a bill so grotesque in its terms, evil in its purpose, and vicious in its possible consequences."[17]

The enactment of this "professor's bill"—the phrase evoked a laugh in the crowded hearing room—meant nothing less than the end of the "constitutional right" of self-medication, which, along with freedom of religion and the press, had been "jealously guarded" since the foundation of the republic. And this tolled the death knell of proprietary remedies. Tugwell had assumed "the ambitious job of Volsteadizing and Carrie Nationizing" the industry. As a result of his measure, the "heavy, cold clammy hand of bureaucracy" would fall upon it. The FDA would turn into a "powerful, sinister machine." Each decision would be "a ukase of a satrap." Drugstores would be "sovietized." Drug advertising would be wiped out in five years.[18]

Much of this fear of dictatorship arose from discretionary powers given in the bill to the Secretary of Agriculture. Particularly worrisome was the clause which let the Secretary make regulations to interpret the bill which, as far as facts were concerned, would have the force of law. Walter Campbell might explain over and again that such a grant of regulation-making authority to an administrative agency had many precedents and that the reasonableness by which such decisions were reached could be tested in the courts. This did not still the oft-repeated cry of imminent czarism. The timing of the bill had something to do with this. There were under consideration other New Deal agencies which caused indus-

[17] *Standard Remedies,* 20 (July 1933), 2; *Oil, Paint and Drug Reporter,* Oct. 9, 1933, FDA Scrapbook; United Medicine Manufacturers of America resolution, cited in *Drug Trade News,* Sep. 18, 1933, FDA Scrapbook; *Standard Remedies,* 20 (Nov. 1933), 5-6, 14; *Advertising & Selling,* 22 (Nov. 9, 1933), 13; H. B. Thompson of the Proprietary Association, Senate Subcommittee Hearings on S. 1944, 172.

[18] The "professor's bill" phrase was that of Dr. James H. Beal, speaking for the National Drug Trade Conference, *ibid.,* 98. *Drug Trade News,* Sep. 18, 1933, Jan. 22, 1934, FDA Scrapbook; *PI,* 164 (Aug. 3, 1933), 37; 165 (Nov. 2, 1933), 6; 166 (Mar. 15, 1934), 78; *Standard Remedies,* 20 (Nov. 1933), 5-6; *New Republic,* 76 (Nov. 8, 1933), 353-55; *Advertising & Selling,* 22 (Nov. 9, 1933), 48.

try to look toward regulatory bodies with suspicion, and, anyhow, for those who did not or would not get the point, the shout of dictatorship was an effective weapon.[19]

It was not only the regulation-making provisions that evoked this cry from the medicine men. Formula disclosure, now as four decades earlier, panicked them. This step, said one editor, was "unreasonable, unnecessary, useless, unjust, and unwise." It would open the door to "piracy," charged another critic, letting every unscrupulous corner pharmacist reproduce and sell any product he desired, to the ruination of the manufacturer. Thus the bill would make "Uncle Sam a thief."[20]

The licensing of laboratories, testified Dr. James H. Beal, spokesman for a coalition of drug groups fighting the bill, would be "a very great menace." Penalties provided in the measure, wrote a spokesman for a proprietary group, were "severe enough to even satisfy a lust for blood." The term "general medical opinion" was much too vague and held dire threats for proprietors. So too did those elastic words which outlawed advertising if it was "in any particular . . . untrue, or by ambiguity or inference create[d] a misleading impression." It mattered not that the drafters had adapted the phrase from a Supreme Court ruling. "There is hardly one piece of [medicine] copy in five," wrote a worried agency man, "at which a zealous snooper could not point the trembling finger of indignant scorn crying 'Ambiguous! Misleading by inference!' "[21]

The "palliative" provision was also dynamite. The "negative advertising" it would require seemed grossly unfair. Proprietary makers should not have to make public confessions from which physicians were protected. "Why not," inquired the attorney for the United Medicine Manufacturers, "require that a sign be put over all doctors' doors saying, 'I do not cure'?"[22]

For all these reasons, there was scarcely a medicine pro-

[19] Senate Subcommittee Hearings on S. 1944, 20-21; Lamb, 291-92.
[20] *Advertising & Selling*, 22 (Nov. 9, 1933), 48; Senate Subcommittee Hearings on S. 1944, 101, 132.
[21] *Ibid.*, 104, 405, 184-94; *Advertising & Selling*, 22 (Nov. 9, 1933), 52.
[22] *New Republic*, 76 (Nov. 8, 1933), 354; *Advertising & Selling*, 22 (Dec. 21, 1933), 32.

prietor throughout the land who did not join in the sentiment that Professor Tugwell's bill should be killed forthwith. Everything after the enactment clause, one witness told the Senate subcommittee, should be stricken out.[23]

The barrage of criticism did not cause the Food and Drug Administration to forsake the field. At the subcommittee hearings, in articles, over the radio, Chief Campbell and his aides insisted on the compelling need for new legislation, explained the provisions of the bill, refuted criticism. Particularly irritating was the proprietors' charge that home remedies would vanish because the bill would wipe out self-medication. If that had been the government's intent, Campbell told the Senators, it could have been achieved by "a single short section" explicitly saying so. What the bill did aim to do was "to make self-medication safe."[24]

To demonstrate that self-medication was not yet safe, Campbell showed the Senators a series of graphic posters, with bottles, labels, advertisements, death certificates attached. Each exhibit pointed up a hazard to life or limb which the FDA could prevent only with difficulty or not at all under existing law. One poster showed before-and-after photos of a comely Ohio woman whose eyeballs had been corroded to total blindness by an aniline eyelash dye. Another tied the horrible death of a Pittsburgh steel manufacturer directly to a proprietary radium water. Still others exposed quack devices, risky reducers, conflicts between controlled label and uncontrolled advertising claims. B. & M. was featured, with a stack of death notices testifying to the sad failure of a horse liniment to cure TB.[25]

The "Chamber of Horrors" was what one reporter dubbed it, and it proved one of the most effective pressures for reform. Like the "Poison Squad" of Wiley's day, this dramatic exhibit caught public attention. Mrs. Roosevelt came to see it in the

[23] Senate Subcommittee Hearings on S. 1944, 172.
[24] Campbell's testimony, *ibid.*, 43-60. John J. McCann of FDA had a private file of mimeographed texts of radio speeches given by FDA officials; Campbell explained the drug provisions in, among other places, *Oil, Paint and Drug Reporter*, Nov. 27, 1933, FDA Scrapbook, and Tugwell wrote not only for trade periodicals but for the *American Scholar*, 3 (Winter 1934), 85-95.
[25] Lamb reproduces a number of the posters.

Food and Drug Administration offices and wrote about it in her column. A set of posters was sent to Chicago for display at the Century of Progress Exposition. Other sets circulated around the country. Time and again Copeland was to wave one of these grim posters on the Senate floor.[26]

"Under present circumstances," Campbell testified before the Senate subcommittee, "a denizen of Central Africa, knowing nothing about administering to the sick, other than that imparted by the practices of a witch doctor, could land in this country, put up an article either of no more therapeutic value than a glass of water or as lethal as strychnine, sell it to the people of this country as a cure for every disease which man might have, and be within the terms of the law."[27]

But neither the Chamber of Horrors nor Campbell's earnest urging could secure enactment of the Tugwell bill. Drug interests and their allies in certain segments of the press, organized into "one of the noisiest and most determined lobbies of modern times," made their great weight felt. Opposition came also from the most responsible elements of the industries to be regulated. Spokesmen for advertising, publishing, fruit growing, food processing, cosmetic making, and pharmaceutical manufacturing appeared before Copeland's subcommittee to condemn the bill. Like the proprietors, each group had particular complaints. Canners, publishers, and advertisers, for example, objected to provisions that would require quality standards for foods and establish grade labeling. Anathema to almost all the industries concerned were the broad discretionary powers given to the Secretary of Agriculture. Copeland himself, when he got around to reading the bill, shared this feeling. Even Walter Campbell was willing to retreat.[28]

Copeland set to work at revising the bill in the light of what he had listened to in the hearings and what he kept

[26] Lamb, 116, 296, 298; Copeland in Senate, for example, on May 16, 1934, *Cong. Record*, 73 Cong., 2 ses., 8958.

[27] Senate Subcommittee Hearings on S. 1944, 44.

[28] Sternsher, 231; the Senate Subcommittee Hearings were a primary sounding board for this opposition. Copeland's opinion in *Cong. Record*, 73 Cong., 2 ses., 8957; Campbell's in *Foods, Drugs, and Cosmetics: Hearings before a Subcommittee of the Committee on Commerce, United States Senate, . . . on S. 5* (74 Cong., 1 ses., 1935), 358-59.

learning in almost daily conferences with representatives of the affected industries. Never before, he told his Senate colleagues, had he suffered "so many worries and so much trouble." At last he produced a version he believed "sane, sensible, workable," and on it the entire Committee on Commerce held new hearings in late February and March 1934. The revised draft, in Walter Campbell's judgment, was not as good as at first but nonetheless "desirable." His view and that of the makers of proprietaries were still far apart. Spokesmen for two of the three proprietary trade associations—the Proprietary Association and the United Medicine Manufacturers of America—had made their wishes frankly known at the hearings, as had several individual proprietors. The modifications in Copeland's draft, while embodying some of their suggestions, had not improved the bill at all, most of them felt. In some ways, indeed, the new version was even more threatening to them than the original Tugwell draft. "The forbidden list of diseases has jumped from 34 to 42 in a few weeks," noted the UMMA's counsel, "making it possible for one to forecast the life expectancy of self-medication under this proposed law with almost mathematical certainty." Proprietors still favored the 1906 act, modestly revised, or, if some more thorough measure should pass in time, they felt it ought to be one of their own devising. Their version, as Campbell saw it, would provide the industry "extraordinarily solicitous consideration" and would provide the public "very much less protection than it now has."[29]

If the medicine proprietors were not satisfied with Copeland's new draft, neither were the representatives of Consumers' Research. Kallet had considered even the first version of only half-hearted help to consumers and, at the hearings, had rebuked Copeland for giving health talks on a radio program sponsored by a yeast firm which used suspect testimonials

[29] Copeland in Senate, *Cong. Record,* 73 Cong., 2 ses., 1934, 2728-29; *Foods, Drugs, and Cosmetics: Hearings before the Committee on Commerce, United States Senate, . . . on S. 2800* (73 Cong., 2 ses., 1934), 58-62, 131-43, 199-208, 390-401, 468, 606. Campbell is cited at 606 and Clinton Robb, UMMA counsel, at 132. The proprietary interests favored the bill drafted by Dr. J. H. Beal and introduced by Representative Black of N.Y., Cavers, 10; *N.Y. Herald-Tribune,* Aug. 17, 1934; *Standard Remedies,* 21 (June 1934), 12-13.

from foreign physicians. In view of these circumstances, Kallet said, the hearings should be "reconvened under a new committee and an unquestionably impartial chairman." The committee's "procommercial bias," Kallet charged at the second hearing, had "emasculated" the original version. "The subsequent career of the bill," he added scornfully, "should be recorded in political textbooks as a case history of how legislation supposed to protect the public against the depredations of business is made." Consumers' Research forces, therefore, favored the bill's defeat as ardently as did the medicine makers and, like them, had a bill introduced into Congress embodying their own extreme views.[30]

Copeland brought a still further revised measure from the hearings to the Senate calendar. FDA men hoped that it would pass, and their moods alternated between optimism and gloom. "You have conducted a masterly retreat," wrote a law professor who had helped in the initial drafting process, "and have kept the principal vantage points." In mid-May, amid an atmosphere of tension, the bill got to the floor for an hour's debate. "Senators," Copeland warned his colleagues, "the wrath of thousands will come down upon the heads of those who willfully prevent the passage of the bill." But the measure was passed over and no more was heard of it before the session ended.[31]

Before the next Congress opened, proprietary spokesmen leveled angry charges at the FDA. The agency was "sulking." Irked at the "severe trimming" which their pet bill had received, a trade journal asserted, officials, "in a blind fury . . . immediately started to swing the club at the heads of those who were mainly responsible for thwarting their plans."[32] Larger appropriations and a favorable political climate were permitting more rigorous enforcement than in the twenties, and proprietors were far from pleased.

[30] Senate Subcommittee Hearings on S. 1944, 355-56; Senate Committee Hearings on S. 2800, 276-314.
[31] *Cong. Record* (73 Cong., 2 ses.), 4567-73, 8955-67, quotation at 8967; Cavers to Crawford, Mar. 24, 1934, "Legislation, 1927-40 Bills," FDA Records, RG 88, NA; Crawford to Cavers, May 18, 1934, "Correspondence on Legislation."
[32] *Drug and Cosmetic Industry*, Sep. 1934, FDA Scrapbook.

At the beginning of the 74th Congress, in January 1935, Copeland reintroduced his bill. Now it bore marks of further change as a result of the Senator's continuing conferences with interested parties. The medicine makers had won some concessions on label claims—the bill gave "too big a present to the pain-killers," one FDA friend felt—but the changes were not sufficient to woo them from a bill of their own. Should the proprietary-sponsored measure pass, observed another FDA ally, "only a kind providence" could "protect the consumer." Such a contingency, however, seemed hardly likely, and, indeed, Copeland maneuvered so adroitly that his "hybrid mixture" that came back to the Senate in March after new subcommittee hearings still impressed an FDA spokesman as "a splendid bill." At this juncture Franklin Roosevelt sent his first words to Congress on the theme. They were by no means a command. The President expressed his "hope" that legislation might be enacted to protect the "honest enterpriser" against "evaders and chiselers" and to "provide a bulwark of consumer confidence throughout the business world."[33]

The debate on Copeland's measure was extensive and acrimonious. While the makers of proprietary medicines flooded the Senate with telegrams and letters, vigorous efforts were made on the floor to amend the bill in those respects most desired by the proprietors. The "heart of the opposition," as Copeland termed it, lay in two attempts, one, to substitute the Federal Trade Commission for the Food and Drug Administration as the agency that would supervise food, drug, and cosmetic advertising; the other, to reduce the multiple seizure authority of the FDA not only below the level of Copeland's bill, but even below that of the 1906 law.[34]

For over 20 years, the FTC had maintained some control

[33] Text of bill, S. 5, a number it was to bear until its final passage in 1938, in *Cong. Record* (74 Cong., 1 ses.), at 100; Cavers to Crawford, Jan. 8, 1935, Milton Handler to Crawford, Feb. 25, 1935, and Crawford to Cavers, Mar. 16, 1935, "Correspondence on Legislation"; *Christian Science Monitor*, Mar. 5, 1935, FDA Scrapbook; FDR's message, *Cong. Record*, 4262. From this point on, Copeland had the constant help of his technical adviser, Ole Salthe, who had served as director of food and drug work while Copeland was health commissioner of New York City.

[34] The Senate debate continued for a week in early April and then

over false advertising, and Commissioner Ewin L. Davis had come before two of the committee hearings to state firmly that the Commission did not want to relinquish its monopoly. In Davis' desire, all proprietary groups staunchly concurred. Copeland was not persuaded. The deplorable condition of nostrum advertising, he told his Senate colleagues, was a sound argument for giving authority to the FDA. Since the FTC had performed inadequately, since the Raladam decision had limited its purview to cases involving injury to competitors, and since FTC procedures were slow and penalties weak, the FDA should take on the job. Food, drug, and cosmetic advertising was, after all, an inevitable extension of labeling, and the FDA, unlike the FTC, had the scientific staff to arrive at all the necessary decisions.[35]

A test on the FTC issue did not arise at once. Senator Bennett Champ Clark, who came from the state in which Listerine was made, talked of offering an amendment, but did not do so. Regarding multiple seizures the problem was immediate. Senator Josiah W. Bailey presented, and the Senate accepted, amendments that left proprietary drugs virtually immune to the most effective weapon FDA had possessed for clearing the market quickly of threatening nostrums. A critic had once called the seizure action of no value, like the arrest of a murderer's revolver after it had killed its victim. On the contrary, the FDA held, seizure was comparable to arresting the murderer's bullet in flight before it reached its intended victim.[36]

Throughout the twenties, the Proprietary Association had offered unceasing objections, and to eliminate or circumscribe multiple seizures had been one of its main goals. To accomplish this aim had been an expressed purpose of all proprie-

---

again in late May. *Cong. Record* (74 Cong., 1 ses.), 4734-38, 4748-50, 4840-51, 4858-69, 4900, 4905-20, 4982, 4989, 5018-25, 5093, 5099, 5137-40, 5215-34, 7963, 8162-63, 8341, 8350-56. Copeland refers to "the heart of the opposition" at 5022. *Wash. Daily News,* Apr. 2, 1935, FDA Scrapbook.

[35] Senate Committee Hearings on S. 2800, 231-40; Senate Subcommittee Hearings on S. 5, 109-15, for Davis' appearances. One expression of Copeland's view of this is in *Cong. Record* (74 Cong., 1 ses.), 5023.
[36] *1935 Report of the Food and Drug Administration*, 16.

tary groups at hearings on the various versions of the Copeland bill.[37] Now during debate concerted pressure was brought. Copeland was convinced that a plot existed to destroy or emasculate his bill.

"There is, in effect," the Senator said, "a conspiracy on the part of these patent-medicine men—and some of them are sitting in the gallery right now as I speak—seeking to defeat the bill. Then there are certain newspaper interests who are so afraid that they will not be permitted any more to run the vile advertising which I have exhibited, who are so afraid that their dividends will be affected by this attack upon their revenues that they are here in force, and possibly, though I pray not, they may have influence enough to beat the bill."[38]

Copeland poured out his bitterness and scorn on "the patent-medicine advertiser and manufacturer, the vilest man on the face of the earth," as he sought in vain to prevent the weakening of the multiple seizure authority. And when he failed—the vote on the Bailey amendment was 44 to 29—Copeland said that, as far as he was concerned, the bill was dead. But Copeland rallied from his despair, conferred with Bailey and Clark, got the best compromise he could, and on May 28 saw his much-patched measure pass the Senate.[39]

The pure food and drug bill was by now so transformed from the draft that first had borne his name that Tugwell, now Under Secretary of Agriculture, could scarcely recognize it. Consumers' groups were angry at Copeland's yielding. "Ironically," a Consumers' Research spokesman said, the Senate bill was "a more adulterated and misbranded product than anything marketed" by the industries which were supposed to be controlled. By passing the bill, charged Kallet, the Senate had "made itself, knowingly or not, an accessory to thievery and murder." Representatives of the women's organizations which had banded together to press for an adequate law did not use such strong language, but they were disap-

[37] *Standard Remedies*, 10 (June 1924), 12; 12 (June 1926), 21; 14 (May 1927), 22; Cavers, 13-15; Senate Committee Hearings on S. 2800, 206, 390, 468.

[38] *Cong. Record* (74 Cong., 1 ses.), 5025.

[39] *Ibid.*, 5023, 5231, 8350-56; *N.Y. Jnl. of Commerce*, Apr. 10, 1935, FDA Scrapbook.

pointed. Opponents of the original bill, said the spokesman for the American Association of University Women, had "drawn the teeth they feared," and she summed up the details of the weakening process:[40]

"The list of incurable diseases for which so-called 'cures' can not be sold has been cut from forty-two to nine.

"The restriction against advertising a mere palliative as a cure has been removed.

"Standards of strength for germicides and antiseptics have been eliminated. . . .

"There are no minimum fines; fines have been reduced.

"Protection against cumulative poisons, stimulant-depressants and sedatives has been removed. . . .

"Weakening administrative changes have been made.

"There is the shocking restriction of multiple seizures to those products only that are 'imminently dangerous to health.' "

Trade circles were saying the Senate bill was not unlike the draft which had been sponsored by the Proprietary Association. Indeed, the key weakening amendments had been transferred into Copeland's document from that draft. So it was not surprising that the Proprietary Association's general counsel should term Copeland's measure "fair and reasonable" and urge its prompt passage by the House.[41]

Within the Food and Drug Administration it was hard to get "enthusiastic" about the bill. Nonetheless, Campbell and his aides would not protest the erosion process too strenuously —if only the House could somehow soften the impact of the Bailey amendment circumscribing multiple seizures. Gross deception, Campbell suggested, as well as imminent danger, should be actionable.[42]

[40] *Christian Science Monitor*, May 29, 1935, FDA Scrapbook; House Subcommittee Hearings on S. 5, 505, 523, 386.

[41] *PI*, 171 (June 13, 1935), 71; Ruth Lamb to Mrs. Helen Woodward, Jan. 31, 1938, FDA Decimal file .062, F&D Act Gen May-June 20, 1938, Federal Records Center, Alexandria; *N.Y. Jnl. of Commerce*, June 7, 1935, FDA Scrapbook. The Institute of Medicine Manufacturers, another proprietary trade association, was still not happy.

[42] Crawford to Cavers, May 29, 1935, and Crawford to William Cantrell, Aug. 26, 1935, "Correspondence on Legislation"; Campbell before House Subcommittee Hearings on S. 5, 86, 98.

During the summer a House subcommittee held lengthy hearings. Virgil E. Chapman, a Kentuckian, was chairman, and he set about the task with the President's wishes for good speed. The same old ground as in the Senate hearings was retrod, but with a different step. Copeland had debated points with witnesses from industry, but not sharply, nor had he sought to inquire into their backgrounds. Chapman equipped himself ahead of time with information on those who came to testify and on the products they represented. Suavely and cleverly, he used these facts as the basis for penetrating probing.[43]

Lydia Pinkham's daughter and granddaughter were in the hearing room while Chapman posed for the company's attorney embarrassing questions the latter seemed not prepared to answer. Reading a purported formula for the Vegetable Compound, the Congressman asked the lawyer if it was a "fair analysis."[44]

"I do not know, sir. I cannot answer your question."

"Does the alcohol in it have any effect?"

"Well, I think so, of course, Mr. Chairman. I think alcohol —I believe in the use of small doses of alcohol."

What, Chapman queried, was the medicine good for?

"It is a beneficent product, sir, for women and women's trouble. Beyond that, I do not know. I never took it."

Chapman inserted into the record a pink slip signed by the Pinkham Company suggesting that the Compound might be very hard to buy if a new food and drug bill was passed, and urging that a letter be mailed immediately to the reader's Congressman opposing the measure. "We are trying," the pink slip read, "to stop this bill from becoming law." Was the Pinkham Company, Chapman asked, "responsible for that propaganda?"

"Mr. Chairman," the attorney replied, "it is the first time I have ever seen or heard of the pink slip."

Chapman read also two versions of multigraphed letters which the pink slip would aim toward Washington. "The

[43] *Ibid., passim.*
[44] Lamb, 298; House Subcommittee Hearings on S. 5, 240-50. The Pinkham attorney was Hugh H. Obear.

women of America will show you," one of them stated, "that you cannot deprive them of Lydia E. Pinkham's Vegetable Compound without hearing from us at election time." The letter also disparaged competing remedies made by other members of the Proprietary Association.

Chapman also brought out in questioning one of Senator Bailey's constituents, Smith Richardson, head of the company that made Vick's Vaporub, that Richardson had modified his labeling under Food and Drug Administration pressure rather than risk multiple seizures for implying, during an epidemic, that his ointment might prevent pneumonia and the flu. Richardson had just told the House subcommittee that his company had sent a letter to 2,100 newspapers favoring the Copeland bill "providing there be no tampering with the Bailey amendment."[45]

An evasive but most revealing witness, under the Kentucky Congressman's dogged questioning, was William P. Jacobs, who, it turned out, wore at least five proprietary hats. He made a medicine. He ran an advertising agency. He operated Jacobs' Religious List, responsible for placing advertising in a long string of church papers published throughout the South. He served as publicity chairman for the United Medicine Manufacturers of America. And he was executive vice-president of the Institute of Medicine Manufacturers.[46]

Jacobs was slow to admit that there was personal advantage in these multiple connections, although he did agree, under Chapman's prodding, that he had solicited UMMA members for advertising placed in the religious press. Likewise, Jacobs denied threatening the press with loss of advertising should a new food and drug bill pass, although he did confess to writing letters to newspapers and radio stations describing the kind of law he favored.

"You held out to them," said Chapman, "that there was a 'Sword of Damocles' hanging over their heads in the form of this bill pending in Congress, and if this bill became a law the 'Fasteeth' and 'Lydia E. Pinkham's Vegetable Compound' with

[45] Ibid., 341-56.
[46] Ibid., 189-92, 660-94. One of Jacobs' five hats, his UMMA publicity chairmanship, was not mentioned at the hearings. Lamb, 304.

18 percent alcohol would not advertise with them any more. Is that correct?"

"I was not quite that fluent, Mr. Chairman," Jacobs replied.

Nor would Jacobs admit to knowing that medicines advertised in his religious papers had been in serious trouble with the Food and Drug Administration for claiming efficacy in treating such things as snakebite, ulcers, and cancer.

"Don't you think," Chapman asked, "that before you insert advertisements in these religious journals, along in the same columns or parallel columns with hymns and prayers, and lessons from the Bible for the children, you ought to know what is in these products . . . ?"

"If that rule, Mr. Chairman, were applied to all newspapers and advertising," Jacobs answered, "there would be no advertising."

Such unawareness seemed difficult for Chapman to grasp.

"You know," he stated, "that many a person, when he picks up that church paper, believes it is second only to the Bible, and believes everything in it even down to the advertisements of Calotabs and 666."

But Jacobs would not confront this paradox.

"You are a good salesman . . . ," he told Chapman in reply, "I wish we had one as good as you are."

What Congressman Chapman found out by his keen questioning made him an enthusiastic convert to the cause of a strong law. When he became aware that the major proprietors were all for speeding the Senate bill through the House, Chapman withstood the pressure. Rumor had it that an effort was made but failed to get enough Congressional signatures to discharge the committee and bring the bill to the floor. Chapman opposed haste. More education was needed, he believed, both among House members and among the broader public. Peeved that the press had paid so little attention to his lively hearings, the Kentucky Congressman looked into the possibility of using motion pictures and the radio.[47]

The FDA, hopeful that a more rigorous bill than Copeland's might emerge because of Chapman's enthusiasm, itself

[47] Cavers, 16-17; Crawford to Cavers, Aug. 30, 1935, "Correspondence on Legislation."

sought to quicken public interest. Ruth deForest Lamb, who handled public relations for the agency, published a book. Dedicated to the women's organizations which had provided the FDA unflagging support, *American Chamber of Horrors* summed up the case for a strong new law. It described once more, with poignant case histories, the evils which could not be touched and sorrowfully narrated the way in which a good bill had been pummeled into an indifferent one by the relentless blows of its enemies. Miss Lamb's conclusion was not defeatist: there were both optimism and exhortation in the title of her concluding chapter, "There's Going to Be a Law!" Proprietors who had reached the point of espousing almost the same bill as the FDA were shocked at Miss Lamb's lion-like attack. "All of which clearly indicates," asserted a trade paper, "that the Administration does not give a damn for the industry or its cooperation." If the FDA was renewing its efforts for a measure stronger than the bill that had passed the Senate, elements of the drug and cosmetic industry were drumming up new antagonism to a measure even as restrictive as that.[48]

Chapman's campaign of education among his fellow Congressmen was only partially successful. Nine months after the hearings a substitute food and drug bill was brought into the House. It contained some restoration of the multiple seizure powers which had been weakened by the Bailey amendment in the Senate bill. But it gave sole control of food, drug, and cosmetic advertising to the Federal Trade Commission. Such a disposition was in accord with the desires of proprietary groups, but this was not the compelling reason for the change. Several members on the House committee in charge of the bill were antagonistic to the Food and Drug Administration for actions it had taken against powerful fruit-growing interests in their districts. Tugwell especially was blamed for what apple growers considered an arbitrary and needless order sharply reducing the amount of spray residue permissible on apples going to market. Even more important, FTC chairman Ewin Davis was a former member of the House and made the most of this old school tie in his very effective testimony before the House subcommittee. Chapman had fought the move to de-

[48] *Drug and Cosmetic Industry,* Mar. 1936, FDA Scrapbook; Lamb, 323.

prive the FDA of advertising control in committee and argued against it in "Additional Remarks" appended to the House Report. His effort, however, was in vain. The committee majority went all the way with the FTC.[49]

President Roosevelt notified the Speaker that he wanted action before the waning session ended. The rules were suspended and, after only 40 minutes of debate, the bill was passed. To ensure this result, House leaders had pledged themselves not to yield on the FTC issue in conference with the Senate. And, though other issues were reconciled between the two conflicting versions, the House conferees stood firm on this, even when Copeland said he would rather see the bill die than agree to this change. Finally Copeland phoned the White House. One of the President's secretaries reported that Roosevelt preferred to have the FDA in charge of advertising, but he would not veto the bill solely because control was given to the FTC. A last-minute compromise was tried: the FDA would be given jurisdiction over advertising relating to health, the FTC over advertising relating to economic cheats. This effort failed when two House conferees objected. Senator Copeland and Representative Sam Rayburn agreed that the conference report of disagreement should stand, but Copeland should present the bill to the Senate including the health-economics proviso. This he did, and the Senate accepted it and sent the amended version to the House.[50]

As the last minutes of the session ticked away, the food and drug issue was stated from two opposing views. As Chapman

[49] Text of the House bill and accompanying majority and minority reports (No. 2755), *Cong. Record* (74 Cong., 2 ses.), 10,237-40, 10,235-36, 10,242. Davis' testimony, House Subcommittee Hearings on S. 5, 631-49; suspicion of Tugwell because of his lead-residue-tolerance decision reflected in *Cong. Record* (75 Cong., 3 ses.), 10,240, 10,243-44.

[50] Crawford to Cavers, June 25, 1936, "Correspondence on Legislation." Earlier in the session Roosevelt had sought to get the House to act. Roosevelt to Sam Rayburn, undated memorandum in the President's hand, Official File 375, Franklin D. Roosevelt Library, states, "Food & Drug Bill. Why not report it out & get it passed." Typed on this memo is a note, Feb. 7, 1936, indicating that Marvin McIntyre, the President's secretary, had learned by phone from Rayburn that he had already begun on the task and would get the bill acted on as soon as possible. The House debate is reported, *Cong. Record* (74 Cong., 2 ses.), 10,235-37, 10,240-44; the Senate action, *ibid.*, 10,514-20.

saw it, the question was: "Will we stubbornly resist this reasonable compromise and thereby deny the consuming millions of American people the protection to which they are entitled?" But Representative Carroll Reece, who, like Commissioner Davis, came from Tennessee, phrased the matter differently: "If you want to place the advertising under Dr. Tugwell and give him a whip lash not only over business, but over the press of this country, vote for the motion made, but if you want to give it to the Federal Trade Commission, a quasi-judicial body, vote against it." "The printed Record," an observer wrote, "can give you no idea of the boos and catcalls that greeted the mention of Dr. Tugwell's name or the cheers for Ewin Davis."[51]

Rayburn fought the trend. "There might be a little lobbying around here by some people," he told the House, "but there is nobody who has lobbied around this Capitol on any bill in the 23 years I have been in Congress more than the members of the Federal Trade Commission have lobbied on this bill. . . ." When the vote was taken, the score stood: Tugwell and the FDA, 70; Davis and the FTC, 190. So the bill died.[52]

"Peculiarly enough," wrote Charles Crawford, "the worst enemies of the legislation originally, the patent medicine group, are in no wise responsible for the defeat of the measure." The bill had reached a form which the large proprietors were willing to accept. Also, as prior to 1906, the protracted agitation over a national bill had spurred states to action. New laws much more rigorous than old ones were passing state legislatures, and from state to state their terms were different. Proprietors were becoming almost eager to assume greater obligations under a new national law, since it would tend to bring harmony among state practices.[53]

Some advocates of reform were rather more pleased than grieved that this particular version of the battered food and drug bill had gone down to defeat. Copeland's "willing hand,"

[51] *Ibid.*, 10,677; Ruth Lamb to Mrs. Helen Woodward, Jan. 31, 1938, FDA Decimal file .062, F&D Act Gen May-June 20, 1938, Federal Records Center, Alexandria.

[52] *Cong. Record* (74 Cong., 2 ses.), 10,679-80.

[53] Crawford to Cavers, June 25, 1936, "Correspondence on Legislation"; *Drug and Cosmetic Industry*, July 1936, *Drug Trade News*, Mar. 1, 1937, and *Ntl. League of Women Voters News Letter*, July 23, 1937, FDA Scrapbook.

asserted a consumer's periodical, had been guided by the lobbies to create a "legislative monstrosity." This very same word
expressed the view of the American Medical Association. The
AMA had played a less active role in working for a new law
than prior to 1906. Almost as critical as industry of the Secretary of Agriculture's potential "dictatorship" under the Tugwell bill, the AMA appreciated later modifications of the administrative provisions at the same time that they deplored the
simultaneous weakening of controls over drugs. The AMA's
legislative counsel, Dr. William C. Woodward, had appeared
at every hearing to present the doctors' point of view. Both in
his corporate and in his personal capacity, he was a firm foe
of quackery: as health commissioner of Boston he had once
launched an attack on B. & M. By the time of the House hearings, Woodward objected to the way in which drug controls
had been "whittled away and undermined." This same note
was sounded in a *Journal* editorial in May 1936. "The first
bill introduced," the editorialist wrote, "has been subjected to
a sort of plastic surgery in the legislative operating rooms
which has resulted in a specimen not even resembling the
original model and utterly deficient in many particulars. Altogether the result is an asthenic, chinless and impotent monstrosity."[54]

Not until 1938 did the House of Representatives again
bring to vote a comprehensive food and drug bill. In the
meantime, however, they settled the imbroglio over advertising. The House vote had made clear the sentiments of that
body, and a bill was prepared bolstering the scope of Federal
Trade Commission control over food, drug, and cosmetic
advertising. Chapman and Copeland, in their respective
Houses, fought the bill but, realizing that it had the votes to
pass, sought to equip it with stronger sanctions to deter would-
be violators. As the bill stood, only advertisers who could be
proved guilty of fraud or who vended commodities inherently

[54] *Consumers Union Reports*, June 19, 1936, FDA Scrapbook. Dr.
Woodward's testimony appears in Senate Subcommittee Hearings on
S. 1944, 46-67 (a written statement); Senate Committee Hearings on
S. 2800, 349-89; Senate Subcommittee Hearings on S. 5, 153-69; House
Subcommittee Hearings on S. 5, 298-321. *JAMA*, 106 (1936), 1902;
109 (1937), 74B.

dangerous need fear more than an order telling them to cease and desist their false advertising. But the attempt to add fines failed, largely because the FTC did not want them. The amendment to put more teeth into the bill, said Representative Lea, after talking with an FTC representative, "would, in effect, convert the Federal Trade Act . . . into a criminal statute primarily as to advertisements. . . . This is not the practical way to deal with business men."[55]

Thus the FTC won its jurisdictional contest with the FDA, securing in the Wheeler-Lea Act the kind of advertising control measure its members desired. The Secretary of Agriculture urged the President to veto the bill, but he did not.[56]

With the controversial advertising issue settled, one major deterrent to revision of the 1906 law was gone. A second obstacle, the presence of Tugwell in the Department of Agriculture, disappeared when the Under Secretary quit the government to become vice-president of a molasses company.[57] A third handicap was also reduced. Public interest, despite the Chamber of Horrors and the activities of women's groups, had remained tepid. Now it came to a quick boil.

Headlines the country over broke the news of a mounting death toll from "Elixir Sulfanilamide." The report was especially disturbing since sulfanilamide had been widely heralded in the press as a miracle medicine, a chemotherapeutical breakthrough. In this case, nothing was wrong with the sulfa, but in another respect a terrible mistake had been made. The chief chemist at a small pharmaceutical plant in Bristol, Tennessee, seeking for a liquid dosage form, had hit upon the solvent diethylene glycol. Unaware of reports describing the compound's toxicity, the chemist had tested his new concoction for appearance, fragrance, and flavor—but not for safety.

[55] Cavers, 18-19; Charles Wesley Dunn, in *Wheeler-Lea Act: A Statement of Its Legislative Record* (N.Y., 1938), reprinted all pertinent material from the *Congressional Record*. Congressman Lea's statement appears in House Report No. 1744 (75 Cong., 3 ses.), 406.

[56] Henry A. Wallace to D. W. Bell, Acting Director, Bureau of the Budget, Mar. 17 and Mar. 19, 1938 (carbons), FDA Decimal file .062, F&D Act Gen May-June 20, 1938, Federal Record Center, Alexandria. A draft of a proposed veto message was enclosed which, it appears, was prepared by Crawford.

[57] Sternsher, 322.

Production began both in Bristol and in the firm's Kansas City plant. Nearly 2,000 pints of the viscous pink liquid were made, and on not one label was the solvent named.[58]

Nearly two months later, the FDA heard a rumor that deaths were occurring in Oklahoma from some sulfa compound. Investigation quickly revealed the terrible truth. Only a technicality made the drug misbranded and let the FDA take action: all elixirs, according to the *Pharmacopeia*, must contain alcohol, and this "Elixir" did not. The agency threw its entire staff into the task of tracking down and seizing the poisonous medicine. Most of the 93 pints which had reached patients had been prescribed by doctors. Some, however, had been sold over the counter by druggists to customers whom they did not know, largely because of publicity praising sulfanilamide's effectiveness in treating gonorrhea. Displaying great patience and ingenuity, Food and Drug inspectors, aided by state and local authorities, managed to account for 99.2 per cent of all "Elixir Sulfanilamide" produced. In South Carolina, one bottle, not yet empty, was found on the very grave of an "Elixir" victim, tossed there by the bereaved in accordance with an ancient local rite.

Death from diethylene glycol is protracted and it is painful. The "Elixir," according to FDA calculations, brought death to at least 107 persons, many of them children. One of the most poignant documents in the whole record of food and drug legislation is a letter written to Franklin Roosevelt by the mother of one of the victims. She told how her child, a little girl of six, had died in agony, and begged the President to get a law so that other families would not have to suffer as hers had done. With the letter she sent a picture of her daughter's smiling face.

The chemist who concocted the "Elixir" took his own life. The doctor who owned the company—during the unfolding

[58] *Report of the Secretary of Agriculture on Deaths Due to Elixir Sulfanilamide-Massengill* (Sen. Document No. 124, 75 Cong., 2 ses.); *1938 Report of the Food and Drug Administration*, 13; *1939 Report*, 23-24; FDA Notices of Judgment 28324, 29751, 29752, and 30776; James Harvey Young, "The 'Elixir Sulfanilamide' Disaster," *Emory University Qtly.*, 14 (1958), 230-37; the chemist's suicide is reported in Kenneth G. Crawford, *The Pressure Boys* (N.Y., 1939), 73.

tragedy he had told the press, "I do not feel that there was any responsibility on our part"—paid a fine of $26,100, the highest ever levied under the 1906 law. The public, shocked into a new awareness that the law had loopholes, urged Congress to remedy the fault.

But there still were problems. A rift had developed between Copeland and the President. Differing with Roosevelt on many policies, Copeland had refused to attend the 1936 Democratic convention and had spent much of the campaign touring the Holy Land. Later he fought FDR's plans for expanding the Supreme Court. The President came to hope that someone other than Copeland might lead the Congressional effort in behalf of food and drug reform. Responding to one of Dr. Harvey Cushing's several letters urging Roosevelt's support for a vigorous law, the President replied in December 1936: "My difficulty is a political one. I hope to have someone other than your medical colleague, Dr. Copeland, handle it at the coming session. Enough said!"[59]

Tugwell, in first broaching the subject of a new law to Franklin Roosevelt, had reminded the President that the first law had been enacted during Theodore Roosevelt's administration, and the second Roosevelt had not been indifferent to the continuing attempt to secure revision. Except for his one message to Congress, however, his own efforts to help the cause occurred behind the scenes. Initial opposition from many industrial groups and powerful segments of the press was so heated that the President, for political reasons, let Tugwell shield him and bear the brunt of the bitter attack. Within the government, too, the marked differences in judgment about how far the new law should go forced upon the President the role of reconciler. At one point fairly early in the game, Roosevelt's private secretary noted in a memorandum, "President suggests having Rex Tugwell and Copeland together to fight it out. The President will sit in and hold the sponge." Later, when the FDA–FTC dispute over control of advertising became a troublesome problem, Roosevelt called in Tugwell and Davis

[59] *Wash. Daily News*, Jan. 4, 1937, and *Wash. Star* [Feb. 24, 1937], FDA Scrapbooks; *N.Y. Times,* Feb. 24, 1937; Roosevelt to Cushing, Dec. 28, 1936, President's Personal File, Roosevelt Library.

for a joint—and futile—conference. From time to time, the President brought pressure to speed Congressional action or to influence its direction. When, in a personal letter or phone call, he expressed a personal opinion, his weight was thrown toward strengthening rather than weakening the draft being considered at the time. He urged Senator Bailey, for example, not to destroy the FDA's multiple seizure authority, the President's letter, indeed, being a verbatim copy of a draft prepared for him by Tugwell. But the food and drug bill never received from Roosevelt the staunch support he gave to other measures. His difficulties with Copeland obviously made it harder for the President to make effective what interest he had. Things reached the point where reporters joked Roosevelt about his ignorance concerning the legislative status of the Senator's bill.[60]

Another obstacle had developed by 1937. A new provision had appeared in the House committee draft which came close to reducing food and drug controls to an absurdity. It was the work mainly of the apple growers, still fearful that the FDA would be too stringent in policing insecticide spray residues. The clause would set up such an endless chain in the appealing of FDA regulations to the district courts that the agency would be reduced to impotence. The Secretary of Agriculture informed the House of "the department's considered judgment that it would be better to continue the old law in effect than to enact [the new bill] with this provision." The Attorney General concurred, and a minority of the House committee felt the same. But in June 1938 the House of Representatives passed the measure with the offending clause remaining.[61]

[60] Sternsher, 225, 230; M. A. LeHand to Marvin McIntyre, Feb. 28, 1934, O.F. 375, Roosevelt Library; Roosevelt to McIntyre, Feb. 9, 1935, ibid.—Roosevelt's appointment book shows that the Tugwell-Davis conference took place on Feb. 14; Tugwell to Roosevelt [Apr. 1935], ibid.; Roosevelt to Bailey, Apr. 26, 1935, ibid.; Press conference, March 10, 1936, Press Conferences, vol. 7, p. 185, Roosevelt Library.

[61] The majority and minority views are given in Food, Drug, and Cosmetic Act, House Report No. 2139 (75 Cong., 3 ses.), the minority report citing the Secretary of Agriculture. The Attorney General is cited, Cong. Record (75 Cong., 3 ses.), 7892. Debate and passage are given, ibid., 7773-99, 7889-7903.

Once again, as two years before, Senate and House conferees met to try to reconcile their differences. "Frankly," wrote Charles Crawford, "I do not feel very optimistic because it looks like the worse rather than the better provisions of the two bills are to be combined in the Conference Committee." But the debacle of 1936 was not repeated, and Crawford's gloomy presentiments were not fulfilled. To the committee Copeland took his associate and former food and drug aide, Ole Salthe, who had sought advice from FDA officials as to which of the differing provisions might be best calculated to serve the consuming public. Regarding some matters, Salthe was provided with written compromise provisions that would make the measure, as Campbell and Crawford saw it, a better bill. In the committee it soon became apparent that the conferees were willing in general to accept Copeland's judgment as to which provisions to adopt. When disputes arose, the Senator called upon Salthe to present and explain the way he would resolve the matter. As a result, the list of suggestions Salthe took with him were accepted almost without exception. The judicial review provision was modified to make it much less objectionable. The multiple seizure authority was somewhat restored. "Had the Committee adopted the alternatives to the provisions Salthe proposed," Crawford later wrote, "the resulting bill would have been worthy only of veto."[62]

As it was, the Senate quickly approved the conference report, and the House, after hearing another round of objections from the apple growers, also voted for the bill. On June 25, 1938, President Roosevelt added his signature. At long, weary last, the fight was over. The Food, Drug, and Cosmetic Act was one of the last major domestic measures enacted during the New Deal.[63]

Tugwell the terrifying was gone from government. He viewed the final bill as "a subverted thing," the result of "a cause . . . betrayed." Copeland the compromiser was also gone. Driving himself too hard, he had collapsed on the Senate

[62] Crawford to Milton Handler [June 1938], FDA Decimal file .062, F&D Act Gen June-July, Federal Records Center, Alexandria; Crawford on Salthe, *F&D Rev.*, 36 (Oct. 1952), 201.
[63] *Cong. Record* (75 Cong., 3 ses.), 8731-38, 9087-9101, 9616.

floor and died on the last night of the session, never knowing whether or not the President with whom he had squabbled would sign the measure that had been his main preoccupation during his last five years. Walter Campbell, Chief of the Food and Drug Administration, was still around. He had done his best, initially and through all succeeding stages, to secure as strong a measure as practical politics would permit. Two months before the bill was passed, writing to a man who had fought hard for legislation before 1906, Campbell said, "I believe that if Doctor Wiley and you, prior to the passage of the present [1906] act, had taken the position that only a perfect bill would be accepted, we might not even now have as good a law as we do have." Now he was not jubilant, but neither was he so despairing as his former ally and superior. "Five years of legislative consideration," he wrote in his 1938 report, "have produced a measure that will unquestionably afford greatly increased public protection even if it does not contain all of the provisions its advocates have urged."[64]

Misbranding provisions relating to proprietary medicines were markedly stronger than in Dr. Wiley's now superseded law. Many Tugwell bill clauses, indeed, had survived in the 1938 law with only moderate change. Any false and misleading statement in the labeling of a remedy was now banned; no longer need the government prove fraudulent intent with respect to therapeutic claims. False labeling included not only erroneous positive statements but also the failure to reveal germane facts, especially the omission of warnings in circumstances when medication might be hazardous. Drugs dangerous to health when used according to directions were outlawed. A significant step was taken in the direction of formula disclosure for non-official drugs. The common names of all active ingredients were required upon the label. In addition, for a list of potent drugs and habit-forming narcotic and hypnotic substances, quantity and proportion had to be given. Antiseptics must be germicidal. And new drugs—like Elixir

[64] Tugwell, *The Democratic Roosevelt*, 466; *Wash. Post*, June 18, 1938, FDA Scrapbook; Campbell to Robert M. Allen, Apr. 30, 1938, FDA Decimal file .062, F&D Act A (May-Dec.) 1938, Federal Records Center, Alexandria; *1938 Report of Food and Drug Administration*, 1.

Sulfanilamide—must not be marketed until their manufacturers had persuaded Food and Drug officials that the drugs were safe.[65]

The law took account of medical devices. It covered articles aimed at affecting the body's structure or function. It also sought to secure honest labeling on medicines shipped by "doctors" who diagnosed by mail.

The FDA got one new weapon, the injunction, to add to its seizures and criminal actions. Penalties were also stiffened and were made heavier for second offenses and for fraud. Even a first offense might now bring up to a year in prison.

Campbell and his associates set right to work at regulation-making and at enforcing those parts of the law that became immediately effective. To eliminate one of the grimmest exhibits in the Chamber of Horrors, the FDA made its first seizure under the new law. The product was an aniline eyelash "beautifier" of the type that had corroded the eyeballs of the woman from Ohio.[66]

[65] 52 Stat. 1040. Dunn reprints the law, 1-22.
[66] *Detroit Free Press*, July 23, 1938, FDA Scrapbook.

# 9

## IN PURSUIT OF
## THE DIMINISHING PROMISE

*"The purpose of the law is to protect the public, the
vast multitude which includes the ignorant, the unthinking, and the credulous who, when making a purchase, do not stop to analyze."*
—UNITED STATES V. 62 PACKAGES, MORE OR LESS, OF
MARMOLA PRESCRIPTION TABLETS, 1943[1]

WITH their new law as weapon, Food and Drug officials
launched a relentless campaign to make self-medication safe.
It was a sort of cat and mouse game played at tortoise speed.
Full-scale enforcement efforts could not begin at once, for
only part of the law became effective immediately, and Congress had adjourned without appropriating funds to help an
agency, already understaffed, in assuming its new tasks.[2]
When all provisions of the law did go into effect, on the first
day of 1940, less than two years remained before the nation
was plunged into a massive war, a war which forced the Food
and Drug Administration to assume emergency responsibilities and at the same time curtailed its staff and offered quacks
new means of appeal to a disturbed public.

"The manufacturer who attempts to temporize or play hide-
and-seek with the law," wrote James F. Hoge, the Proprietary

[1] 48 Fed. Supp. 878. Court decisions under the 1938 law have been
conveniently reprinted in a Food Law Institute Series, edited by Vincent A. Kleinfeld and Charles Wesley Dunn, each volume entitled
*Federal Food, Drug, and Cosmetic Act: Judicial and Administrative
Record*, with the covering dates, *1938-1949* (Chicago, 1949); *1949-
1950* (Chicago, 1951); *1951-1952* (Chicago, 1953), etc. This case appears in *1938-1949*, 34-44, the quotation at 43.
[2] Walter Campbell to R. M. Allen, July 18, 1939, FDA Records, R.
M. Allen 1936-37-38, Decimal file .062, 1938, Federal Records Center,
Alexandria; *F&D Rev.*, 22 (1938), 147.

Association's counsel, "is going to pay dearly for his fun." Food and Drug officials themselves, through informal conferences with industry leaders, made it crystal clear that they were going to insist on the broadest and strictest interpretation of all sections of the law. Most major proprietors heeded such warnings and scrutinized their labeling. As a result, according to the estimate of a trade editor, 97 per cent of the labels used in the drug industry were modified. Some of these changes were much too modest to suit Walter Campbell and his aides, and they said so bluntly in a circular letter to the industry. Proprietary manufacturers, in their turn, termed FDA regulations issued to interpret provisions of the law too "drastic." Thus an old debate continued. But it was not the products of Mr. Hoge's clients that gave the Food and Drug Administration the most concern. The Proprietary Association continued policing the copy of its members, in 1944 tightening its code of advertising practices, and it sponsored research seeking more than an empirical basis for the botanical ingredients in traditional formulas. By 1947, Charles Crawford, in addressing the Association, could compliment the membership on "an impressive record of the number and extent of improvements you have made over the years." Such commendation did not mean that the FDA would sit idle if, in its opinion, a major proprietor should violate the law.[3]

The FDA's most troublesome antagonists, in the battle to make self-medication safe, were made up of "a small fringe that cannot be catalogued as law-abiding." "In this group," as Crawford defined it, "are some who are clearly dishonest, some who are choice crackpots, and some who are grossly negligent in the conduct of their affairs." Year by year new faces appeared in this rogues' gallery. But some faces reappeared so often before the gaze of Food and Drug regulators as to be almost as familiar as the visages of their own asso-

[3] James F. Hoge, "An Appraisal of the New Drug and Cosmetic Legislation from the Viewpoint of Those Industries," *Law and Contemporary Problems*, 6 (1939), 127; *FDC Reports*, 1 (Feb. 11, 1939), pink 4; (Feb. 25, 1939), pink 1; 7 (Apr. 14, 1945), white 6-7; *F&D Rev.*, 23 (1939), 98; *PI*, 207 (May 19, 1944), 60; Proprietary Assoc., *Code of Advertising Practices* (Wash., 1944); Crawford, "Problems of Compliance and Enforcement under the Drug Law," *FDC Law Qtly.*, 2 (1947), 445.

ciates. It was the "fringe operators," especially the perennials, who, in the words of a federal judge, "outline[d] the limits of action defined by a particular law, then proceed[ed] to operate to the full extent of those limits." Here the cat and mouse game was at its cagiest. The nostrum vendor sought a loophole. The regulator sought to close it by taking the vendor to court. So, case by case and through the years, the exact meaning of the law was spelled out. In the process, the freedom of quackery was vastly circumscribed but not eliminated—the techniques of quackery changed markedly.[4]

With respect to one section of the law, 502(j), there was little that could be legally ambiguous: drugs were misbranded if "dangerous to health" when used as directed in the labeling. Within this danger zone were products against which the Food and Drug Administration had been impotent to act under the 1906 law. Now these hazards to health got top enforcement priority. "Our first search," Walter Campbell said, was for . . . [reducing remedies] containing dinitrophenol." But their manufacturers had heard the word. Although these deadly reducers had been abundant during the fight to secure the law, Campbell's inspectors could find none now. The agency turned to other obesity products containing dangerously potent drugs—including the dried thyroid nostrum named Marmola.[5]

Also in the danger class were powerful pain-killers, proprietaries containing large amounts of cinchophen, aminopyrine, and mixtures of bromides and acetanilid. The FDA warned analgesic manufacturers to adopt labels giving sensible dosage instructions and cautioning against the hazards of overuse. Most heeded, but some did not, and the FDA undertook a widespread program of seizures. Caught in this particular net were major companies, like the Proprietary Association stal-

[4] *Ibid.*; Buffalo District Annual Report, 1951, FDA Decimal file .053, Dept. of Health, Education, and Welfare storage. A 1936 survey of medicine makers in the Los Angeles area revealed that the number of concerns in operation varied from day to day. Western District Annual Report, 1936, FDA Decimal file .053, RG 88, NA. Judge Mathes cited in Los Angeles District Annual Report, 1949, FDA Decimal file .053, HEW storage.

[5] *F&D Rev.*, 24 (1940), 204; *1939 Report of Food and Drug Administration*, 5.

wart Bromo-Seltzer. Its maker protested the FDA's action as "an arbitrary exercise of power" and vowed to fight up to the Supreme Court, but in the end did not. Instead the company consented to a decree of condemnation and changed its formula.[6]

With the war came a shocking revival of an ancient danger, abortifacient pastes. As with dinitrophenol, these corrosive wares were just too hazardous for any use at all: no adequate directions could be written that would make them safe. Cases of death and serious injury mounted. The FDA turned all three of its weapons—seizures, injunctions, and criminal actions—on Leunbach's Paste, Dependon Intra Uterin Paste, Interferin, and others of that ilk.[7]

Other dangerous drugs were seized, like laxatives which did not admit their nature on their labels and purported cures for the drinking habit containing emetine. And section 502(j) gave the FDA power to act for the first time against another threat to the public health, hazardous devices. A preliminary survey on the West Coast turned up such gadgets in fantastic profusion: "pessaries, dilators, nipple shields, breast pumps, syringes of all descriptions, electric insoles, pile pipes, respirators, ear droppers, trusses, catheters, massagers, bust developers, Sea Tangle Tents." The FDA moved to take the worst examples off the market.[8]

The new law required drug labeling to bear "adequate directions for use," and these directions had to include proper warnings to the would-be self-doser. If the drug might be unsafe for children, or hazardous in too large or too long-

[6] Trade Correspondence-2, TC-3, TC-4, TC-14, TC-301, reproduced in Kleinfeld and Dunn, *Judicial and Administrative Record, 1938-1949,* 561-63, 574-78, 687; *1939 Food and Drug Administration Report,* 1; 1940 *Report,* 15; 1941 *Report,* 15; *Business Week,* Mar. 18, 1939, 8; *F&D Rev.,* 24 (1940), 35; Bromo-Seltzer, FDA Drugs and Devices Notice of Judgment [DDNJ] 81. Reports by the FDA District chiefs indicate the large-scale way in which analgesic manufacturers changed their formulas shortly after visits by FDA inspectors. Eastern and Western District Annual Reports, 1939, FDA Decimal file .053, RG 88, NA.

[7] *1942-1943 Report of Food and Drug Administration,* 38; W. R. M. Wharton, "Wartime and Postwar Food and Drug Adulteration," *FDC Law Qtly.,* 1 (1946), 465.

[8] *1941 Report of Food and Drug Administration,* 16-17; Western District Annual Report, 1939, FDA Decimal file .053, RG 88, NA.

IN PURSUIT OF THE DIMINISHING PROMISE

continued doses, or risky if the user was suffering from a
given ailment, the labeling had to say so. For violation of this
provision, the FDA had acted against some of the bromide-
acetanilid proprietaries. Scores of other traditional formulas
on the market, in the view of Food and Drug officials, must be
used with similar restraint if self-medication was to be safe.
To guide manufacturers, the FDA prepared a long list of
warning statements appropriate for laxatives, nose drops,
douches, vermifuges, cough remedies, liniments, pain-killers,
tonics, and other popular proprietary products. The omission
or dilution of such warnings could lead to legal trouble.[9]

The "adequate directions" injunction, the law said, might be
excused if deemed by the FDA unnecessary to protect the
public health, and the agency did issue regulations permitting
some exceptions. Some home remedies—like tincture of iodine
—were so well known that directions would be superfluous. At
the other extreme, some drugs, while extremely useful, were
so powerful—like the new sulfa compounds—that they should
not be taken except under the direction of a physician. Therefore, the regulation stated, such potent drugs could not be
marketed with directions for self-medication, but only with
a label warning against their use except upon the prescription
of a doctor. To guide industry, the FDA announced a list
specifying some of these potent drugs, but the agency made it
clear that others might be included, to be determined in each
case by the cautious manufacturer. In between the mild home
remedies and the potent prescription items lay a border zone
that caused much trouble. For many drugs perhaps safe for
self-medication were also weapons in the physician's arma-
mentarium, and manufacturers began to market these drugs in
both forms. This led to confusion among pharmacists. If a
certain drug was labeled with directions for self-dosage, why
could not the same drug, though bearing the prescription
legend, also be safely sold over the counter? Many pharmacists, FDA surveys revealed, were doing just that. And how
could the pharmacist distinguish, amid the increasing array
of drugs available, which items marked with the prescription

[9] *JAMA*, 115 (1940), 387-88, 937-38; TC-14, Kleinfeld and Dunn,
*1938-1949*, 574-78.

legend might safely—if not legally—be sold direct to customers and which might not? The task was difficult. "In the course of our surveys to uncover dangerous drugs," wrote the chief of FDA's Western District, "it was . . . learned that practically all retail druggists will sell anything a customer asks for and has the money to buy." This problem would vex the Food and Drug Administration for many years to come.[10]

The existence of this border zone did not go unnoticed by the fringe. The prescription legend, some of them decided, might be a shield of safety for them in their promotions. Since the legend was so often honored in the breach, and since they could not label their true intentions without risk, they disguised their nostrums as prescription items and sought to reach the attention of potential customers in other ways. Makers of supposed sex rejuvenators, for example, adopted this ruse. When the FDA announced that there was no specific evidence that dried and ground-up glands had any physiological effect when taken by mouth, promoters adopted the prescription legend and sought to entice buyers in ways less direct. In time the FDA began to plug this loophole, seizing two drugs purporting to be Orchic Substance and Spleen Liquid.[11]

Latent in the "adequate directions for use" section were other and more dramatic judicial adventures. The legislative record was vague as to how elastically Congress had intended to define the clause. Some early commentators held that it applied merely to dosage instructions. But the Food and Drug Administration saw a chance to make of the clause a club to wield against fringe operators. Few who shared in enacting the 1938 law, asserted attorney Hoge less than a decade later, "could have envisaged the faraway destination" section 502(f) would reach.[12]

---

[10] A series of Trade Correspondence items was issued, especially TC-361, *ibid.*, 713-14; Edward B. Williams, "Exemption from the Requirement of Adequate Directions for Use in the Labeling of Drugs," *FDC Law Qtly.*, 2 (1947), 155-65; Western District Annual Report, 1942, FDA Decimal file .053, Federal Records Center, Alexandria; *ibid.*, 1939, FDA Decimal file .053, RG 88, NA.

[11] TC-13 and TC-376, Kleinfeld and Dunn, *1938-1949*, 574, 721; *F&D Rev.* 32 (1948), 282; *FDC Reports*, 16 (1954), white 13-14.

[12] Kleinfeld, "Applicability of the Federal Food, Drug, and Cos-

One of the reasons directions for use might be inadequate, FDA's interpretative regulations asserted, would be the omission of such directions for use "in all conditions for which" the drug—or device—was "prescribed, recommended, or suggested in its labeling, or in its advertising."[13] Recalling their long and frustrating experience with tame labels and venturesome advertising, Food and Drug officials seemed to be seeking by their regulation-making authority to gain a little of the control over advertising they had sought and Congress had denied during the long efforts to expand the law.

The first court test of the regulation involved the regulators with an opponent already well known to them. Chester Walker Colgrove, a Californian who had been in trouble in the courts because of his oil stock and insurance schemes, had turned his attention to petroleum in another way. Owning a well that produced so little oil no company would operate it, Colgrove set up a family corporation to market his petroleum medicinally. A two-ounce bottle of Colusa Natural Oil sold for three dollars with a label recommending its use for treating a variety of skin ailments, including psoriasis, eczema, leg ulcers, and athlete's foot. Colgrove's oil was also put up in capsule form labeled with the same claims. Believing Colgrove's statements and before-and-after pictures to be false and misleading, the FDA moved against him with seizure actions, which he did not contest, and a criminal case. A jury found Colgrove guilty of misbranding and fined him $1,500. An appeal court dismissed this verdict on the grounds that the trial judge had not permitted one of Colgrove's experts to testify about the experimental use of Colusa oil on dogs with mange, and remanded the case for a new trial. But Colgrove pleaded nolo contendere and paid the original fine. He did not, however, stop marketing petroleum. Having moved his therapeutic claims from labels to circulars packed with packages of his nostrum, Colgrove

---

metic Act to Drug Advertising," *FDC Law Jnl.* (1950), 48; Maurice L. Stewart, "Therapeutic Claims under the Federal Food, Drug, and Cosmetic Act," *FDC Law Qtly.*, 4 (1949), 538; Hoge, "A Significant Aspect of Food and Drug Law Enforcement," *ibid.*, 2 (1947), 49.

[13] These early regulations are cited in Chester W. Colgrove . . . v. U.S., 176 Fed. (2d) 614, in Kleinfeld and Dunn, *1949-1950*, 240n.

now took a new tack. He withdrew entirely any glowing promises from his labeling and contented himself with suggesting that Colusa Natural Oil was "for use in treatment" of psoriasis, eczema, leg ulcers, and athlete's foot.[14]

The government responded by wielding its multiple seizure weapon, and Colgrove fought. Pitted against each other in the trial were a whole host of medical and chemical experts for the government and, for Colgrove, satisfied users, depositions from various doctors, and one live physician from Houston, age 83. Again the government won. Harking back to the McAnnulty rule, Colgrove had argued the existence of a conflict in medical opinion, but the judge could find "no credible or adequate scientific or medical foundation for any claim" that Colgrove's oil would cure the four diseases or would "give relief" or "assist in the treatment of them." Nor did his new-found labeling modesty help him. The phrase "for use in treatment," the judge ruled, in conjunction with the disease names, "would be understood by a person of average intelligence who was suffering from one of the diseases . . . and who was seeking a remedy" as a promise to "cure or alleviate."

Colgrove's next maneuver brought 502(f) squarely into play. He had new labels printed containing directions but no diseases. "Apply to affected parts," the label read, "and rub it in thoroughly morning and night. For open sores saturate cotton pad with oil and bind on by gauze." But there was no mention of what might produce the open sores—no reference to psoriasis, eczema, leg ulcers, or athlete's foot. Colgrove had not forsaken these ailments, however; he had merely moved them to the advertising pages of the nation's press. Indeed, he

[14] The account of Colgrove's litigious career is based on FDA Drugs and Devices Notices of Judgment 380, 381, 1040, 1384, 2087, 2131, 2782, 2833, 2922, 3009, 3045, 3061, 3989; *1949 Food and Drug Administration Report*, 27; *F&D Rev.*, 26 (1942), 161; Western District Annual Report, 1945, FDA Decimal file .053, Federal Records Center, Alexandria; *FDC Law Qtly.*, 2 (1946), 274; and court decisions. The decisions, reproduced in Kleinfeld and Dunn, *1938-1949*, 218-21, and *1949-1950*, 114-20, 237-41, are U.S. v. 9 Bottles . . . Colusa Natural Oil, 78 Fed. Supp. 721; Colusa Remedy Company v. U.S., 176 Fed. (2d) 554, certiorari denied, 338 U.S. 911; U.S. v. Colgrove et al., 83 Fed. Supp. 880; Chester Walker Colgrove . . . v. U.S., 176 Fed. (2d) 614, certiorari denied, 338 U.S. 911.

supplied newspapers with matrices of what he wanted printed and ordered extra copies of the ads to be delivered to dealers who vended Colusa Natural Oil.

Again the government struck, asking a court for an injunction to stop Colgrove from distributing his misbranded petroleum. Directions for use were not adequate, the district attorney argued, citing the Food and Drug Administration's regulations, unless they explained fully how a drug should be taken for ailments specified in advertising. The judge agreed, and Colgrove was enjoined. But he read the injunction decision with the utmost care. In this perusal he found grounds for his next gambit.

It was the case of the substituted conjunction. FDA regulations required labeling to contain adequate directions for use in all conditions for which the drug was "prescribed, recommended, or suggested" in collateral advertising. The injunction, in referring to this clause, had changed the *or* to *and*. So Colgrove went on with his lavish and flamboyant advertising. At the same time he tried to meet the law's labeling requirements by restoring the names of his four key diseases, along with what he obviously hoped might be adequate directions for applying Colusa oil in their treatment. But Food and Drug officials were not persuaded. They sought a judgment holding Colgrove in criminal contempt for violating the injunction. Colgrove was still transgressing section 502(f), they argued, because other ailments than the labeled four were mentioned in the advertising, acne and poison oak, for example. But Colgrove demurred. His advertising may have recommended and suggested his product for acne and poison oak, but being no doctor, he certainly could not have prescribed. And to violate the injunction, the *and* having replaced the *or*, he must be guilty of all three.

Such a feeble and far-fetched defense the court did not accept. Neither "logic nor fairness" required such a narrow definition of "prescribe," the judges said. "Plainly" Colgrove "had intended to be understood as adopting as his own the statements of the doctors and professional dispensers" which he quoted glowingly in his ads. And, in referring to the *and-or* matter, the court commented: "Colgrove was quick to seize upon the discrepancy, and he steered his course so as to sail as closely into the wind as he thought he safely could." Such sailing was typical of Colgrove's whole course—for his involvement with the Food and Drug Administration was not yet done —a course very characteristic of the pseudo-medical fringe.

Colgrove was by no means the only medicine man to test the outer limits of section 502(f). FDA's chief counsel, William Goodrich, once paid a sort of grudging tribute to a woman, Ada Alberty, another "perennial litigant," saying she had served a useful purpose in that her many cases had explored and stretched the "adequate directions for use" clause.[15] Mrs. Alberty's ingenious efforts to market her nutritional wares also helped secure judicial definition of another important section of the 1938 act.

Section 201(m) defined labeling to mean "all labels and other written, printed, or graphic matter" either "upon any article or any of its containers or wrappers" or "accompanying such article." Promoters had grown accustomed to being wary of what they said on circulars packed with their bottles, for the old Sherley Act had covered them. Some proprietors had found a new and safe way to circumvent the Sherley labeling taboo. In packages separate from their medicines, they shipped placards and pamphlets replete with extravagant claims. Dealers displayed the posters, handed out the pamphlets, and sold the medicines. How free was this marketing method to continue under the new law? What did "accompanying" really mean?

At first various courts spoke with differing voices, as Food and Drug officials initiated various cases against Mrs. Alberty and other proprietors. "Accompanying" must be narrowly construed, decided a federal district judge in Wisconsin, in a case concerned with the vitamin products of Royal Lee, another of the FDA's through-the-years antagonists. Words in a criminal statute should not be defined more broadly by courts than Congress intended. Since Congress had seen fit to give advertising to the FTC, labeling under FDA authority should not be defined so as to transgress upon the advertising sphere. Promotional literature shipped separately from Lee's vitamins,

[15] *FDC Law Jnl.*, 8 (1953), 222-23.

the court ruled, even though it was "placed on shelves, display counters, or in window displays" by dealers who sold Lee's wares, did not "accompany" and was therefore not labeling, but advertising.[16]

A federal district judge in nearby Minnesota viewed things differently. Concerned with jugs of a sick-chicken remedy, the the judge ruled that Congress had intended through the 1938 law to expand consumer protection, thus the law, including the word "accompanying," must be construed elastically. Dr. Salsbury's printed matter and his poultry "cure" were interlocking units of a single distribution scheme. It mattered not that pamphlets and drugs were shipped on different occasions, over different routes, arriving at different times.[17]

The conflict in judicial interpretation occurred not only in district courts, but in circuit courts as well. Finally, the Supreme Court was called upon to resolve the issue. Judges in the Seventh Circuit, like the Minnesota judge, had given a broad construction to the law. Health lecturer Lelord Kordel was guilty of misbranding. His separately shipped books and circulars had been displayed on a rack near the counter where his products were sold. It mattered not that some of the books bore a price tag, or that some of them had been sent 561 days later than the drugs. The test of "accompanying" under the law was one of commercial connection—"not of physical contiguity but of textual relationship." On the other hand, judges in the Fifth Circuit sounded like the Wisconsin district judge. A Florida naturopath, Fred Urbeteit, who ran a College of Sinuothermic Institute in Tampa, had shipped 16 Sinuothermic machines—some sold, some rented—to an Ohio chiropractor. Sent separately from Florida to Ohio were copies of a simulated newspaper, "The Road to Health," citing testimonials praising the success of Dr. Urbeteit's methods in treating arthritis and other ills. The machine was mentioned, though not described, pictured, or explained. This literature ended up in the chiropractor's waiting room. The judges could not see that it accompanied the machines. "Accompany means to go

[16] U.S. v. Royal Lee, 40 Fed. Supp. 801, in Kleinfeld and Dunn, *1938-1949*, 443-45.

[17] U.S. v. 7 Jugs . . . of Dr. Salsbury's Rakos, 53 Fed. Supp. 746, in *ibid.*, 64-77.

along with. In a criminal and forfeiture statute the meaning cannot be stretched."[18]

The Supreme Court, in five-to-four decisions, concurred in the Kordel case logic and reversed the Urbeteit decision. "A criminal law is not to be read expansively to include what is not plainly embraced within the language of the statute . . . ," Justice Douglas wrote. But "strained and technical constructions" should not defeat the law's purpose "by creating . . . loopholes in it." The purpose of the 1938 law was to protect the public health. No easy ruse, such as the "sale" of advertising matter (like Kordel's books), should be permitted to circumvent the law. What is required in "accompanying" is to have two transactions "integrated" by "functional standards." The time of shipment of literature and drug or device, relative to each other, is not germane.[19]

So the Supreme Court, in this as in other ways, gave a broad construction to the law. The Food and Drug Administration could thus persevere in fighting fringe operators who continued to devise new ways of keeping their drugs or devices separate from their promises. The literature for an elaborate therapeutic gadget called Color-Therm was typed by a salesman in Oklahoma from an instruction sheet given him in Missouri by the machine's maker. In another instance, an Illinois man bought an intricate device in California and took it home himself by plane to treat his wife. With the machine he got an instruction pamphlet, and more advice came later in printed and letter form from the machine's vendor. The government won both cases. The labeling, courts held, had accompanied the devices.[20]

In a similar spirit, courts aided the Food and Drug Administration by generously construing many other parts of the law

[18] U.S. v. Kordel, 164 Fed. (2d) 913, and Fred Urbeteit . . . v. U.S., 164 Fed. (2d) 245, in *ibid.*, 343-48 and 212-15.

[19] Kordel v. U.S., 335 U.S. 345, and U.S. v. Fred Urbeteit, 335 U.S. 355, in *ibid.*, 382-86 and 249-51. For a critical reaction by the lawyer who handled the appeal for Kordel, see Arthur D. Herrick, "Some Implications of the Kordel Decision," *FDC Law Qtly.*, 4 (1949), 94-104.

[20] U.S. v. 4 Devices, Labeled in Part "Color-Therm," 176 Fed. (2d) 652, in Kleinfeld and Dunn, *1949-1950*, 112-14; Ruth B. Drown . . . v. U.S., 198 Fed. (2d) 999, in Kleinfeld and Dunn, *1951-1952*, 165-71.

so as to rein in the pseudo-medical promoter. Labeling might mean a roadside sign beside an interstate highway. Misleading might mean quoting only favorable parts from medical textbooks while omitting unfavorable words. It might mean deceptive layout: the size of type and the arrangement of text and pictures on the printed page. Or it might signify cautious —indeed true—wording that, hurriedly read, sounded like the promise of a cure. A slight change of labeling since the previous legal encounter, judges said, did not force the government to begin all over again: a summary judgment could be rendered. Nor did a slight change in the name of a product bring about a new case, nor the addition of a new ingredient that made no material therapeutic difference.[21] In ways too numerous to recount, judges adhered to Justice Frankfurter's judgment given in the second case under the law to reach the highest court.

"By the Act of 1938," he said, "Congress extended the range of its control over illicit and noxious articles and stiffened the penalties for disobedience. The purposes of this legislation thus touch phases of the lives and health of people which, in the circumstances of modern industrialism, are largely beyond self-protection. Regard for these purposes should infuse construction of the legislation if it is to be treated as a working instrument of government and not merely as a collection of English words."[22]

The nostrum provisions of the law, then, as seen by the courts, turned out to be more rigorous than even the most ardent—and disappointed—advocates of a strong bill could have anticipated on the day of its passage. Summarizing the situation at the end of a decade of enforcement, one scholar

[21] Maurice L. Stewart, "Therapeutic Claims under the Federal Food, Drug, and Cosmetic Act," *FDC Law Qtly.*, 4 (1949), 536-51; Gold Lax Tonic, Painesville, O., Buffalo Station Annual Report, 1948, FDA Decimal file .053, Federal Records Center, Alexandria; Research Laboratories, Inc. v. U.S., 167 Fed. (2d) 410, in Kleinfeld and Dunn, *1938-1949*, 227-38; U.S. v. Six Dozen Bottles . . . of "Dr. Peter's Kuriko," 158 Fed. (2d) 667, in *ibid.*, 197-99; U.S. v. 17 Cases . . . of Nue-Ovo, in Kleinfeld and Dunn, *1949-1950*, 124-26; Muscle Rub, *FDC Reports*, 16 (1954), 11 white.

[22] U.S. v. Dotterweich, 320 U.S. 277, in Kleinfeld and Dunn, *1938-1949*, 278-85, quotation at 280.

wrote, "The law leaves no apparent loopholes through which the nostrum maker can make unfounded claims."[23] In one sense this assertion was true, but in another sense misleading.

There had indeed been a wholesale flight of false claims from the labeling. It had once been, wrote a district director of the FDA, that a simple survey of packaged remedies in wholesale houses revealed many with suspicious therapeutic promises. This situation was no longer true; such surveys proved futile. To be sure, nothing ever really dies in quackery, and every now and then a new promotion would appear labeled with a grim uninhibited gusto reminiscent of the 19th century. Such, for example, were the Tree of Life General Tonic, the Asthma Aid, the Hair Growing Aid, and other herbal mixtures of Samuel Shokunbi, a West African who had studied at Oxford and Heidelberg, although the only license he held was that of Swedish masseur. Shokunbi's formulas, which made him thousands of dollars a month in the mid-South, came from a popular medical book written by an English doctor who had died in 1640. Such outrageous nostrums earned Shokunbi, in 1950, the most severe first conviction sentence that had ever been handed down under the law—a nine-year prison term.[24]

Despite such an occasional sport from an earlier era, the trend in exaggerated claims was away from the immediate labeling to methods less direct. Collateral advertising, be it pamphlet, newspaper spread, placard, or roadside sign provided one broad avenue, as we have seen, with the Food and Drug Administration traveling in hot pursuit. Another technique, increasingly popular along the fringe, was oral speech. Sometimes the spokesman went out among the people as a spieler or, as the big operators preferred to bill themselves, a "lecturer," talking to those assembled in a crowd. Such pitchmen, the FDA's George Larrick reported in 1948, had increasingly engaged the agency's attention. Long ago, he said, there

[23] *Ibid.*, Introduction, xv-xvi; Stewart, "Therapeutic Claims under the Federal Food, Drug, and Cosmetic Act," 530.
[24] *1946 Food and Drug Administration Report*, 35; Central District Annual Report, 1946, FDA Decimal file .053, Federal Records Center, Alexandria; *F&D Rev.*, 34 (1950), 251, 265; DDNJ 3297.

had been the "Konjola Man," who moved from one drugstore to another talking to little informal groups. More recently, spielers had been vending their wares through variety stores, booming their pitches over public address systems. The big timers rented an auditorium for a week or two, advertising in advance their course of lectures—the first one usually free, the rest for a fee—in the press or by direct mail. All kinds of showmanship—including scantily clad girls—sought to increase the lure. Lecturers, under FDA pressure, had abandoned labeling claims, had even ceased sending circulars to health food stores selling their wares. Now the vogue, Larrick said, was to recommend the products from the lecture platform. Some lecturers managed to take in $25,000 a week in fees and sales.[25]

Equally popular was the door-to-door approach. Teams of salesmen were recruited to ring door bells, bringing their pulverized alfalfa and complex vitamin and mineral mixtures into the parlors of America. Under Food and Drug Administration pressure, the immediate labeling approached rectitude. No claims were printed on the bottles. But what the salesman said, after assessing the health worries of those he chatted with, might reach the outer limits of exaggeration. His product might cure cancer, relieve arthritis, mend a broken leg. Or it might merely prevent the common cold. "You eat food to make blood," one salesman told a would-be customer. "You send down junk, your body will be junk. Your body will wind up in the junk pile. You send down vital elements that are needed, you're okay. Whenever you get your body normalized, you won't have no condition. You can't even take a cold. I don't care how you're exposed to freezing temperature, wet feet and cold feet, you'll never take it if you get your blood stream up to par."[26]

Food and Drug inspectors knew what was going on, for they posed as customers and caught the fleeting words of doorbell ringers with tape recorders. Such tapes helped them win cases in court, for judges agreed that oral promises were "ad-

[25] Larrick, "Some Current Problems of Enforcement," *FDC Law Qtly.*, 3 (1948), 26-65.
[26] Joseph R. Bell, "Let 'em Eat Hay," *Today's Health*, 36 (1958), 24.

vertising" and therefore adequate directions for use must be printed in the labeling.[27] It was hard for a promoter to devise labeling that could demonstrate how alfalfa taken daily for several months could cure a serious disease. But how could a small staff of inspectors police the impromptu utterances of thousands of salesmen blanketing the country? In any case, in the nutrition field, some assertions could be made, very persuasive to ill-informed listeners, which might be dubious but did not contravene the law.

For with the change in techniques of reaching the public, promoters of drugs and devices for self-treatment also modified the kinds of therapeutic promises they made. They moved into the gray areas where medical science had not yet won major victories—arthritis and the common cold, for example— or where scientific opinion had not yet fully crystallized as to the certain path a person should follow to retain or regain his health. The greenest pasture in this respect was nutrition, the relation of diet to health.

Of great advantage to promoters in this field was a list of 31 allowable claims listed in a sort of legal truce negotiated in 1951 between the FDA and one of the major distributors of food supplements, after a protracted and bitter battle in the courts. Vended by some 15,000 door-to-door salesmen, Nutrilite contained vitamins, minerals, alfalfa, watercress, and parsley. Its early promotion centered on a pamphlet written by the president of the company, a Stanford University Ph.D., offering it as a cure for most non-infectious ailments, including asthma, ulcers, eczema, arthritis, and mental depression. In successive editions, claims were toned down. But the FDA considered Nutrilite a major imposition on the public, especially the doctrine that the average American diet lacked essential protective ingredients, and sought by seizures, injunction, and criminal indictment to drive the product off the market. Nutrilite fought back and gained a significant weapon while taking a deposition from Oscar R. Ewing, administrator of the Federal Security Agency. (The FDA had been moved into the Agency from the Department of Agriculture in 1940.) Part of

[27] *Ibid.*; *F&D Rev.*, 31 (1947), 219; DDNJ 2405, concerning the products of health lecturer David V. Bush.

the FDA's evidence regarding the state of the national diet had come from Ewing's 1948 report to the President on *The Nation's Health*. In questioning Ewing, the Nutrilite attorney cited from this report the opinions of some experts that dietary deficiencies still existed in America. Did Ewing agree? He answered that he did. The Food and Drug attorney got into the record the fact that Ewing was no physician and could not speak in this field with authority. But a delicate contretemps had arisen. Should the case come up in court, the Nutrilite lawyers could demonstrate a conflict between the FDA's position and that of their chief. This development, perhaps, played some part in the FDA's desire to compromise rather than risk losing the suit. More fundamental was the desire to draw as quickly as possible some kind of line between promotional claims that were permissible and those that were not, in a very complicated field. A long trial and inevitable appeals, even if victory should be forthcoming, would mean delay. And nutritional nonsense was expanding in the market.[28]

Hammered out after long negotiations, the Nutrilite consent decree would have been hard for the average door-to-door salesman of nutritional supplements to comprehend, let alone follow. The average customer, in attempting to read it, might have been at an even greater loss to catch its fine distinctions. A paragraph on vitamin C illustrates the problem: "If it is claimed that a deficiency of vitamin C leads to dental caries, anemia, defective teeth and gums, sponginess of the gums, pyorrhea, some gum infections, loss of appetite, and local hemorrhages of the mucous membranes of the nose, mouth, gums and about the face, it shall be explained (1) that these symptoms could occur only when the daily intake of vitamin C is less than the minimum daily requirement over a prolonged period, (2) that these conditions, while they may be concomitant signs of a vitamin C deficiency, do not of themselves prove

[28] U.S. v. 91 Packages . . . "Nutrilite Food Supplement," 93 Fed. Supp. 763, in Kleinfeld and Dunn, *1949-1950*, 189-90; Mytinger & Casselberry, Inc. v. Oscar R. Ewing, 87 Fed. Supp. 650, in *ibid.*, 256-65; Oscar R. Ewing . . . v. Mytinger & Casselberry, 339 U.S. 594, in *ibid.*, 275-80; U.S. v. Mytinger & Casselberry, in *ibid.*, *1951-1952*, 204-13; *FDC Law Jnl.*, 6 (1951), 473; Lester L. Lev, "The Nutrilite Consent Decree," *ibid.*, 7 (1952), 56-69; DDNJ 3381, 3382, 3383.

a vitamin C deficiency, and (3) that these symptoms are non-specific and may be caused by any of a great number of conditions or may have functional causes."[29]

Whatever the complex nature of nutritional science, this was not the sort of language, these not the caveats, that door-to-door salesmen were accustomed to using. Nor did they all adopt them. Even deeper trouble with nutritional nonsense lay ahead.

Another trend along the fringe, in the migration from claims on labeling, brought the development of "clinics." Shrewd operators sought to avoid battles with the Food and Drug Administration by withdrawing from interstate commerce, setting up treatment centers, and enticing the sick and frightened to come to them. A new wave of state food and drug laws had been enacted in imitation of the 1938 act, but many had loopholes and most were ill enforced. In any case, the clinic operator sought to evade their terms—and federal law as well—by pretending to the legitimate practice of one of the licensed health professions. Unscrupulous physicians, osteopaths, naturopaths, and chiropractors either ran the clinics or were hired by lay operators to diagnose and treat. Some of these schemes relied on impressive electrical devices, like Urbeteit's Sinuothermic machine. Others dispensed drugs and pseudo-drug products: dried vegetables, glandular extracts, vitamins, and minerals, sometimes labeled "food" in an effort to impart to them an ethical aroma. The prescribing even of the horns and hoofs of animals was not unknown.[30]

In seeking to combat this kind of quackery, the Food and Drug Administration occasionally uncovered an interstate angle that gave it jurisdiction. But cases were extremely difficult and costly to develop. And victories that were won caused later opponents to fight the FDA with even greater determination. In the late 1940's, the agency discovered that a greater

[29] U.S. v. Mytinger & Casselberry, in Kleinfeld and Dunn, *1951-1952*, 204-13, quotation at 209.

[30] Western District Annual Report, 1943, FDA Decimal file .053, Federal Records Center, Alexandria; Kansas City District Annual Report, 1949, FDA Decimal file .053, HEW storage; *Business Week*, Nov. 12, 1938, 24, 29; Melvin E. Mensor, " 'SNAFU' in State Food Laws," *FDC Law Jnl.*, 12 (1957), 690-704.

proportion of its cases was being contested, in part because of the heavier penalties provided in the 1938 law, compared with 1906, in part because already convicted promoters knew that convictions for second or third offenses meant larger fines and longer prison terms.[31]

If penalties were severe enough to force fringe operators to fight when challenged, penalties were nonetheless too weak to frighten disreputable promoters into abandoning their lucrative schemes. Prison sentences, given in only a small proportion of convictions, were short, and more often than not suspended if the violator abstained from resuming his illegal operation for a probationary period. Fines were too small to be a true deterrent. In 1950 the average fine for all food and drug cases terminated was $565.[32]

Other handicaps hampered the Food and Drug Administration in fighting quackery. Its resources were not sufficient for the magnitude of its task. During the first 18 years under the 1938 law, the agency handled a fifth more cases of all types than it had handled during the 32-year span of the 1906 law. But this was not enough. The staff of the FDA grew only modestly as the years went by—and sometimes diminished, as certain members of the appropriation committee in the House regarded some FDA enforcement actions with disfavor. At the same time the industries to be surveyed and regulated kept expanding. When Walter Campbell resigned in 1944, to be succeeded by Paul B. Dunbar, a trade periodical noted Campbell's greatest achievement as commissioner: how much he could get done on such a small appropriation. The paucity of funds continued. At the 1953 inspection rate, Commissioner Larrick stated, it would take the agency ten years to give just one inspection to every food, drug, and cosmetic establishment—not counting retail stores—doing a substantial business in interstate commerce.[33] Medical quackery was a part of this

[31] Eastern District Annual Report, 1947, FDA Decimal file .053, Federal Records Center, Alexandria; *F&D Rev.*, 32 (1948), 1; N.Y. District Annual Report, 1949, FDA Decimal file .053, HEW storage.

[32] Francis E. McKay and Benjamin Frauwirth, "The Penalty Provisions of the Federal Food, Drug, and Cosmetic Act," *FDC Law Jnl.*, 6 (1951), 575-92.

[33] William W. Goodrich, "Judicial Highlights of 50 Years' Enforce-

total complex of business, and it got a high priority in the enforcement plans. But there were not enough inspectors to do the exhaustive job required. As with other crime, the amount of quackery varied inversely with the amount of enforcement time devoted to it.[34] The Food and Drug Administration performed yeoman's service, but pseudo-medicine continued.

Something of the massive effort required of the FDA in preparing a major case is illustrated by its contest with Marmola. During the Congressional hearings, this thyroid-extract reducing remedy had been mentioned as an egregious example of the dangerous drugs which the old law could not keep off the market. Other regulatory agencies had had their try, but obesity was not a disease within the purview of the FDA's labeling control. With the new law, Marmola was one of the first proprietaries against which the FDA began to develop evidence, and in several ways the case turned out to be significant.[35]

Marmola promotion, in the wake of its 1931 Supreme Court victory over the Federal Trade Commission, had become especially cocky, its pamphlets referring disparagingly to "silly gossip about harmful ingredients."[36] The Commission's defeat in this case, indeed, became a key argument for giving control of drug advertising to the FDA. Seeking to reverse this major

---

ment," *FDC Law Jnl.*, 11 (1956), 75; chart "Enforcement: Personnel and Appropriations, Fiscal Years 1941-56," accompanying mimeographed text of Jan. 27, 1955, address by Bradshaw Mintener, "Industry and the Food and Drug Administration"; *Business Week*, May 6, 1944, 33-35; Larrick, "Our Unfinished Business," mimeographed text of Dec. 8, 1954, address.

[34] 1955 *Annual Report of the U.S. Department of Health, Education, and Welfare* (FDA), 171.

[35] The discussion of Marmola is based mainly on the FDA case record, Interstate Office Seizure No. 48304-D, DDNJ 1251, which includes newspaper clippings on the trial and a helpful ms. summary of the testimony by K. W. Brimmer, M.D., entitled "Michigan's Marmola Menace." The district and circuit court decisions were U.S. v. 62 Packages, More or Less, of Marmola Prescription Tablets, 48 Fed. Supp. 878, and 142 Fed. (2d) 107, in Kleinfeld and Dunn, *1939-1948*, 34-44 and 107-10; the Supreme Court denied certiorari, Raladam Co. v. U.S., 323 U.S. 731. Also useful was the Marmola folder, AMA Dept. of Investigation.

[36] Marmola pamphlet in "Advertisements of Medicinal Preparations and Devices, 1933-7," FDA Records, RG 88, NA.

loss, the FTC issued in 1935 a new complaint against Marmola, this time making sure that injury to competitors as well as to consumers was amply demonstrated. In the hearing Edward Hayes once again defended the proprietary that had supported him so well for more than three decades, his testimony bolstered by that of a Detroit physician telling the tale of a lazy beagle. After chasing rabbits for half an hour, the doctor said, the hound fell to the ground exhausted. But on a diet of the thyroid glands of sheep, the beagle revived, two months later winning a blue ribbon in the Canadian trials. This and more human testimony did not save Hayes from a cease and desist order, issued in 1937. But Marmola appealed, and in the same month in 1941 that the Food and Drug Administration action went to trial, won another victory over the FTC, when a circuit court adjudged the cease and desist order void.[37] Hayes could not know this cheering news, or appear as witness in the FDA trial. He had died in 1939.[38]

Marmola labeling had been somewhat toned down with the passage of the 1938 law, recommending its four tablets a day "*only* as a treatment for adult fat persons whose excess fatness is caused by hypothyroidism . . . but who are otherwise normal and healthy." But its main gospel was the same. Science had dispelled the old notion that "laziness or gluttony" were the sole reasons for excess weight. The "basic cause" was a "deficiency" in the body, which Marmola's half grain of desiccated thyroid would counteract. From person to person the speed of weight loss would vary, but "a moderate rate of reduction" was best. There might be side effects, for all drugs could produce in some susceptible persons "unpleasant or harmful" symptoms. If this occurred, the circular advised, stop taking Marmola until the symptoms disappeared, then resume with half the former dose. The labeling disavowed explicitly that it was diagnosing; only physicians could do that.[39]

[37] FTC Docket 2406; In the Matter of Raladam Company, 24 *FTC Decisions* 475 (complaint and order); Raladam Co. v. FTC, 123 Fed. (2d) 34 (circuit court decision).

[38] W. B. Simmons memorandum, Feb. 27, 1940, in FDA file, Interstate Office Seizure No. 48304-D.

[39] DDNJ 1251.

Believing Marmola dangerous and even its more cautious claims false and misleading, the FDA seized 62 packages that had been shipped from Detroit to LaCrosse, Wisconsin. To make its case in court, the FDA employed the opinions of expert scientists, a mail inquiry of physicians, evidence from clinical trials, and sad instances of women whose use of Marmola had brought disaster.

At the trial in Madison before a judge, 19 notable scientists —drawn from private practice and such institutions as the Mayo Clinic and the universities of Wisconsin, Michigan, and Chicago—challenged Marmola's basic theories. Obesity did not result, they said, from an underactive thyroid gland. Undue weight was gained simply by taking into the body more calories through food and drink than the body expended through work or the output of heat. Nor did the thyroid hormone, necessary to normal life, exert any direct effect upon the fat deposits of obesity. Indeed, some people with hypothyroidism—too small an output of the hormone—were very thin, and some with hyperthyroidism—too great an output— were too fat. For the layman who was accumulating unnecessary pounds, therefore, to diagnose his own problem as hypothyroidism and start taking Marmola was ridiculous.

It was worse than ridiculous, the experts testified, it was a dire threat to health. For hyperthyroidism was a disease, dangerous in itself and in its possible consequences. Small doses of desiccated thyroid might actually act as a tonic, increasing appetite and therefore weight. Large enough doses to cause weight loss could achieve this result only by producing the disease of hyperthyroidism. From person to person, the border of danger would differ, since the metabolic rates of individuals differed. No lay person could himself know when the amount of thyroid he was taking had reached the point of threatening his physical reserves. These factors of safety in his kidneys, nerves, pancreas, blood vessels, and heart might reach severe depletion because of excessive thyroid while a person still looked healthy and felt fine. The Marmola dosage was enough, the medical scientists said, to activate latent diabetes, spur on borderline pellagra, precipitate incipient tuberculosis, cue a severe emotional disturbance, or bring on—especially in an overweight person—a heart attack. Even without these direst of results, the symptoms of hyperthyroidism were grim enough: vertigo, nausea, headache, nervousness, trembling, palpitation, labored breathing, menstrual suppression.

Ninety-eight per cent of some 2,000 members of the American College of Physicians who answered a mail inquiry arranged by the FDA believed that the indiscriminate use of two grains of thyroid a day—the recommended Marmola dosage—for a period of one to two months posed danger to health. Some of the government witnesses had sought to induce experimentally a carefully controlled hyperthyroidism. A fifth of the patients in the experiment developed distressing, and sometimes hazardous, symptoms, with dosages of two daily grains of desiccated thyroid or less. In some cases injury resulted from dosages as low as one-fifth, or even one-tenth, a grain a day.

What had occurred in the clinic, under the most cautious controls, also took place within the large number of Marmola's customers, who used its thyroid extract in the random way customary among those practicing self-dosage. Six women, serving as government witnesses, gave from the stand their tragic testimony.

One Chicago woman of 24, growing up in an unhappy home, had weighed 165 pounds by the time she was 18. Called "Fatty" and subject to the crude jokes and ostracism of her schoolmates, she had sought to remedy her plight. Secretly purchasing Marmola, she used it according to directions, but without a very great restriction on her eating. Thus, although she began to vomit occasionally and developed dizziness, headaches, and muscular pains, she lost very little weight. After three months she decided on an even more rigorous regimen. Taking five Marmola tablets a day, she cut her breakfast to a cup of coffee and a piece of unbuttered toast, her lunch to a bottle of pop. She ate no supper at all. Her spells of vomiting increased, and at last she began to lose weight rapidly. After seven months, when her stepmother discovered what she was doing and forbade further use of Marmola, the girl's weight was down to 90 or 95 pounds. Even without more thyroid extract, her weight continued to plummet, reaching

[ 213 ]

a low of 50 pounds, and her unpleasant symptoms continued. At the time of her testimony in court, though having gotten her weight back up to 70 pounds, she still was very ill.

When the young woman had finished her story, noted a Food and Drug medical officer, there was "not a dry handkerchief in the house."[40]

Marmola had its own medical experts who challenged the validity of the case made by the government's witnesses. Thyroid in the Marmola dosage was safe, they argued, and would cause no permanent damage. The symptoms of hyperthyroidism were admittedly unpleasant, they said, but transitory, and not too high a price to pay for the reduction of excess weight by people who lacked the will power to diet.

Besides defending its tablets, the Marmola company sought in its case to attack both the Food and Drug Administration and the new law the Administration was seeking to enforce. The agency was trying to use the law, a trial brief argued, to secure "bureaucratic" powers over the public's "inalienable right" of self-medication. This power grab was being undertaken in cooperation with the group that would profit most from its success, the "inner circle" of the American Medical Association. Should the FDA prevail in its interpretation of the law, "the proprietary medicine industry . . . must ultimately go out of business and the general public must henceforth obtain all of its medicaments by virtue of a special dispensation in the form of a doctor's prescription, if at all. Gone forever are the days of the family medicine chest. . . ."

In any case, Marmola's promoters insisted, the 1938 act was unconstitutional. Its provisions were too uncertain and indefinite, permitting unwarranted search and seizure, and unlawfully delegating legislative powers to an agency within the executive branch.

Fifteen months after the taking of testimony, the district judge delivered his decision. In this first court test of the 1938 law's constitutionality, he thoroughly explored the issues and found no conflict between the law's provisions and the Constitution. Nor did he agree with the Marmola contention that

[40] Undated Karl W. Brimmer memo, in Interstate Office Seizure No. 48304-D file.

the act, or the FDA's interpretation of the act, was aimed at the elimination of self-medication. The law "was enacted to make self-medication safer and more effective," he ruled, "and to require that drugs moving in interstate commerce be properly labeled so that their use as prescribed may not be dangerous to the health of the user." Marmola was not so labeled. "The substantial portion of the public, after reading the labeling . . . ," the judge said, "would conclude that Marmola is a safe and efficient remedy for obesity, which is not a fact." Testimony by the government witnesses had been most persuasive. In Marmola there was "an inherent and potential danger that may reasonably be expected to attend its use when one considers that it will be used by the strong, the weak, the old, the young, the well, and the sick, without first having a physical examination or a diagnosis of their condition by a competent physician."

The 1938 act had not been passed to safeguard "experts," the judge stated, rendering another judgment significant for the future application of the law. "The purpose" was "to protect the public, the vast multitude which includes the ignorant, the unthinking, and the credulous who, when making a purchase, do not stop to analyze."

Such a purchaser had been the young woman from Chicago, whose pitiful testimony had so impressed the court.

So 62 packages of Marmola, seized by the government, were condemned under the law. The circuit court in due course affirmed this decision, and the Supreme Court, by denying certiorari, let it stand. While the district judge was still weighing his judgment, the Supreme Court had already looked at Marmola advertising and found it bad. Reversing the circuit court's decision in the Federal Trade Commission case, the highest court restored the Commission's cease and desist order.[41] Following up its part of this double victory, the Food and Drug Administration attacked Marmola throughout the country with multiple seizures.[42]

Four years had elapsed between the initial seizure of Marmola and the Supreme Court's denial of certiorari ending the

[41] FTC v. Raladam Company, 316 U.S. 149.
[42] DDNJ 1252.

case. Uncounted thousands of dollars had been expended, and hundreds of hours by legal and medical experts. The victory was one measure of the skillfulness of the Food and Drug Administration's preparation. During the trial a medical specialist paid tribute to the government's case. "This is better," he said, "than a post graduate course on thyrotoxicosis."[43] Such elaborate and careful preparation was required for all the major contested cases—Colusa Oil and Nutrilite, Kordel and Urbeteit. With personnel short and resources scanty, the FDA could in any fiscal year work up only a relatively few important cases in the fringe area of self-medication. Many promoters of dubious drugs and devices were left to wait their turn.

[43] Undated Karl W. Brimmer memo, in Interstate Office Seizure No. 48304-D file.

# 10

# TWO GENTLEMEN FROM
# INDIANA

---

*"And the striking thing about it is that all the time these defendants operated this institution they knew there was no cure for diabetes; they knew the only treatment for diabetes was insulin and a restricted diet, free from sugar. Yet, notwithstanding that knowledge, in their avarice and greed for wealth, they wrongfully advised these trustful patients, and, as a result, they suffered damage and injury, and some have gone to an early grave."*

—UNITED STATES V. DR. CHARLES F. KAADT (KAADT DIABETIC INSTITUTE AND KAADT DIABETIC CLINIC), DR. PETER S. KAADT, AND ROBERT S. BENSON, 1948.[1]

---

IN 1923 the Canadian physician Frederick G. Banting was awarded a Nobel prize for the discovery of insulin and for the first successful use of this hormone in treating patients afflicted with diabetes. Soon thereafter, an Indiana doctor marketed a starkly different treatment for the same disease. The achievement of Banting and his associates offered the hope of something approximating normal life for men, women, and children hitherto doomed to a hazardous existence and, quite frequently, to rapid death. The achievement of Charles Frederick

[1] Judge Patrick T. Stone while sentencing in the district court, *Transcript of Record in the United States Circuit Court of Appeals for the Seventh Circuit, No. 9617, The United States of America, Plaintiff-Appellee, vs. Dr. Charles F. Kaadt, Defendant-Appellant; No. 9618, The United States of America, Plaintiff-Appellee, vs. Dr. Peter S. Kaadt, Defendant-Appellant; Appeals from the District Court of the United States for the Northern District of Indiana, Fort Wayne Division* (Indianapolis [1948]), 725-26.

Kaadt and his physician brother snatched that hope away from many diabetics who responded with pathetic eagerness to their delusive promises.

A decade after the enactment of the 1938 law, the Food and Drug Administration, bolstered by favorable court decisions, began action aimed at sending to prison these two gentlemen from Indiana. The Kaadt case illustrates the specious "clinic" as an evasionary maneuver to circumvent the new law. It shows too how the old in quackery persisted into the new day: the rapid progress of medical science had not eliminated the renegade physician, nor had a major breakthrough associated with that progress, like the discovery of insulin, stopped heartless efforts by charlatans to prescribe for diseases newly controllable by scientific treatment. The Kaadt case also reveals how various agencies—the FDA, the Post Office Department, an alert press, the American Medical Association, the Better Business Bureau, a state medical licensing board—could, when the need was great enough, combine their efforts into a united attack against the most egregious quackery.

Diabetes had long been a quack favorite. "In connection with no disease," wrote a physician in the year the first food and drug law went into effect, "is quackery in and out of the profession more rampant." In that era, life expectancy for those who became ill with the disease averaged about five years—for children about two. This was short enough to be deeply disturbing, yet long enough (as compared with death from an acute infection) to give the quack a chance to make his appeals heard. In its earlier stages, diabetes does not produce much pain or suffering, a situation useful to the quack, since pain tends to drive the ailing to regular practitioners. In its absence self-medication seems a plausible course of action. The orthodox treatment for diabetes also aided the quacks, for it required a complete and often irksome change in previous routines of life. An obscure and complex metabolic disorder, diabetes, before insulin, could be treated only with a regimen of hygiene and severely circumscribed diet, both as to quantity and kinds of food. Although semi-starving lengthened the life expectancy, patients often rebelled against its limitations and yielded to the quack's promise of an easier way.[2]

Even after Banting's notable discovery, diabetes therapy often required rigorous dietary restrictions, and the insulin itself established a new routine against which the impatient might rebel. The only method of introducing insulin into the body was by hypodermic injection—in the early years by several injections a day. Quacks, in playing on fear of the needle, struck a responsive chord. Thus, even after Dr. Banting's achievement, there was plenty of room for Dr. Kaadt's appeals.

Kaadt had secured his M.D. degree in 1902 from the Keokuk Medical College. Three years later he moved to Indiana, beginning a general practice in Fort Wayne. Soon he was supplementing his fees with a salary for serving as division surgeon for a railroad, a post he held for over 30 years. In the mid-1920's other doctors in the Midwest began to hear of Kaadt's "wonderful new treatment" for diabetes. It was, he asserted, an "absolute cure." The formula, Kaadt told his patients, was secret, "disclosed" to him "by an old European woman." Perhaps a new promise of a new cure, announced at this time, was more than ever alluring. Popular optimism engendered by Banting's discovery—as so often happens in quackery—helped Kaadt by conditioning would-be customers to a more hopeful prognosis. Kaadt's sales, at any rate, began to grow.[3]

"It is not necessary to use insulin . . . ," he wrote an inquirer. "It is not necessary to diet. . . . The length of treatment varies from three to seven months depending on the severity of the case. I have patients who took the treatment several years ago and as yet show no return of the disease." Kaadt sold his treatment by mail, without seeing his patients, and a $5 bottle contained enough medicine to last for 20 days.[4]

Dr. Kaadt was a member of his local medical society, and in

[2] Thomas B. Futcher, "Diabetes Mellitus," in William Osler, ed., *Modern Medicine: Its Theory and Practice* (Phila., 1907), 789-96, quotation at 794; Howard F. Root, "Prognosis in Idiopathic Diabetes Mellitus," in Robert H. Williams, ed., *Diabetes* (N.Y., 1960), 645-46; *N&Q*, I, 459.

[3] *Indianapolis Better Business Bureau Bulletin*, 19 (Mar. 1947) and 20 (Feb. 1948), in Kaadt file, AMA Dept. of Investigation; *Transcript of Record*, 628; JAMA, 97 (1931), 479.

[4] Cited in *ibid.*

1930 an official of the American Medical Association, prompted by letters of inquiry from physicians, wrote asking what the miraculous medicine contained. No answer came back. A year later, a second letter brought a reply but no formula. His results with his remedy, Kaadt said, had been "gratifying," but he would postpone an announcement until he could prove his claims, since his "experience with this disease, its cause and treatment" was "so widely different from the general opinion of the profession." When he had complete records of several hundred cases, he would submit a paper.[5]

Kaadt's cases accumulated but, of course, no paper came. His "Diabetic Laboratories" became the "Kaadt Diabetic Institute"; his personal replies to inquirers expanded into a pamphlet and advertising in such journals as *Home Circle Magazine* and the *Pathfinder*. In 1932 the Food and Drug Administration cited Kaadt, alleging that his "Diabetic Ferment Treatment" was misbranded. At a hearing in Chicago, Kaadt boasted that his formula cured 90 per cent of all cases. To avoid trouble, however, he would remove all claims for diabetes from his labels. This he did, and the FDA did not go on with the case. The label change did not hamper Kaadt's business in the least. Customers, whether they came in person or shopped for health by mail, had been persuaded to try Kaadt's formula before they ever saw his label.[6]

Four years later, Dr. Kaadt established new and larger headquarters, moving his Institute westward from Fort Wayne to the village of South Whitley. There a capacious inn, built for the carriage trade, had fallen victim to the depression. The two-story building of brown brick, with its large lobby, its ample dining room, its well-appointed kitchen, and its numerous guest rooms, provided a perfect site for treating diabetic patients, if mail prescribing should prove hazardous.[7]

The Post Office Department had, indeed, received a com-

[5] *Ibid.*

[6] *Ibid.*; information furnished by the Post Office Dept.; FDA file, Interstate Office Seizure No. 19-331H, FDA Records, RG 88, Federal Record Center, Alexandria. An ad appeared in the *Pathfinder*, Oct. 3, 1936.

[7] *Indianapolis BBB Bull.*, Mar. 1947.

plaint from one of Kaadt's customers and had launched a test case. An inspector, using an assumed name, had answered an advertisement, returned a case history sheet with symptoms vaguely stated, and submitted a sample of sugarless synthetic urine concocted by a Food and Drug Administration chemist. Back came Kaadt's answer that the urine contained sugar and that he would accept the case for treatment. The inspector sent his money, and Kaadt mailed his medicine. Analyzing the yellow-brown cloudy fluid, the Food and Drug chemist gave his verdict: it was essentially saltpeter—potassium nitrate —dissolved in vinegar. These ingredients were not only useless in treating diabetes; saltpeter, especially in the quantity prescribed by Kaadt, would irritate the gastrointestinal tract and the kidneys, already overworked in diabetes, and lead to the most serious complications.[8]

Saltpeter was no new ingredient in diabetes quackery. A central characteristic of the disease was the body's inability to utilize carbohydrates properly, leading to sugar excretion in the urine. Doctors had developed chemical color tests of the urine as an indication of the presence of diabetes and, when insulin was being used, as a clue to the effectiveness of the insulin dosage. The test was simple and impressive, and quacks turned it to their advantage. The trick was to fool the diabetic into believing that the nostrum was decreasing the sugar in his urine and thus promoting a cure. Diuretics increased the quantity of urine and also diluted it. This resulted in a lighter color when the test was made, even though the total amount of sugar excreted daily in the greater quantity of urine might be larger than before. The diabetic, believing from the evidence of his own eyes that he was better, might instead be worse. Ninety-five per cent of the quack remedies for diabetes, estimated the AMA's Dr. Arthur Cramp, were diuretics. Such was the action of saltpeter.[9]

If this form of deception was his intent, Dr. Kaadt did not hint at it in his literature. Indeed, he rather frowned on testing the urine for sugar. "It would be better for you," he had

---

[8] Information furnished by Post Office Dept.
[9] *N&Q*, II, 183-84; III, 42, 44; Cramp, "Some Diabetes 'Cures' and 'Treatments,'" *Hygeia*, 13 (1935), 916-20.

written a patient some years before, "so long as you are feeling good not to have any tests made as it only puts you on the wrong track and will interfere with you getting well." Still and all, his medicine contained a great deal of saltpeter.[10]

Dr. Kaadt did not subscribe to the orthodox explanation of diabetes, that the "islands of Langerhans" in the pancreas failed to produce enough insulin to regulate, in the liver and muscles, the use of carbohydrates derived from digested food. Instead he blamed the disease on digestive failure, the "faulty fermentation," mostly in the small intestines, of sugars and starches. This theory was fantastic, reported the FDA to the Post Office, so a citation was issued Dr. Kaadt's Institute to show cause why his venture should not be declared fraudulent and denied use of the mails. The Indiana doctor went to Washington.[11]

With Dr. Charles to the Post Office hearing went his brother, Peter Kaadt. Also a physician, Peter had received his medical degree from the Rush Medical College in Chicago in 1895. After some years of practice in the Midwest, he had moved to Portland, Oregon, where he had added to his doctoring the teaching of anatomy in a dental college. In 1938 Dr. Peter had temporarily left his practice to help Dr. Charles, whose health was not robust, and so was on hand for the three days of testimony before Post Office officials. The upshot was a stipulation —signed during the same week in which the new Food, Drug, and Cosmetic Act became law—in which Charles Kaadt avowed the complete discontinuance of any use of the mails to promote his home treatment.[12]

The doctor did not lock the door of his South Whitley Institute. He did, however, revamp his methods of doing business. He abandoned the mails as a method of communication and resorted to telephone and express. That is, he strove to do so. When money to pay for some of his turbid fluid reached him by letter, he mailed it back, advising the diabetic sender to

[10] *JAMA*, 97 (1931), 479.

[11] Kaadt pamphlet, *Of Great Interest to Diabetics*, in FDA file, Interstate Office Seizure No. 19-331H; information furnished by the Post Office Dept.

[12] *Ibid.*; the stipulation date was June 20, 1938. Biographical data on Peter Kaadt, *Transcript of Record*, 593-96, 635, 667.

place his order by phone and remit payment by express. This use of the mails to advise customers to use a differing route, postal authorities decided, was a violation of the stipulation. Dr. Charles was indicted and tried in a federal court in Fort Wayne.[13]

The need to prove fraudulent intent proved to be the stumbling block in the Fort Wayne courtroom. The government presented experts on diabetes to describe the hazardous unorthodoxy of the Kaadt treatment. A boy of 12 testified that Dr. Charles had never examined him, but had diagnosed and prescribed only by mail. To the father's worried inquiry, Kaadt had replied, "Your son is taking too much insulin!" Four days after receipt of this letter, the boy had collapsed from lack of insulin in a diabetic coma. Another witness, who testified from a stretcher, died of diabetes—unknown to those in court —while the prosecutor was engaged in summing up. But Dr. Kaadt's parade of satisfied users to the witness stand was also impressive. When the jury returned from their deliberations, they found that Dr. Kaadt was guilty on only one of the six counts in the indictment. The judge, partly on technical grounds, partly from persuasion, voided the guilty verdict and granted a motion for a new trial. "It is hard to conceive," he said, "that the defendant devised a scheme to defraud and had the intent to defraud in the face of these witnesses who honestly believe in the efficacy of the treatment."[14]

The new trial did not take place. Because of the death of witnesses and the expense a retrial would involve, the case was dismissed. Dr. Kaadt did not tempt fate by resuming use of the mails. He seemed, indeed, to grow more cautious than ever. Inquirers received a printed letter in which he frankly confessed that a Post Office Department ruling prevented his mailing the detailed information they had requested. "It is compulsory that I examine my patients," he wrote, "so if you can conveniently do so, and care to, come to the Institute."[15]

Patients came in such increasing numbers that Kaadt's brown-brick building could not hold them all for the three

[13] Information furnished by the Post Office Dept.
[14] Ibid.
[15] Ibid.; Indianapolis BBB Bull., Mar. 1947.

prescribed days of initial treatment. They scattered out into dozens of South Whitley homes, where housewives went into the room-renting business. As many as a hundred new patients arrived daily from all parts of the country. Such a patient load, even though each hopeful diabetic took but a brief span of Dr. Charles' time, was arduous, and the doctor was 70 and not in good health himself. In 1944 Dr. Peter closed down his Oregon practice and came to South Whitley to lend a hand.[16]

Peter could not help Charles evade the reckoning that was soon to come. In May 1946 a Pittsburgh physician, president of the American Diabetes Association, wrote a letter of complaint to the AMA. The Kaadts' counsel to diabetics, he said, was shocking and the results grim. He had records on 17 patients who had been treated at South Whitley, 12 of whom had later been admitted to hospitals as emergency patients in diabetic coma. Five of the 17 had died. This concrete evidence strengthened the resolve of officials of the Indianapolis Better Business Bureau. Long active in the crusade against quackery, the Bureau had been assembling a file on the brothers Kaadt. In June 1946 the BBB sent an investigator in the guise of a patient to the establishment—now called a Clinic—where he was interviewed so hurriedly by Dr. Charles that he was not even asked his name. Diagnosed as diabetic and sold medicine for home treatment, the investigator went straight from South Whitley to a reputable clinic. Tests showed, of course, that he did not have the disease.[17]

With such evidence in hand, the BBB petitioned the Indiana Board of Medical Registration and Examination for a revocation of Charles Kaadt's license to practice medicine. His methods of treating diabetics, the petition charged, amounted to "gross immorality" and violated the medical practice law.[18]

Long before a hearing date set by the Board, Dr. Charles had left the Clinic, never to return as dispenser of diabetic drugs and diets. He sought help for his own pernicious anemia at the Johns Hopkins Hospital and then went to Tennessee for further treatment. Peter stayed on in South Whitley. He closed the Clinic but, in the same abode, pursued a private

[16] Ibid.; Transcript of Record, 595.
[17] JAMA, 131 (1946), 251; Indianapolis BBB Bull., Mar. 1947.
[18] Ibid.

practice for diabetes sufferers. The nature of this practice was revealed by another undercover investigator, an observing reporter for the *Indianapolis Star*, who gave the citizens of Indiana a patient's eye view of what went on in the ex-Clinic.[19]

Robert Johnson, absolved by a specialist of having diabetes, showed up at the Kaadt establishment as Robert Cook. He told a waitress, who between meals took his personal history, that he had lost ten pounds in six months and that his mouth was dry. A nurse showed him where to put his two-a-day specimens of urine, although he was not questioned for diluting one specimen with tap water, another with shaving lotion. When he inquired as to his condition, a nurse who neither knew nor asked his name quickly responded: "Oh, you're just fine." Nor was he chided for failing to take the prescribed medicine with two of his meals.

Johnson was sent to a rooming house to spend the night. "They only keep those with gangrene or the blind ones at the institute," his landlady told him. His meals were eaten at the main building, where menus contained such sweets—taboo on strict diabetic diets—as ice cream, chocolate cake, and vanilla pudding. The medication beside each plate consisted of black pills and brown pills and a glass of the traditional Kaadt stand-by, a reddish brown acidy liquid.

"You just see . . . [Dr. Kaadt] once," a nurse told Johnson, "the night before you leave."

Johnson joined other patients outside Kaadt's office.

"Wait your chance," the nurse counseled, "and then just crowd your way in."

"Dr. Pete"—as his staff called him—looked "benevolent" to the reporter. Conservatively dressed, tall and erect, Kaadt had white hair, shell-rimmed glasses, "nobly large nostrils and a large mouth." His eyes told Johnson nothing but that the doctor was tired—another patient told the reporter that Kaadt had dozed off during their consultation. Kaadt's voice was "hoarse and petulant." After studying the reporter's history sheet and listening to his protest that he did not have

[19] *Transcript of Record*, 597-98. The *Star* series of seven articles appeared Sep. 10-16, 1946.

diabetes, the doctor said: "You probably have a mild case. You should snap out of it pretty soon if you watch your diet."

Then, despite the pretense of individual prescriptions for individual patients, Kaadt marked a diet sheet for Johnson to conform in every respect with all the others he had marked that day. And even though the reporter's take-home medication was stamped with individual numbers to show that it was only his, the prescription had been secured from the prescription room by a taxi driver in less than five minutes.

For his basic three-day treatment—board, room, medicine at meals, and a short conversation—Dr. Peter charged Johnson $30, plus another $30 for the 90-day supply of medicine taken home. Since patients were then coming and going at the rate of 50 a day, according to a nurse's estimate, Kaadt's daily gross was $3,000. A later calculation presented in court, based on the quantities of raw materials Dr. Peter ordered, placed the monthly gross at $60,000.[20]

At the ex-Clinic, Johnson had met patients from all over the country. Most of them, he felt, rather enjoyed being sick. But this did not excuse Kaadt, who had advised many true diabetics to cut down on their insulin. To patients seriously ill, Johnson wrote in the *Star*, South Whitley was a "profane Mecca." Diabetics were offering up "this gift of life, their insulin, to the easy glory of a medical entrepreneur."

Charles Kaadt was still in Tennessee when the Indiana Board of Medical Registration met to weigh the charges brought against him by the Indianapolis BBB. His lawyers first sought a postponement of the hearing, then permission for him to resign his license, but in vain. The BBB began to present its witnesses: Kaadt patients who had gone into coma after abandoning insulin for his $30 gallon jugs of vinegar-saltpeter mix—which cost him 90 cents. The evidence proved so incriminating that, before it was all given, Dr. Charles' attorneys threw in the towel. He would consent, they said, to a "cancellation" of his medical license "with prejudice," and would promise never again to practice in Indiana.[21]

[20] The $60,000 estimate was made by the district attorney in his summing up at the trial. *Indianapolis Star*, Apr. 15, 1948.
[21] *Indianapolis BBB Bull.*, Mar. 1947.

On the same day as these hearings, the Board began proceedings aimed at canceling the license of Peter Kaadt. Unlike his younger brother, Peter was still at work. Nor did he give in so easily. Peter fought the Board and, when he lost, appealed to a state circuit court and won. The evidence, the judge ruled, was insufficient to convict Peter of "gross immorality" in his medical practice. Thus Peter Kaadt was given a year's grace in which to continue prescribing saltpeter and vinegar, before the Indiana Supreme Court, early in 1948, reversed the circuit court, vindicated the Board, and forbade Peter to practice as physician within the state.[22]

"We feel," the Indianapolis Better Business Bureau had charged, "that the case of the Kaadt Diabetic Institute . . . involves by far the largest and most reprehensible operation of its kind in the United States." The denial of the Kaadts' right to practice medicine was an important victory. But was it enough? Officials of the Food and Drug Administration thought not. Armed with court decisions expanding the definition of labeling to make it seem broad enough to cover the Kaadt methods, the FDA had been gathering evidence for many months before the Indiana Supreme Court handed down its decision. Two weeks later, the Kaadt brothers and their Clinic superintendent were indicted on seven counts of violating the 1938 law. The case was tried in Fort Wayne during April 1948.[23]

It was no problem to establish that Kaadt's medicines had crossed state lines. Customers testified to receiving jugs sent from South Whitley, and an FDA inspector introduced in evidence a stack of waybills, with Dr. Charles' name as sender, demonstrating that both medicines and pamphlets—the labeling—had been shipped to various states by railway express.[24]

The main task of the United States attorney and his assistants was to persuade the jury that the Kaadt medicines were misbranded, that statements in the pamphlets were false and misleading in suggesting that the medicines possessed efficacy

[22] *Ibid.*, Mar. 1947 and Feb. 1948; *Indianapolis Star*, Mar. 28, 1947.
[23] *Indianapolis BBB Bull.*, Mar. 1947; FDA file, Interstate Office Seizure No. 19-331H; *Transcript of Record*, 1-28 (the indictment). The dates of the trial were April 5-14.
[24] *Transcript of Record*, 45, 94-95, 105, 132-33.

in treating diabetes. In one pamphlet Dr. Charles had offered "real hope" for the "possibility of recovery" through "a treatment, which is free from prolonged or continuous dieting, with internal medicine, taken by mouth, and without the necessity of absence from home, work, or business." The majority of patients, he wrote, resume "a normal diet within two or three weeks." Kaadt's dietary doctrines, according to another leaflet, included the view that "among the things most diabetics have been taught to avoid but which in many cases are beneficial are: ice cream, cakes and pies, milk and cream, all citrus fruits. Honey (clover or buckwheat only). In fact most anything that is made of sugar that has been *thoroughly cooked.*"[25]

That the Kaadts had followed these theories in practice was the burden of many witnesses. The South Whitley waitresses—as the *Star* reporter had observed—served diabetic patients with sweet desserts. There was even *uncooked* sugar on the table. Dr. Charles, before his retirement, had reiterated and expanded his dietary notions in lectures to his patients. One diabetic boy of 13, Leonard Schulist, had taken rough notes. At the trial, two years later, Leonard was asked to read the notes to the judge and jury.[26]

"Honey is best," he read. "You can use it. . . . You can . . . eat all you want. . . . Boiled sugar is safe. . . . You can drink whiskey. . . . It is good for diabetes. . . . Smoking does not affect diabetics in any way."

"Read it out louder," the boy was asked.

"No beer, positively. . . . Anger is bad for diabetics."

"Anger?" the judge asked.

"Yes," said Leonard, and continued puzzling out his notes. "Never be nervous. . . . All sugar that has been boiled can be eaten by diabetics. . . . Insulin is cause of bloating. . . . Not due to pancreas. . . . Not due to shock. . . . You should always have sugar in urine."

"Read that again," the district attorney said.

"You should always have sugar in urine . . . ," Leonard complied. "If you don't eat enough, you do still feel hungry,

[25] *Of Great Interest to Diabetics; Transcript of Record,* 5-12.
[26] *Ibid.,* 103, 134, and (for Leonard's testimony) 397-98.

eat more. . . . Don't ever get [a] blood sugar [test], it is dangerous. . . . The less insulin, the better. . . . No can go on diet, can't be done. . . . It is dangerous. . . . If you have one, throw it away."

Leonard had gone home from the Clinic and thrown his diet away, his mother testified, biting her lips to hold back the tears. He had also, on the advice of one of Dr. Kaadt's nurses, cut down on his insulin. Not long afterward, at a birthday party, the boy had eaten ice cream and cake.[27]

"In the morning," Mrs. Schulist said, "I went to call Leonard for school, and he appeared lazy and didn't care to get up."

"What did you do then?" the government attorney asked.

"I thought I would get him a glass of milk, and he began to throw up, and went back to lie down. So I thought I would let him miss school that day, which he never had done before; and in the afternoon he seemed to be more lazy and in a stupor, sort of. And my husband left for work, and he told me to call him if Leonard did not feel well. . . . I told him I would call him, but I didn't call. I saw Leonard was sleeping; I thought he would be all right. He was flushed. I knew something was wrong. I thought, well, I will wait until my husband comes home; he will know what to do."

"What happened then?"

"He began to breathe heavy, and just then, when my husband came, he said, 'Call his doctor.'

"I said no, no, because he is taking this treatment he is supposed to have some kind of reaction.

"He said, 'Take the urine test,' which I did. I got the solution which was given me [at the Kaadt Institute]. I said, 'It doesn't show anything. It is just like the urine would be if I didn't put anything in it.'

"He said, 'Put more solution,' which I did; he said, 'Put more urine in.' I did that. It didn't show anything.

"He said, 'Take the regular test.' So I took the Benedict and Clini-Test. They both showed he had an awful lot of sugar in his urine."

"Was Leonard taken to the hospital?" the district attorney asked.

[27] *Indianapolis Star*, Apr. 9, 1948; *Transcript of Testimony*, 391-92.

"Around one o'clock at night we called the ambulance, took him to the hospital immediately."

"Is Leonard taking the Kaadt treatment today?"

"No."

"Is he taking insulin today?"

"Yes, sir."

"How is he getting along today?"

"Wonderful. He is growing fast. He is brilliant in school."

Leonard's physician, Dr. William Lefevre, affirmed that it had been diabetic coma that had brought the boy unconscious to the hospital, that with the resumption of insulin and proper diet Leonard's diabetes was under good control. The doctor did not speculate on the damage that had been done during Leonard's lapse from the proper regimen.[28]

Dr. Lefevre was but one of a number of medical specialists, testifying for the government, who stressed that the abandonment of proper treatment was the most hazardous feature of the Kaadt advice. Dr. Henry T. Ricketts, head of the diabetes clinic at the University of Chicago, described for the jury in layman's language the disastrous chain of events unloosed when injections of insulin were stopped or reduced below the needed amount. Without insulin, he said, the diabetic cannot derive nourishment from any food containing sugar or starch. The sugar in the blood rises higher and higher and finally "spills over into the urine, like water going over a dam." Since the body cannot use starches and sugars, it must rely for heat and energy on proteins and fats. This is the reason that rapid weight loss is a symptom of diabetes. Eventually the breakdown of fats exceeds the body's ability to handle it. Acid by-products, especially diacetic acid and acetone, build up in the blood faster than they can be excreted through the urine. These acids, Dr. Ricketts testified, "are toxic; they poison the tissues of the body, and particularly the tissues of the brain; and the liver, and the kidneys." The diabetic patient "develops shortness of breath; he gets nauseated, he vomits; he becomes very dehydrated; he excretes large volumes of urine . . . ; and he goes into a stupor, and the stupor deepens into coma. Unless he is given insulin, he dies."[29]

[28] *Ibid.*, 377.    [29] *Ibid.*, 325-26, 331-32.

Some diabetics, especially older people, Dr. Ricketts stated, can control their disease by careful dieting without insulin. But if they break the taboos, they confront great danger. The hazard of a coma is always present, and less dramatic long-range complications—infections, cataracts, hemorrhages in the retina of the eye, deterioration of the entire vascular system— are certain to develop.[30]

The venerable Elliott Proctor Joslin of Boston, the nation's leading authority on diabetes, made the same point. A slight, balding man of great dignity, Dr. Joslin stood on the witness stand for two hours as he discussed the disease to which he had devoted half a century of research. Diet, exercise, and insulin, he said, were the proper treatment, and he added, "To say one word against following treatment straight through to the end, that is terrible; that is terrible."[31]

The Kaadts had gone further at South Whitley than to discredit the orthodox treatment for diabetes. For this treatment they had substituted Dr. Charles' medication. Government witnesses explained the irrelevance, the positive harmfulness, of the Kaadt approach.

What patients had taken home with them from the Clinic, Food and Drug chemists testified, were four things.[32] One was a ferric chloride solution for testing diacetic acid in urine. If the patient showed diacetic acid, Dr. Ricketts was asked, did that mean his diabetes was at a dangerous stage?[33]

"Yes, decidedly so," the physician answered. "It is the stage just before coma."

Could a patient—like Leonard Schulist—be a severe diabetic and not necessarily reveal diacetic acid at the time of using the Kaadt test solution?

"That is true. If people have disease of the kidneys it may be the urine will not contain diacetic acid, even though the blood contains large amounts."

The second item on the Kaadt prescription list was a vegetable laxative pill, the third an enzyme "Digestive Tablet."

[30] *Ibid.*, 330-34.
[31] *Ibid.*, 421-51; *Ft. Wayne Journal-Gazette*, Apr. 9, 1948.
[32] Testimony on FDA chemical tests, *Transcript of Record*, 171-230.
[33] *Ibid.*, 328.

Neither would help the diabetic, government witnesses said, and overuse of laxatives was a hazard in itself.[34]

Last and central in the Kaadt therapy was the liquid Dr. Charles had relied on for more than a score years, now slightly changed. A starch-digesting enzyme had been added, but to FDA chemists the $30 gallon jug consisted essentially of vinegar and saltpeter. Indeed, all digestive power of the enzyme was destroyed by the acid in the jug before it reached the stomach.[35]

As a treatment for diabetes, the government experts agreed, the Kaadt concoction was "of absolutely no value." Vinegar had no therapeutic purpose, testified an Indiana University biochemist, R. N. Harger, and saltpeter was the only active drug in an "incompatible" mixture. Even saltpeter, long used as a diuretic, had been dropped from that "druggists' and doctors' bible," the *Pharmacopeia,* as "practically valueless." There were positive hazards to its overuse, including "distress of the stomach and intestines . . . , irritation of the kidneys . . . , changes in the blood . . . , giddiness and nausea, and irregular heart action." Taking the Kaadt mixture as directed, Dr. Harger asserted, could well lead to a considerable overdose. In fact, the biochemist concluded, the whole Kaadt therapeutic system was "perfectly ridiculous."[36]

This same judgment was expressed by Dr. Barach of Pittsburgh, who had earlier raised the alarm in the *JAMA.* Nothing in the Kaadt treatment could help the diabetic state. "I would vouch for every member of our association," he added, "one thousand specialists in diabetes, that they would confirm what I have said."[37]

The government sought to establish that, despite the Kaadt avowal of individual prescriptions for each patient according to his need, each customer got the same kind of jug of vinegar and saltpeter mixed by guesswork in the same big barrel in the basement. Nor did Dr. Charles or Dr. Peter know many exact details about the ailments of their patients. A brief medical history, often taken by an unskilled employee, several urinalyses, a short conversation, did not add up to the

[34] *Ibid.,* 176, 221, 242-43.     [35] *Ibid.,* 174, 180-81, 218.
[36] *Ibid.,* 232-34, 238, 241, 262.     [37] *Ibid.,* 404.

"thorough examination" claimed in Kaadt promotion. Dr. Charles, indeed, had sometimes been curt.[38]

"When I got in there to Dr. Charles," one woman testified, "I tried to talk to him about my condition. He didn't talk at all about diabetes, or anything. He talked about his trip to Florida in an airplane."[39]

Case history testimony the prosecution presented with telling effect. Besides the sad tale of Leonard Schulist, government witnesses described for the jury, in all their shocking details, five other encounters between diabetic patients and the Kaadts. One witness, Eleanor Swanson, had, at the age of eight, forsaken for three years her doctor to place reliance in the Kaadts. She gave up insulin, ate pie and cake, and made nine trips from Cedar, Michigan, to South Whitley. Disaster came in the form of diabetic cataracts. Six operations had been required to remove the lenses from Eleanor's eyes. At one point in the testimony, she took off her thick glasses while the district attorney held up a glasses case 12 feet away. Eleanor could not see it; she could see the lawyer himself only as a vague outline. Never without her glasses, Eleanor's doctor testified, would the 14-year-old girl be able to see again. Never, he added, had he seen cataracts develop in a juvenile diabetic who was faithful to proper treatment.[40]

Two of the prosecution "witnesses" against the Kaadts were not present in Fort Wayne to testify, for they were dead. Their widow and widower spoke for them.[41]

Satisfied users who took the witness stand in defense of the Kaadts lacked the effectiveness of the prosecution's "injury" witnesses like Eleanor Swanson. They had no doctors to bolster their own assertions of remarkable recovery. And during cross-examination their evidence sometimes came close to backfiring. A retired furniture salesman credited the Kaadt treatment with improving his eyesight. "I always had used glasses," he said. "I can read and write without them now." But when a government attorney held objects 15, 10, and 5 feet from the salesman, he could not tell what they were. Another

---

[38] *Ibid.*, 57, 93, 109, 147, 151.     [39] *Ibid.*, 119.
[40] *Ibid.*, 293-94, 297; *Indianapolis Star*, Apr. 8, 1948.
[41] *Transcript of Record*, 353-55, 312-17, 321-25.

defense witness, a checking clerk in an automobile plant, credited $300 worth of Kaadt's medicine for his recovery from an aggravated diabetic state. "I haven't an ache or a pain," he said, "feel perfect." But a company doctor took the stand to show the jury a urine test given that very afternoon, revealing a four-plus urine sugar reading, dangerously high. The clerk's eye symptoms, moreover, were so suspicious, the doctor had already made an appointment with an eye specialist.[42]

None of the three medical witnesses presented by the defense was a diabetes expert. Neither, of course, was Dr. Peter Kaadt, and his testimony in his own behalf was one of the high points of the case. Dr. Charles sat the trial through, a small scrawny man, showing little interest in what went on, now and then placidly dozing. He had been very sick, he told a reporter, and could remember hardly anything.[43]

Dr. Peter spent hours in the witness chair. Tall, broad-shouldered, and erect, he sat with his glasses perched on his forehead, and answered questions in a slow, low, patient voice, constantly stroking his chin with the index finger of his left hand.[44]

When he took charge at South Whitley, Peter Kaadt said, he had eliminated some of his brother's practices with which he did not agree. He had ended the Clinic and engaged only in private practice. He had dispensed medicine only by individual prescriptions, and, unlike earlier procedure, had kept a file of prescriptions written. He had stopped prescribing by mail, accepting bed patients, and treating children. He had destroyed thousands of pamphlets, not because they were illegal, but because he "didn't like them from an ethical standpoint." He had played down the diacetic acid test, opposed alcoholic drinks, and treated insulin with more respect than had his brother.

Still and all, Dr. Peter believed in the efficacy of the therapeutic system which Dr. Charles had developed. He would

[42] *Ibid.*, 459, 467, 479-92, 701-705; *Ft. Wayne Journal-Gazette*, Apr. 9, 1948.

[43] *Transcript of Record*, 530-58, 575-89; *Ft. Wayne News Sentinel*, Apr. 13, 1948.

[44] *Ibid.*; *Indianapolis Star*, Apr. 13, 1948; Peter Kaadt's testimony in *Transcript of Record*, 593-679.

not flatly call it a "cure" for diabetes. "I have had patients," he told the judge, "who were apparently cured for three years after I had treated them. Now, whether you call that a cure, or not, I don't know."

Had he ever told a patient he could cure diabetes?

"Absolutely never; no; that is not an ethical thing. No honest physician would do that."

Dr. Peter's theory of diabetes was that the disease was "of nervous origin, because the sympathetic nervous system controls all of the secreting glands of the body."

"It can follow shock," he elaborated, "it can follow injuries; sorrow; people that have financial difficulties, or family troubles. . . . It is not only the pancreas, it is all of the glands of the body. The pituitary is invariably a factor. . . . Then, as I say, the thyroid gland, the adrenal glands, the sex glands, they are all involved.

"Now, when you have anything that causes a depressed condition through the sympathetic nervous system, all of the secretions are retarded, not only the islands of Langerhans, all the secretions of the liver, or the stomach, or the intestines, and the pancreas."

What it all seemed to boil down to came out in the cross-examination.

"Will you state," Dr. Peter was asked, "whether or not it is your belief diabetes is due to poor digestion and if you treat the patient for digestion you can restore him to health?"

"That has been my experience," he answered. "It is not only a deficiency of insulin; it is a deficiency of all the digestive secretions."

Both the acetic acid in the vinegar and the saltpeter, Peter Kaadt asserted, reinvigorated the digestive process by stimulating glandular secretions, although he admitted it was "rather difficult to explain" how. Most diabetics, he insisted, lacked hydrochloric acid in their stomachs, and the acetic acid could serve the same function of sparking "those alkaline glands that empty into the duodenum." The saltpeter, containing potassium, also replaced a deficiency in the body's potassium suffered by diabetic patients taking insulin. It performed this therapeutic function, Dr. Peter insisted, without harm. "I have never seen potassium nitrate have any poisonous effect," he said.

The standard treatment for diabetes was wrong, Peter Kaadt charged, the weighing of diets, the daily testing of urine. "And what does that do to the patient? It keeps them depressed. That is what we don't want to do. I tell my patients, 'Don't weigh your diet.' I don't even want them to examine their urine every day, by golly. I tell them I would rather they didn't do it at all, but if they want to do it every couple of weeks or so, that is sufficient."

Such were the incredible medical views of Dr. Peter Kaadt, who considered himself an expert on diabetes but thought it "questionable" that Elliott Proctor Joslin was. The prosecution's cross-examination was merciless. Peter was forced to admit that he was a member of no medical society, that, indeed, his license to practice had been revoked. He had written no paper on diabetes, performed no animal or clinical research. Ideas presented in his direct examination, he had to agree, conflicted with ideas expressed at the Post Office hearing and in his testimony before the state medical board. Claiming expertness in diabetes, he could not define some of the elementary terms. He did not know how many calories there were in a gram of carbohydrate, or in a gram of protein, or in a gram of fat. "Oh, we don't pay much attention to calories," he testified. "I don't think that is of any consequence." He admitted he did not know how to make a blood sugar test, or a glucose tolerance test, or a test for basal metabolism.

It was a devastating performance, and Peter Kaadt left the witness stand, wrote a reporter, "apparently near breakdown."[45]

In the summing up, a defense attorney called the Kaadt brothers "modern-day Christopher Columbuses," and compared them with history's misunderstood scientists—Lister expelled from the London medical society, Pasteur stoned in the streets of Paris. A more apt comparison, replied a district attorney, was with the witch doctor. The monuments erected to the Kaadts, he said, were "all in the form of tomb stones." "Christopher Columbus," another government lawyer ob-

[45] *Indianapolis Star*, Apr. 14, 1948.

served, "didn't lose his sailing license for gross immorality in sailing a ship." And bitter reference was made to $30 a jug and 30 pieces of silver.[46]

The jury found the three defendants guilty on all counts, recommending leniency for the Clinic superintendent. A mistrial had been narrowly averted only because the foreman, suffering an attack of angina, bravely remained at duty until the jury agreed. When the verdict was read, the Kaadt brothers "sat as if dazed, unbelieving." Peter "half rose from his chair, then slumped back again."[47]

The sentencing came three weeks later. Charles Kaadt walked into the courtroom, but Peter, who had suffered several heart attacks since the trial, was wheeled in on a hospital cot, where he lay motionless under a pink spread. "These men . . . ," their lawyer pleaded, "have reached the winter of life, if not the closing days of life. They have no previous conviction and if ever defendants deserved the utmost consideration, I submit, Your Honor, it is these men."[48]

Judge Patrick T. Stone—who had also presided over the Marmola trial—was not completely unmoved, but he remembered other unfortunates who had appeared in the courtroom during the trial.

"It has taken years of effort on the part of the United States Attorney and the Food and Drug Department," he said, "to bring you defendants to the bar of justice, to answer for your crimes. The proof submitted to the jury as to your guilt was overwhelming. I am satisfied that for many years you have engaged on a wide scale in a sordid, an evil and a vicious enterprise, without the slightest regard or consideration for the patients that consulted you, seeking relief from diabetes. These patients were innocent and hopeful, but so gullible. They poured out to you their savings, hoping and believing that you would cure them of their ailment.[49]

"And the striking thing about it is that all the time these defendants operated this institution they knew there was no cure for diabetes; they knew the only treatment for diabetes

[46] *Ibid.*, Apr. 15, 1948.
[47] *Transcript of Record*, 720-21; *Indianapolis Star*, Apr. 15, 1948.
[48] *Ft. Wayne News Sentinel*, May 4, 1948; *Transcript of Record*, 725.
[49] *Ibid.*, 725-26.

was insulin and a restricted diet, free from sugar. Yet, notwithstanding that knowledge, in their avarice and greed for wealth, they wrongfully advised these trustful patients, and, as a result, they suffered permanent damage and injury, and some have gone to an early grave.

"You have brought disrepute to your profession, disgrace and dishonor to you and your family. . . .

"If these men were younger men, I would not hesitate to impose the maximum sentences possible in this case. I shall give to them something they withheld from their patients, that is, just a little human consideration for their condition of health."

So, instead of the seven-year sentences they might have received, Charles and Peter Kaadt were each fined $7,000 and sent to prison for four years. It was indeed the winter of Dr. Peter's life. Released because of illness before his prison term was over, he died in 1951. Dr. Charles served out his term and died in 1957. An effort by Peter's wife to continue a surreptitious distribution of the medicine was cut short by her accidental asphyxiation in a motel. Even to the end Kaadt disciples had been pitifully faithful to the infamous vinegar-saltpeter mix.[50]

[50] *Ibid.*, 726-27; DDNJ 2578; *Indianapolis Star*, Feb. 8, 10, 24, 1949; FDA file, Interstate Office Seizure No. 19-331H; *Ft. Wayne Journal-Gazette*, Dec. 27, 1948; Oliver Field, AMA, to author, Jan. 5, 1961. The Kaadts had appealed the district court verdict and lost in the circuit court. U.S. v. Dr. Charles F. Kaadt and Dr. Peter S. Kaadt, 171 Fed. (2d) 600, in Kleinfeld and Dunn, *Judicial and Administrative Record, 1938-1949*, 388-93.

# 11

## THE GADGET BOOM

*"To call this a radio, you might as well call it a cat."*
—TOBIAS G. KLINGER, ASSISTANT DISTRICT ATTORNEY, IN HIS
SUMMING UP, UNITED STATES OF AMERICA V. RUTH B.
DROWN, 1951[1]

IN early April of 1948, Mrs. Marguerite Rice of Blue Island, Illinois, observed that a small lump had formed in her right breast. Very disturbed, she went to see her family doctor. He gravely told her that the lump might be cancerous and urged an immediate trip to the hospital so that a biopsy might establish an accurate diagnosis. But Mrs. Rice did not go. She telephoned her husband, an engineer and vice-president of a suburban corporation, who was in California on business. In a day or so Rice and his wife talked with each other again. He agreed with her decision to stay away from the hospital. There might not be need to go. "I [have] found," he said, "a new miracle."[2]

The miracle was a "Radio Therapeutic Instrument" that banished the need for operations, which Rice had heard about from a business friend. Its inventor was a Dr. Ruth B. Drown, whose laboratories were in Hollywood. Rice phoned for Mrs. Drown and learned that she was temporarily in Chicago. As soon as he got back home, Rice took his wife to Mrs. Drown's hotel for consultation.[3]

Mrs. Drown was a brisk, commanding woman in her mid-

---

[1] Transcript of testimony in the case of U.S.A., Plaintiff, vs. Ruth B. Drown, an individual, Defendant, in the U.S. District Court, Southern District of California, No. 21639-Criminal, p. 1036. This typewritten document, in the FDA archives, is cited below as "Drown transcript."

[2] FDA file on Drown Radio Therapeutic Instrument, Interstate Office Seizure No. 60-624K, FDA Records, Washington; Drown transcript, 50-51.

[3] *Ibid.*, 37-40.

50's, with angular features and a contralto voice. Learning from the Rices the disturbing reason for their visit, she took a drop of Mrs. Rice's blood upon a small piece of blotter and placed the blotter in the slot of a small black box. After twisting a series of knobs on top of the box, while rubbing her finger across a rubber plate, Mrs. Drown told the Rices what her diagnosis revealed. The lump in Mrs. Rice's breast was not a cancer, but was caused by a fungus growth that had spread through the digestive system to the liver. Moreover, Mrs. Rice was suffering from gall bladder trouble, a kidney that had ceased to function, and a deficiency of hydrochloric acid. These maladies were capable of cure within five months, Mrs. Drown said, by means of her Radio Therapeutic Instrument. She suggested that Mrs. Rice go for treatment to a Chicago doctor, Findley D. John, who used this instrument in his practice. For this encouraging counsel, Rice gave Mrs. Drown a check for $50.[4]

Daily Mrs. Rice made the 20-mile journey from Blue Island into Chicago for treatment at Dr. John's office. His therapeutic device looked much like the diagnostic device in Mrs. Drown's hotel room. Two wires ran out from the machine, each with a metal electrode at the end. On one of these Mrs. Rice was directed to place her feet; the other she put upon her stomach. After several weeks of treatment—costing $200—Mrs. Rice found the daily journey too taxing to continue. She need not keep coming, Dr. John informed her. "Just stay at home," he said, "and we can treat you by radio wave. That's what's wonderful about the Drown machine; it's just as effective when the patient is miles away as when he or she's here."[5]

So Mrs. Rice stayed at home, and Dr. John, with a drop of her blood on blotting paper, continued the treatments by remote control. When Mrs. Drown again visited Chicago, she confirmed her first diagnosis and urged the need for continuing therapy, expensive though it was. A month later, with a new bill of Dr. John's for $350, Rice wondered if it might not be cheaper to own his own machine. Again in California, he went to the Drown Laboratories and, for $423.07, bought a Drown Radio Therapeutic Instrument, which he took back on

[4] *Ibid.*, 8; FDA file 60-624K.    [5] *Ibid.*; Drown transcript, 25.

the plane with him to Illinois, along with an "atlas" of "rates," or dial settings, for his wife's ailments.[6]

So Mrs. Rice, with a black box in her own home, followed directions carefully, setting the nine dials as specified and spending many hours with her feet on the metal plate at the end of one wire, the other electrode on her stomach. When not giving herself direct treatment, she engaged in distant therapy, clamping her blotter with blood between the electrodes. Thus she was able to sleep and to do her shopping, while the Drown instrument operated 24 hours a day.[7]

Despite such fidelity, Mrs. Rice's health did not seem to improve. After four months of home treatment, she communicated her anxiety to Mrs. Drown. Back came another assortment of dial settings, determined by a Hollywood–to–Blue Island diagnosis made possible by the dried drop of Mrs. Rice's blood in Mrs. Drown's machine. Writing to thank Mrs. Drown for the new numbers, Rice sought new reassurances. "Does the checkup show any improvement . . . ?" he asked. "There is a new lump forming in the breast. Does this show in your checkup? Is there any indication that cancer is present?"[8]

The reply was prompt. There was "improvement indicated," wrote Mrs. Drown, and the new lump was "congested lymphatic." Mrs. Rice's "condition has never been cancerous but any lump can cause it if let go long enough without proper treatment." Mrs. Drown would "do all I can but Mrs. Rice must realize if she's to get well she must swing her attention on to the work and put every effort forth. . . ."[9]

It was hard to pursue therapy more zealously than 24 hours a day. But Mrs. Rice persevered for three more months. The Drown treatment, however, seemed to do no good. Indeed, the breast condition seemed definitely worse. Rice phoned to Hollywood for counsel. "We suggest," came Mrs. Drown's reply, "that Mrs. Rice have the breast removed if she feels that she is not getting hold of the trouble with our treatment. She can treat the condition afterwards on the instrument."[10]

This was the first intimation from Mrs. Drown during the

[6] *Ibid.*, 8, 10, 13, 24; FDA file 60-624K.
[7] Drown transcript, 24-27.  [8] *Ibid.*, 16-18; FDA file 60-624K.
[9] Drown transcript, 17-18.  [10] *Ibid.*, 18-19.

year and a half of Mrs. Rice's treatment that a malignant condition might exist. To the Rices this realization was shocking enough in itself. Its dreadful import was driven home with devastating force by a new factor. Simultaneously with the arrival of Mrs. Drown's letter came a condemnation of the Drown instrument in the *Chicago Tribune* as unmitigated quackery.[11]

Frightened and angry, the Rices sought medical attention in New York City. Before going east, however, Rice got in touch with the Bureau of Investigation of the American Medical Association and told of his wife's experience with Mrs. Drown. The AMA notified the Chicago office of the Food and Drug Administration, which immediately sent an inspector to talk with the Rices.[12]

This was by no means the first time the FDA had heard of Ruth B. Drown. For a number of years the agency had been concerned about her gadgets and others of similar ilk. Device quackery was ancient in America, but not until the 1938 law did the FDA secure authority to act against it. From early days, stretching gadgets had been marketed to increase height, compressing gadgets to remold breasts, fumigating gadgets to cure catarrh, skull-capping gadgets to restore hair. The main currents of device quackery in American history, however, had flowed from electromagnetism and electricity. This began in the late 18th century amid public curiosity over such enterprises as Mesmer's therapeutic seances in Paris and Franklin's kite experiments in Philadelphia. Dr. Elisha Perkins of Connecticut produced the first widespread mania with his metallic tractors, "gleaned up," said his state medical society in ousting him, "from the miserable remains of animal magnetism." It was Perkins' theory that his small gold and silver points—the first medical item patented under the Constitution—would, when stroked across the body, draw off a noxious electrical "fluid" which accumulated in the tissues and caused disease.[13]

Some of Perkins' many successors also sought to heal by

[11] *Ibid.*, 53; FDA file 60-624K; *Chicago Tribune*, Aug. 4, 1949.
[12] FDA file 60-624K.
[13] Young, *The Toadstool Millionaires*, 16-31; Jacques M. Quen, "Elisha Perkins, Physician, Nostrum-Vendor, or Charlatan?," *Bull. Hist. Med.*, 37 (1963), 159-66.

# THE EVOLUTION OF A LABEL

How the manufacturers of Swamp Root found it necessary to eliminate the grosser falsehoods from their labels when the Food and Drugs Act went into effect.

The British labels of to-day are practically the American labels of six years ago!

Here are the British and American labels of 1912. *Compare them.*

## AMERICAN LABELS

## BRITISH LABELS

Falsehood 1
Falsehood 2
Falsehood 3
Falsehood 4

Falsehood 5
Falsehood 6
Falsehood 7
Falsehood 8
Falsehood 9
Falsehood 10
Falsehood 11
Falsehood 12

" I might say that it [Swamp Root] consists chiefly of sugar and water colored with caramel...."
— *Dr. L. F. Kebler, Chief of Div. of Drugs, Department of Agriculture.*

Therapeutic claims on proprietary medicine labels grew more restrained under the impact of the 1906 law. This American Medical Association poster shows how. See ch. 3. Food and Drug Administration photograph no. 88-GS-1 in the National Archives.

By fighting the government in the courts, the makers of Dr. Johnson's Mild Combination Treatment for Cancer won from the Supreme Court a verdict that the 1906 law did not apply to therapeutic claims on labels. This decision forced Congress to plug the loophole with the Sherley Amendment of 1912. See ch. 3. The medicines are FDA photograph no. 88-GS-4 in the National Archives; the advertisement appeared in *Park's Floral Magazine* [...]

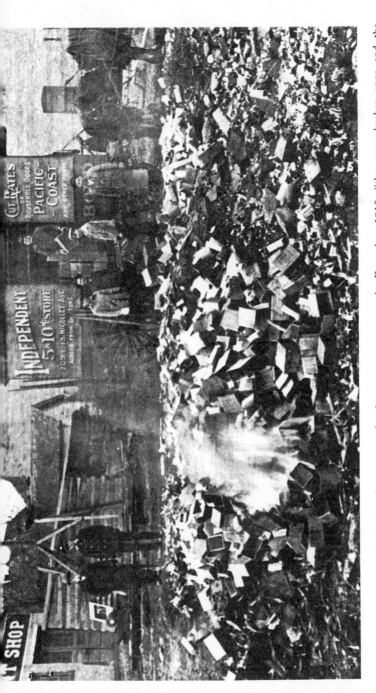

As a U.S. marshal, a food and drug inspector, and a fireman watch, 539 boxes and 322 cartons of Microbe Killer go up in flames, condemned to destruction by the court in the first seizure of a nostrum contested under the Sherley Amendment. "It was taken from the warehouse," the St. Paul inspector wrote in December 1913, "the cases broken open and the bottles and jugs smashed and the cases and cartons were burned." See ch. 3. Photograph in Bureau of Chemistry General Correspondence, Record Group 97, courtesy of National Archives.

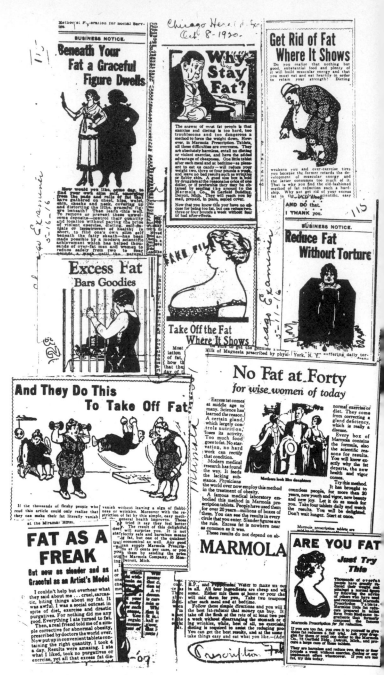

This montage of newspaper ads, from the AMA Department of Investigation files, extols Marmola, a reducing remedy that contained thyroid extract and thus posed grave danger to health. The Post Office Department, the Federal Trade Commission, and the Food and Drug Administration all went to court to try to curtail the hazard. See chs. 6 and 9. Photograph courtesy of AMA.

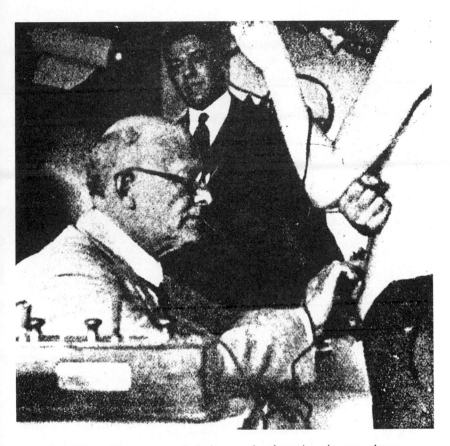

Dr. Albert Abrams, one of device quackery's major pioneers, shown "diagnosing a patient's condition from a blood specimen by means of resistances boxes and abdominal reflexes of a boy reagent." See ch. 7. This illustration appeared in the *Scientific American*, 130 (June 1924), 383, and is reproduced by permission of that journal.

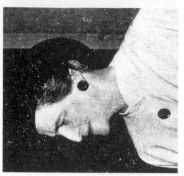

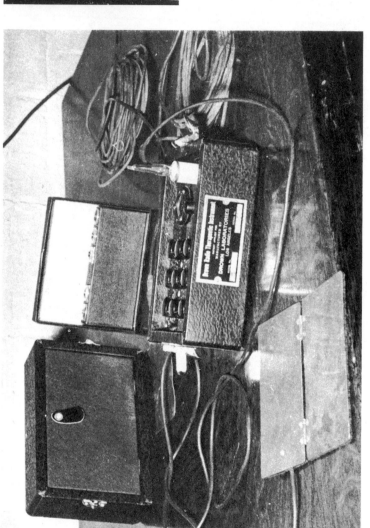

Mrs. Ruth Drown's Radio Therapeutic Instrument savored of the Abrams tradition. One witness at Mrs. Drown's trial for violating the 1938 law said she would trust the instrument to penetrate the Iron Curtain, should she be hurt in an accident in Moscow, to diagnose the extent of her injuries and send healing rays from Hollywood. See ch. 11. Both photographs courtesy of AMA, the one of Mrs. Drown from an undated *Journal of the Drown Radio Therapy.*

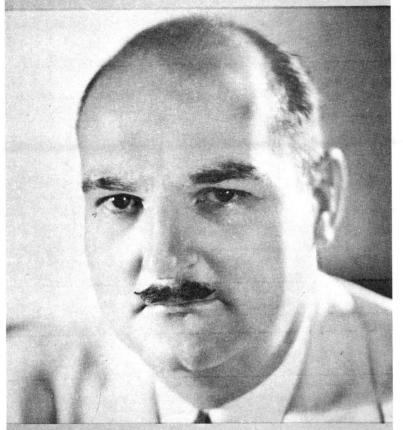

Hohensee was one of a host of nutritional lecturers who sought to
frighten Americans about the adequacy of their food supply and then
sell them special foods, vitamin supplements, kitchen gadgets, and
books of dietary advice. See ch. 16. Cover of a direct mail brochure
in the author's possession.

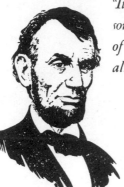

"It is true that you may fool all of the people some of the time; you can even fool some of the people all of the time; but you can't fool all of the people all of the time."

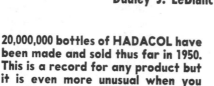

*"You were right, Mr. Lincoln,"*

says Senator Dudley J. LeBlanc

**20,000,000 bottles of HADACOL have been made and sold thus far in 1950. This is a record for any product but it is even more unusual when you consider that HADACOL is advertised in only 22 states.**

**Advertising has sold the first bottle of HADACOL to many folks; HADACOL is a very meritorious product and the results it has obtained have made possible the sale of these 20,000,000 bottles in 10 months.**

**Faith has been an important factor in the development of HADACOL — faith made possible its creation and the faith the American people have placed in my product has been responsible for its growth. I pledge to the American people that the faith they have placed in HADACOL will never be violated.**

**Truthfully,**

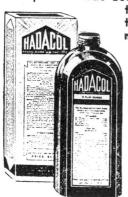

DUDLEY J. LeBLANC, President
THE LeBLANC CORPORATION

# HADACOL

Hadacol, promoted by Louisiana state senator Dudley J. LeBlanc, provided one of the gaudiest proprietary booms of the 20th century. Getting "right" with Lincoln was just one of LeBlanc's promotional stunts in behalf of his tonic. He also revived the old time medicine show and blew it up to gargantuan proportions. See ch. 15. This advertisement appeared in the *Atlanta Journal* for November 11, 1950.

getting bad electricity out of the body; others sought to cure by putting good electricity in. For a century and a half, the magnetic belt was vended to do the latter, mostly, in its many gaudy versions, aiming to restore "vital power" missing from middle-aged males. A "voltaic belt" of 1890 could do much more: besides improving health and posture, it could comb the hair, press the clothes, and promote a luxuriant mustache —all in 30 days. These belts were joined by countless other items of therapeutic apparel circling the human frame— electromagnetic wrist-bands, cravats, anklets, elbow pads, necklaces, head-caps, corsets, all sold with claims that their electrical input would cure dread ailments.[14]

As the utility of electricity became more stunningly apparent to Americans during the ongoing Industrial Revolution, so too did the utility of electricity increase for quacks. Pill-pushers appropriated the names of both telegraph and telephone. And schemers with a modicum of mechanical skill built gadgets of increasing complexity, appropriating the glamor of those amazing but mystifying machines which Edison and other inventors were introducing.

One of quackdom's early Edisons was Hercules Sanche, who marketed first the Electropoise and then the Oxydonor. Each was a sealed metal cylinder, and to one end was attached an uninsulated flexible cord ending in a small disc, to be attached to wrist or ankle with an elastic band. "The Electropoise," Sanche said, "supplies the needed amount of electric force to the system, and by its thermal action places the body in condition to absorb oxygen through the lungs and pores." The main difference between the Electropoise and the Oxydonor was that the latter cost $35 instead of $10. Their commercial success bred countless imitators, one of them the Oxypathor. This gadget merits an honored place in the history of anti-quackery, for in 1915, after a long and hotly contested legal battle, the Post Office Department had won a criminal fraud case against its maker, the first victory against a quack

[14] Gerald Carson, *One for a Man, Two for a Horse* (N.Y., 1961), 33-35; *Printers' Ink: Fifty Years, 1888-1938* (N.Y., 1938), 84; *A Treatise on the Application of John M. Tesch & Co.'s Electro-Magnetic Remedies* (Milwaukee, 1866); Boston Electro-Pathy Institute broadside, 1859, in the American Antiquarian Society.

device, offering the hope of at least some control over outrageously fraudulent gadgets if promoted by mail.[15]

Do-it-yourself healing, however, although a large-scale enterprise, came to be overshadowed in the mechanical device field
by a system wherein practitioners manipulated the gadgets.
Reputable medicine, as the 20th century proceeded, turned
more and more to diagnostic and therapeutic instruments, and
so too did quackery. By 1915, when the Oxypathor case was
won, Albert Abrams had already entered upon his fabulous
career. In the decades that followed, it was Abrams' imitators
and heirs—Ruth Drown among them—who constituted the
most significant school of device quackery in the nation.[16]

Device quackery preyed on the same widespread credulity,
fear, and desperation which permitted all other forms of
quackery to flourish. Gadgets could possess certain kinds of
persuasiveness denied to drugs. One was the power to shock.
A New York "clinic" early in this century treated young men
who were led to believe they might be suffering from syphilis
or the dire consequences of self-abuse. The patient sat naked
upon a sort of toilet throne, his bare back resting against a
metal plate, his scrotum suspended in a whirling pool. The
plate and pool were linked by wire to a battery. No frightened
sufferer could question the rigor of this therapy. Further,
gadgets could appeal to several of the senses. The Violetta,
vended as useful in 86 ailments, ranging alphabetically from
abscess to writer's cramp, impressed itself simultaneously
upon the hearing, seeing, smelling, and feeling of its user. A
small, high-voltage generator, ionizing the air in a hollow
glass head, the Violetta buzzed and crackled, produced a
bluish glow, exuded ozone, and with its sparks tingled and
warmed the skin.[17]

Devices permitted quacks to display their customary ambiv-
alence toward orthodox medicine. Relying for impressiveness

[15] N&Q, I, 295-301; II, 706-13.
[16] On Abrams, see above, ch. 7; K. L. Milstead et al., "Quackery in
the Medical Device Field," in *Proceedings, Second National Congress
on Medical Quackery* [1963] (Chicago, 1964), 30-39.
[17] Champe S. Andrews, *A Century's Criminal Alliance between Quacks
and Some Newspapers* (N.Y., 1905), 7-8; Violetta folder, AMA Dept.
of Investigation. The author has a working Violetta model in his possession.

in part on the alleged kinship of their gadgets to known and respected instruments like the x-ray and the electrocardiograph, quacks also promoted their machines at the expense of reputable medicine by boasting of their druglessness. A public uneasy about huge doses of calomel, which might cost them teeth and even jawbones, as in America's "heroic age" of medication, a public disturbed about thalidomide, as in the mid-20th century, paid heed to the bragging of the drugless healer. "Electricity," he said, ". . . will do more for you than all the drugs ever compounded."[18]

In the year that Abrams reached his ascendancy, Sinclair Lewis noted in a novel, "[Babbitt] had enormous and poetic admiration, though very little understanding, of all mechanical devices."[19] Whatever special advantages device quackery might have, its fundamental force has come from the combination of admiration and incomprehension that so many Americans have shared with Babbitt. Here in the heartland of mechanization, equipment of enormous complexity, with flashing lights and wiggling dials, could send voices through the air, direct accumulating cars through an assembly line, detect and shoot down planes. Why not also cure disease?

The end of World War II saw an upsurge of device quackery. Radar and television excited public interest. Onto the market poured a vast quantity of surplus electrical equipment, easy to get and cheap for fashioning into awesome contrivances. The Food and Drug Administration, ending its wartime responsibilities, was closing in on some of the major areas of drug quackery, using its new powers under the 1938 law, thus prodding some quacks to try machines. Concerned also about mechanical devices, the FDA found many of them hard to attack, since many of the most insidious—like those of Mrs. Drown—were in the hands of chiropractors, osteopaths, and M.D.'s licensed by the states. The right of a licensed practitioner to determine what therapy was best for his patients was not one to be transgressed lightly, and this legitimate safeguard for the reputable physician was shielding many licensed "quacks."[20]

[18] N&Q, II, 721.   [19] Lewis, Babbitt (N.Y., 1922), 68.
[20] Central District annual report, 1946; Los Angeles Station annual

Mrs. Rice's sad circumstances gave the FDA an opportunity it had long been looking for. Up to this point officials had not been able to launch a case against her Radio Therapeutic Instrument, first of all, because Mrs. Drown had made changes in successive models. A seizure action might encounter difficulty in court if the model seized was different—even slightly and irrelevantly different—from the model in production. Also, so tightly knit was the circle of Mrs. Drown's disciples that the task of seizing an instrument that had traveled in interstate commerce was hard to accomplish. Practitioners using the device in their practice were understandably not cooperative with agents from the FDA. Disillusioned and chastened, the Rices were willing to let their experience be used for the protection of others, even at the cost of placing their most private misfortunes upon the public record. They permitted the FDA to seize the black box, so ill-fated for them, and the various brochures, diagnostic charts, and letters which constituted its labeling. The FDA filed a libel against the Radio Therapeutic Instrument, charging that it was misbranded. Mrs. Drown did not contest the action, and the court condemned the device. The FDA continued assembling data that might permit a criminal action against the box's maker.[21]

The AMA had also known of Mrs. Drown before Rice came to relate his terrible tale. As early as 1941 a warning had appeared in the *Journal*. Rice's story caused the AMA to send a physician to interview Mrs. Drown when next she came to Chicago. There he met another woman, prominent in the city's social and educational circles, a devoted champion of the Drown approach to health. But none of his looking and listening persuaded the doctor that Mrs. Drown's ideas or apparatus possessed the slightest therapeutic value. The AMA undertook to oust from membership M.D.'s—like Dr. John—who employed the Drown gadgetry and to call into question the licenses of Drown practitioners in Illinois.[22]

report, 1947; Western District annual report, 1948, FDA Decimal file .062, Federal Records Center, Alexandria; Div. of Regulatory Management annual report, 1952, FDA Decimal file .053, HEW storage, Washington.

[21] FDA file 60-624K; DDNJ 3059.

[22] *JAMA*, 116 (1941), 888-89; Drown file in AMA Dept. of Investiga-

Sorely tried, with worse expected, Mrs. Drown consented to engage in an amazing trial by ordeal. She agreed to demonstrate the power of her medical machines before the assembled scientific talent of the University of Chicago. Mrs. Drown may have entered upon the venture with reluctance; certainly the Chicago scientists did. Neither party had much choice. Urging Mrs. Drown to the test was her influential pro tem champion, the woman with whom the AMA investigator had visited at the hotel. She was a member of the University's cancer board, hopeful that a vindication of Mrs. Drown's devices by reputable scientists would serve suffering humanity. University administrative officials, including Chancellor Robert M. Hutchins, also believed—although for different reasons—suffering humanity would profit by the test. The groundwork was laid by the eminent physiologist Anton J. Carlson, so often an expert witness for the FDA. A committee of physiologists, surgeons, physicians, photographers, and radiologists conducted the test, headed by Paul C. Hodges, professor of radiology. The professors insisted upon—and Mrs. Drown agreed to—the strictest of scientific controls and full publicity for all results.[23]

On the last day of 1949 Mrs. Drown sought to show the professors how her machine could take an x-ray by remote control. The husband of the woman who had arranged the test lay elsewhere in the city, recovering from a fracture in the neck of his left femur. A drop of his blood on blotting paper was present in the test room. Could the Drown machine use this blood to take a radio photograph of the state of healing in the hip? She tried. The results were poor, she admitted, probably because the machine was out of line and the developing and fixing chemicals had been improperly mixed. In one shot, however, Mrs. Drown claimed that she could make out the impacted fracture. The Chicago scientists could see no difference at all between the "successful" and the unsuccessful shots. The film images that impressed Mrs.

tion, especially Dr. F. T. Jung memo, Sep. 9, 1949; *Chicago Tribune*, Feb. 21, 1950.

[23] Mimeographed "Report of Committee Appointed to Investigate Claims of Mrs. Ruth Drown," in FDA file 60-624K; *Chicago Tribune*, Jan. 26, 27, 28, 1950.

Drown were "simple fog patterns produced by exposure of the film to white light before it had been fixed adequately."

That same afternoon, Mrs. Drown's diagnostic instrument went on trial. From ten patients whose state of health had been established, the Chicago scientists had extracted blood. As she had earlier done for Mrs. Rice, so now Mrs. Drown sought to do for the unknown: determine their ills. The procedure was protracted. During the entire afternoon she managed to accomplish only three diagnoses. The first patient, she asserted, after an hour of probing, was suffering from a cancer of the left breast which had spread to the ovaries, uterus, pancreas, gallbladder, spleen, and kidney; she was, moreover, blind in her right eye, not producing ova, and afflicted with reduced function of some 15 organs in her body. When the tedious test was over, Dr. Hodges reported the University's findings: the patient was, to be sure, a woman; her affliction was tuberculosis of the upper lobe of the right lung.

Mrs. Drown's second diagnosis was equally sweeping—and included improper functioning of both a uterus and a prostate! In fact, the male patient's principal complaint was severe high blood pressure. Mrs. Drown had termed that normal.

The third case, according to the Drown instrument, was especially grave, probably cancer of the prostate with spread to nearby organs and bones; prognosis was poor. According to Dr. Hodges, however, the patient was a healthy young male physician on the hospital staff.

After these "spectacular failures"—as the scientists' report termed them—Mrs. Drown proceeded to the third grim phase of the University of Chicago trials. Two anesthetized dogs, one a control, were placed on an operating table. A physician nicked the femoral artery of both dogs, then ligated the artery in the control animal. As blood from the test animal poured out over the table and onto the floor, the doctor predicted death within 10 to 15 minutes unless he likewise tied the artery or unless Mrs. Drown's hemorrhage control device, set up in the next room, fulfilled its promise.

"Mrs. Drown stood in the doorway watching her animal bleed," Dr. Hodges reported. "From time to time we asked whether she thought her experiment was working, and reminded her that she was the one to decide whether or not a ligature was to be applied." Finally she said to tie the artery. The "fiasco" was over. Mrs. Drown's erstwhile champion, who had arranged the tests, was "all but weeping."

Ruth B. Drown's next great trial came 20 months later in Los Angeles, in the United States District Court. Her misbranding of the device which Rice had carried back to treat his wife, the government charged, was a criminal violation of the 1938 law, since the Radio Therapeutic Instrument could not perform the healing miracles claimed for it. The list of allegedly false claims culled from Mrs. Drown's promotional brochures was long and bold. Her machine, she had asserted, would eliminate lumps in the breast and prevent cancer from them. It would also cure such divergent ailments and conditions as tipped uterus, an extra kidney, low function of the testicles of a six-year-old boy, heart trouble, loss of speech and memory, and on and on.[24]

Nor was there any truth, the government charged, in the theories advanced by Mrs. Drown to explain her alleged cures. Her instruments, she had written, "tune[d] into the human body on the same principle as the commercial radio tunes into sound." As Einstein had stated, the universe contained one common source of energy. And everything in the universe, according to the Drown gloss, had "its own individual rate of vibration"—each organ, each gland, even each disease. The Drown instruments, using the body's "electromagnetic force," could tune in on the glands and organs, assaying their functioning, determining disease, and healing. Mrs. Drown's therapeutic instrument directed the total body energy of a patient through the machine back to the diseased part at the same vibratory rate that had been discovered during diagnosis for the ailing organ. "This steps up the vibrations in that particular area. Through the process of metabolism constantly going on in the body, the new cells which form will come in at the higher or normal rate and the diseased cells will automatically fall away. . . ."[25]

[24] DDNJ 4029.
[25] *Ibid.*; Drown transcript, 13-16. Many of the statements were taken from a brochure, *The Drown Radio Diagnostic Therapeutic Photographic Instruments.*

All this, the government charged, was nonsense.

Mrs. Rice was not in Los Angeles to help the government present its case in a court room filled with Mrs. Drown's loyal supporters. By the time Mrs. Rice had stopped using the Drown device, her cancer was inoperable. She was now too weak to accompany her husband on his sad journey to California. As the first prosecution witness, Rice told the judge and jury of his family's misadventures with Drown therapy, of Mrs. Drown's promises that were not fulfilled.[26]

After this sobering prologue, the prosecution sought to show why, on scientific grounds, Mrs. Drown's gadgets could not diagnose or heal. A parade of experts, under the able questioning of assistant district attorney Tobias G. Klinger, challenged her claims and pooh-poohed her theories.

A radio engineer for the Federal Communications Commission, Robert J. Stratton, told the jury what the Drown device really was, taking the apparatus apart for their scrutiny. It consisted of a box, he said, with a bakelite panel for a top, which contained an entire electrical circuit of a very simple sort, a wire connecting two blocks, each of a different metal. The principle of galvanic action, Stratton said, had long been known; two dissimilar metals in contact with each other generate a very small voltage which registers on a sensitive microammeter inserted in the circuit, like that on the Drown device.[27]

"What would be the function of a human being," Klinger asked Stratton, "if he had the German silver on his solar plexus and the block tin . . . under his feet?"

"It would just complete the circuit," the engineer replied. "Just a piece of wet sponge could do the same thing."

The dial settings on the nine knobs, Stratton asserted, were utterly irrelevant. No more meaningful was the insertion into the slot of dried blood on a blotter: the slot was in no way linked to the galvanic circuit.

Was there any resemblance, the engineer was asked, between the Drown device and a radio?

Both devices contained wire, he answered. That was their

[26] Drown transcript, 20-63; FDA file 60-624K; Tobias G. Klinger, "Conflict with Quackery," *FDC Law Jnl.*, 8 (1953), 779.
[27] Drown transcript, 85-97, 239-65.

only similarity. Nor did Mrs. Drown's gadget send forth radio waves.

Stratton's testimony was buttressed by that of an atomic physicist, Moses Greenfield, professor of radiology at UCLA. There was nothing in Mrs. Drown's instrument, he told the jury, that could measure electrons or measure or pick up radio waves or radioactivity of any kind. Even for completing a galvanic circuit, Greenfield testified, a person was not very satisfactory. "The only difference," Greenfield said, "between using the human body and, let us say, a salt solution would be that the human body does a rather poor job and salt solution . . . a rather good job."[28]

The assistant dean of the University of Southern California Medical School, Homer C. Lawson, demonstrated with a compass that, despite Mrs. Drown's assertions, there is no magnetic field surrounding the human body. And he insisted that, despite her protestations, each gland in the human body did not possess its own peculiar individual atomic vibrations.[29]

Physicians, concerned more directly with the therapeutic than the electrical aspects of the Drown devices, continued the prosecution's attack. The machines were "perfectly useless," would do "no conceivable good," would be "laughable if . . . not so dangerous." So spoke Dr. Elmer Belt, urologist and member of the California Board of Health. The danger came, he said, in treating diseases such as cancer by "any hocuspocus method." Delay was "equivalent to writing a sentence of death for the patient."[30]

From the University of Chicago the government brought Dr. James W. J. Carpender, a radiology professor who had been present on the disastrous afternoon when Mrs. Drown had sought to diagnose three patients from three spots of dried blood and had three times failed. And from Chicago also came Mrs. Rice's current physician to tell the jury that the lump in Mrs. Rice's breast was still there.[31]

Mrs. Drown's defense against the prosecution's case began long before her first witness sat in the witness chair. It was implicit in the cross-examination of the physicists and physi-

28 *Ibid.*, 184-236.      29 *Ibid.*, 466-95.
30 *Ibid.*, 104-83.       31 *Ibid.*, 427-65, 274-75.

cians who testified against her. From Texas Mrs. Drown had brought a genial, chatty, easy-going attorney, E. B. Simmons, not inexperienced in suits involving chiropractors. What Simmons seemed to be about in his leisurely cross-examination was to impress the jury with the inexpertness of scientific experts and the misunderstood merit of Mrs. Drown. He strove to find gaps in the medical knowledge of the doctors on the stand and engaged in long excursions into medical history, asking physicians countless details about which they were understandably ignorant. When the court asked Simmons what he was seeking to demonstrate, the lawyer replied, "It would show this, that if . . . [the doctors] do not know much about their own profession, they might not know too much about hers."[32]

Simmons' history lesson had another aim, to furnish Mrs. Drown with honorable antecedents. Had there not been women of humble birth, Madame Curie, for example, who had made momentous scientific discoveries? Had there not been a long parade of notable scientists who had suffered ridicule and persecution from their scientific contemporaries, only to be vindicated in the future? Did not Dr. Faraday successfully perform an experiment in 1833 that Dr. Price had tried in 1783 before the Royal Society without success? "Even a chiropractor's demonstration"—as at the University of Chicago—"might fall flat, might it not?"[33]

Still through the medium of cross-examination, Simmons strove for other points: that the government witnesses had not used the Drown instrument for therapeutic purposes under the inventor's tutelage; that recognized principles of physics might be legitimately restated in Drownian terms; that Mrs. Drown's theories were not more farfetched or mysterious than those involved in getting a man's image on a camera film or a wireless photograph from Korea to New York.[34]

Nineteen of the defendant's patients—including several teachers—took the stand in her behalf, avowing marvelous cures or benefits from the Drown therapy in a whole host of diseases and conditions. One loyal supporter was Mrs. Patia

[32] *Ibid.*, 116, 147, 211-16, 312, 319-20, 392.
[33] *Ibid.*, 214, 479-80.   [34] *Ibid.*, 484, 221-32, 314-16, 450-55.

Power, who asserted that during World War II she had constantly given remote treatment to her Marine transport pilot son—Simmons' questions made it obvious that she meant Tyrone—and "in his over two years of service he never went to sick bay once."[35]

And no more fervent champion could any beleaguered practitioner have than Mrs. Eleanor Allen.[36]

"We don't call it 'a box,'" Mrs. Allen testified. "We call it 'an instrument,' an instrument played by a master artist."

She credited the instrument with saving her from pneumonia when she was in Atlantic City by healing rays aimed in her direction all the way from Hollywood. Should she be in a terrible accident, she said, in Moscow, the rays of the machine would penetrate the Iron Curtain, diagnosing the extent of her injuries and producing a cure. Mrs. Drown's device "is not black magic," her champion argued. "It is science."

Such was the ardent testimony of faith in Mrs. Drown presented in court by the chairman of the school board for Los Angeles.

Several defense experts—one M.D., two chiropractors, and the inventor of a helicopter—spoke in behalf of Mrs. Drown's theories, but none of the men still used her instrument professionally.[37]

As final witness for the defense, Mrs. Drown took the stand in her own behalf. Simmons led her along a long, long trail of autobiographical apologia.[38]

She had been born in Colorado, Mrs. Drown said, and had come to California in 1919. After a year of study at an osteopathic college in Missouri, she had transferred to the Los Angeles Chiropractic College, completing her degree and receiving a California license. Since then she had engaged in "extensive post-graduate work." Her interest in radiation dated from 1919, when she made a crystal radio.

"When I first was making the radio," she testified, "I was working for the Southern California Edison Company and

35 *Ibid.*, 500-841, Mrs. Power, 821-41.
36 *Ibid.*, 772-89.
37 *Ibid.*, 519-44, 555-601, 717-71.
38 *Ibid.*, 842-1027 for Mrs. Drown's direct testimony and cross-examination.

was then required to repair all of my machinery in my department. I had four years and a half of training of repairing machinery. . . ."

With this electrical background, Mrs. Drown said, she
learned of the intriguing views of Albert Abrams. She went to
the office of an Abrams-oriented doctor "and worked as a nurse,
first, and was studying diagnosing, and I diagnosed for four
doctors for two years, just experimentally, taking their cases
that were difficult to handle and learning as I went along."

Her own ideas began to diverge from those of her precep-
tors, she said, and in 1923 she began research in earnest, working "continuously." "My every day, my every night," she said,
"has been a study." At first she used her invention only to diagnose. Then she discovered, to her amazement, that she could
take photographs over long distances and also relieve disease.
Through 22 years, she had diagnosed or treated over 17,000
cases. She did not make claims to cure, as that was unethical.
But the only cases in which she had been unable to get results
were "when the patients came too late."

"I will ask you," Simmons questioned, "if in all the cases that
you have diagnosed and treated whether or not Mrs. Rice is
the first one who has ever complained?"

"In all the 22 years," the defendant answered, "she is the
first case that has ever been turned in against us."

Mrs. Drown was suspicious of the Rice machine that sat in
the courtroom. Even though the defense had stipulated it *was*
the instrument Rice had bought, Mrs. Drown thought it might
have been tampered with, or that there might have been a
switch.

At great length Mrs. Drown expounded on her therapeutic
theories, not forgetting to mention Einstein, and claiming
that her use of blood crystals for healing was cognate to radio,
television, radar, cosmic energy, and the Geiger counter.

What about the University of Chicago trial?

Well, in one of the cases the official report had stated that
Mrs. Drown had diagnosed a condition in the left lung. Dr.
Carpender had testified the same thing. But Mrs. Drown
insisted she had not said the left lung; she had said the right.

"And," Simmons asked, "have you ever said anything else?"

"Never."

"Other than it was the right lung."

"Never."

"Then when the doctor testified the other day that you said it was the left lung, was he right or was he wrong?"

"He was wrong."

And that was all about Chicago.

Mrs. Drown also left the impression through her testimony that applications she had made for patenting her devices were still pending in the Patent Office.

All in all, Mrs. Drown, in the defense image, was a scientist ahead of her time, honored here and there, but by and large as yet misunderstood, even hated, by the jealous members of the medical profession, whom she far transcended in her curative prowess. The government, using a single instance of dissatisfaction out of over 17,000 patients whom Mrs. Drown had served, was aiming its vast power at persecuting a benefactor of mankind.

To shatter this image was Klinger's task in cross-examination. He did so relentlessly, wielding the club of fact.

With respect to Mrs. Drown's alleged electrical experience as machine tester at the Southern California Edison Company, in what department had she in fact worked?

"I was in the addressing department."

At what institutions had she taken her intensive postgraduate study?

She did not mean that she had gone to college, but had engaged in self-study and taken courses at "every [chiropractic] convention that gave them."

Had she ever graduated from an osteopathic college or been granted an osteopathic license to practice?

No, she had not.

Then why had she said so in a sworn affidavit submitted to the Patent Office?

She did not remember. It had been written by her lawyer and she had no doubt signed it not realizing that he had mistakenly put "Osteopathic Physician" in it.

What instruments had Mrs. Drown sought to get patented?

"The photographic instrument was the only one they would let me apply on. . . . They deleted the treatment and diagnosing one . . . [in] 1935 or '36."

Then why was it that the treatment device sold Rice in 1948 bore a name plate including the phrase "Patent Applied For"?

"Most of our plates had them taken off, and if someone got that one, it was an old one and I know nothing about it."

"But that is the one that is in evidence, isn't it?"

"That evidently is. I don't even know. Someone broke into our place and I know nothing about what they got in it."

"It is stipulated to that that is the one Mr. Rice purchased from you."

"But I said I could not be sure, although the instrument was mine, that was the one he bought."

How had Mrs. Drown discovered that her instrument would treat as well as diagnose?

She described her first case dramatically, with a degree of detail she had been unable to summon up respecting the affidavit for the Patent Office.

Klinger then proceeded to point out, in the pages of one of Mrs. Drown's books, an entirely different case, designated as the first she had ever treated.

As merciless as the district attorney's cross-examination was his judgment on the result during his argument to the jury.[39]

"I would say that rarely has a person been so clearly demonstrated in open court to be absolutely untrustworthy, . . . willing to sacrifice truth for expediency. . . . How much more completely can the credibility of a witness be shattered and her testimony impeached?"

Nor was other defense testimony persuasive. User testimony, Klinger told the jury, is "notoriously unreliable, not because people wish to misrepresent the situation but because they do not know it, do not understand it. Just like any of us lay users of drugs . . . , they are not trained to observe, to note, to report scientific data." Referring to Mrs. Power's testimony that her Marine pilot son had avoided sick bay while

[39] *Ibid.*, 1030-59.

receiving remote treatment with the Drown device, Klinger said, "My brother was in the Air Corps for four years, with 30 missions over Berlin, and never has spent a day in the sick bay, and he did not need the machine."

There was, in short, no evidence to bolster Mrs. Drown's "mumbo-jumbo language" against the "spectacular failure" of the University of Chicago trials, "the whole unhappy story of Mrs. Rice," and the combined weight of prosecution scientists that "from every point of view" Mrs. Drown's Radio Therapeutic Instrument was "absolutely and totally worthless."

Lawyer Simmons, explaining the discrepancies in his client's testimony, said that Klinger had gotten "the poor woman confused." In his closing argument Simmons recalled his cast of mistreated scientists who were ahead of their time. But Columbus, Harvey, Semmelweiss, and Billy Mitchell could not help Ruth Drown. On September 24, 1951, after being out some seven hours, the jury declared her guilty.[40]

The case had cost the government, at a conservative estimate, some $50,000. Mrs. Drown's fine for violating the Food, Drug, and Cosmetic Act was $1,000. She appealed the verdict, but the circuit court affirmed the jury's judgment and the Supreme Court would not grant certiorari. While these judicial actions were in process, on November 17, 1952, in Chicago, Mrs. Marguerite Rice died of the cancer which Mrs. Drown's machine had not been able to diagnose or cure.[41]

Thereafter Mrs. Drown was careful to avoid distributing her devices in interstate commerce. She did not, however, cease practicing her pseudo-healing art in her own offices, adding to her total of patients treated through the years until it mounted to some 35,000 men and women. States continued to move with great caution against licensed practitioners who might be employing unethical machines. In 1963, after extensive investigation by the California State Bureau of Food and Drug Inspection, Mrs. Drown was indicted on charges of

[40] *Ibid.*, 1060-95, 1114.

[41] *Ibid.*, 1122; NJ 4029; Klinger, "Conflict with Quackery," 789; FDA file 60-624K. The circuit court decision was rendered Sep. 10, 1952, 198 Fed. (2d) 999, and is given in Kleinfeld and Dunn, *Judicial and Administrative Record, 1951-1952*, 165-71. The Supreme Court denied certiorari, Jan. 19, 1953. Mrs. Rice had died Nov. 17, 1952.

grand theft and attempted grand theft. She died, however, before her case could come to trial.[42]

Albert Abrams had numerous other heirs, and many imitators as well, whose Oscillitrons, Depolarays, Electropads, Neurolinometers, and Radioclasts have awed the ailing and done much mischief. Against their makers the Food and Drug Administration has fought an increasingly vigorous and successful war, to which a significant 1962 court decision has added impetus.[43]

To testify at one of the House committee hearings preceding the 1938 law—back in the days when Mrs. Drown was trying to get a patent—came one of Mrs. Drown's rivals in the medical device field, F. C. Ellis, inventor of the Micro-Dynameter. Ellis was better trained than Mrs. Drown, a graduate engineer from the University of Wisconsin. He had used his ability and expert training in industry and in the Navy. The professional engineer, Ellis told the Congressmen, has revolutionized society. "He wants to do everything on a measuring stick and get things down to a concrete basis where he knows what he is talking about instead of having it all rest on opinions." Physicians, Ellis said, possessed a few precise measuring devices, but not enough. Up to this point in his testimony Ellis sounded like an expert speaking within his realm of competence. Then he swerved off abruptly on a bizarre tangent.[44]

Entering the "virgin field" of medical machines, Ellis said, he had "found a simple instrument based on the very simplest of electrical laws, known and accepted by electrical scientists for hundreds of years." "We make the human body function as a simple electrical cell and measure the current it generates," Ellis explained, permitting diagnosis of virtually every ailment known to man.

[42] Milton P. Duffy, Chief, Bureau Food and Drug Inspections, California Department of Public Health, to author, Sep. 1, 1964; *Life*, 55 (Nov. 1, 1963), 78-81; John W. Miner, Head, Medicolegal Section, Office of the District Attorney, County of Los Angeles, to author, Oct. 20, 1966. Mrs. Drown died Feb. 12, 1965.

[43] Milstead, "Quackery in the Medical Device Field," 30-39.

[44] *Foods, Drugs, and Cosmetics: Hearings before a Subcommittee of the Committee on Interstate and Foreign Commerce, House of Representatives . . . on H.R. 6906 . . . and S. 5* (74 Cong. 1 ses., 1935), 499-505.

If seldom made before Congressional committees, the pitch was not unlike that of most electrical device entrepreneurs. By some quixotic break, a skilled engineer had been converted into a menace to mankind. Nearly three decades later, the Food and Drug Administration managed to win a landmark victory over the Micro-Dynameter. The machine which Ellis had invented, a court decided in 1962, "is not safe for use even in the hands of a licensed practitioner. A device whose labeling claims to be an aid in diagnosing as many diseases as this one, when in fact it is not, is unsafe for use no matter who uses it."[45]

The Micro-Dynameter decision has provided the FDA with a bigger club to swing against the fake machines. So Babbitt and the rest of us are better protected than we have ever been, should our awe and perplexity when faced with therapeutic instruments tempt us to the device quack's door. But we still are vulnerable, and hazard is still at hand. "Despite the success we have had in court in attacking device quackery," FDA Commissioner George Larrick stated in 1964, "so many fake gadgets are still in the hands of practitioners that if we set all of our inspectors at work on nothing else it would take several years to find and take successful action against all of these devices."[46]

Those who would use machines to steal the hope of life from people like Mrs. Rice are still around.

[45] U.S.A. v. Ellis Research Laboratories, Inc., 300 Fed. (2d) 550 (1962).
[46] George P. Larrick to author, Apr. 21, 1964.

# 12

## THE CHEMOTHERAPEUTIC
## REVOLUTION

---

*"When an untrue or misleading health claim is de-
liberately, fraudulently or pretentiously made for a food,
drug, device or cosmetic, this is quackery. . . .*

*"It matters not whether the quackery is practiced by
the witch doctor or the licensed medical practitioner;
the Indian medicine man or the pharmacist; the proprietary drug manufacturer or the prescription drug
manufacturer; . . . the health lecturer . . . [or] the
doorstep diagnostician . . . —it is still quackery."*

—DR. KENNETH L. MILSTEAD, 1963[1]

---

THE quarter century following the enactment of the Food,
Drug, and Cosmetic Act of 1938 witnessed a revolution in
the drugs which doctors prescribed for ailing patients. So vast
was it in scope, so significant in repercussions, this revolution
ranks as one of the major events in medical history. Its side
effects for self-medication were bound to be enormous.

That same sulfanilamide, whose disastrous mixing with a
poisonous solvent had led to the "new drug" provision in the
1938 law, heralded the day of miracle drugs. Sulfanilamide
fulfilled the hope of Paul Ehrlich, early in the century, for a
specific drug to combat bacterial infection. While important
discoveries had been made—insulin for diabetes, the use of
liver extract to treat pernicious anemia—efforts between 1915
and 1935 to duplicate the specificity of Ehrlich's pioneer anti-
syphilis drug had proved discouraging. The 1920's were "dol-

[1] Milstead, "Enforcement of Antiquackery Laws," *Jnl. Amer. Pharmaceutical Assoc.*, ns 3 (Sep. 1963), 458.

drum years" in chemotherapy. Many authorities spoke of the outlook as barren.[2]

But sulfanilamide, with its amazing ability to conquer various staphylococcal and streptococcal infections, renewed hope. Franklin Roosevelt, Jr., desperately ill with a "strep" infection, was given the drug and quickly recovered. In the previous decade, Calvin Coolidge's son, under similar circumstances, had died. Hundreds of Americans, like young Roosevelt, survived previously fatal infections when treated with sulfanilamide, a product of German and French research. Other sulfonamides followed in the years ahead, drugs so effective that the original sulfa became obsolete.[3]

With World War II came penicillin. In searching for drugs to combat infections in war wounds, British scientists turned back to the accidental discovery of Alexander Fleming in 1928. Fleming had observed that a common mold, contaminating his culture plate of staphylococcal germs, had killed the germs. But he had been unable to concentrate the beneficent lethal force exuded by the mold. In the early war years, Howard Walter Florey and his associates succeeded somewhat better. Growing the mold on broth in outmoded bedpans, they managed to isolate a very small quantity of penicillin for a clinical trial. In February 1941 a London policeman, gravely ill with an infection, was given the drug. He rallied remarkably, but the drug supply ran out. The patient relapsed and died. New supplies of penicillin, tediously prepared, proved, with children, the drug's lifesaving potency. Florey came to the United States, seeking help in getting penicillin mass-produced.[4]

Major American pharmaceutical manufacturers were ready for this challenge. Their own growing research potential had been quickened by the demands of the 1938 law's "new drug" requirements. Research staffs were expanding to provide the safety data demanded by the Food and Drug Administration before it would permit a new drug to be marketed. Know-how was increasing with respect to synthetic techniques and pro-

[2] Shryock, *The Development of Modern Medicine*, 438-39.
[3] Donald G. Cooley, *The Science Book of Modern Medicines* (N.Y., 1963), 19-21.
[4] *Ibid.*, 22-24.

duction methods. Under governmental sponsorship, a crash program succeeded in making penicillin cheaply and in large quantities. From 29 pounds produced in 1943, the output expanded until sufficient supplies were available for the Normandy landings of the Allied invasion forces. During the war, as Austin Smith, a president of the Pharmaceutical Manufacturers Association later observed, the American pharmaceutical industry came of age.[5]

In the postwar years penicillin, first isolated and then synthesized, was made by the hundreds of tons. Penicillin was followed by other antibiotics, by anti-malarials, synthetic vitamins, new and improved vaccines, steroid hormone-like compounds, antihistamines, tranquilizers, and other potent therapeutic agents. Dickinson W. Richards, a Nobel laureate, has summed up the impact of these new drugs on health: "the long way that we have come toward control of streptococcal, pneumococcal, even staphylococcal infections, of Gram-negative infections of many varieties, of syphilis, gonorrhea, tuberculosis, malaria, plague, yellow fever, cholera, typhus and typhoid, poliomyelitis and measles, towards the partial relief of arthritis, asthma, lupus, skin affections, nervous and mental diseases of many forms, and so on down the line. In addition, there are the new and most useful agents to control particular aspects of acute or chronic illness, such as the anticholinergic drugs in gastrointestinal diseases, and the antihypertensive drugs, and the remarkably effective new diuretics."[6]

Life expectancy at birth in the United States had been 60 years in 1937, when sulfanilamide appeared. By 1956 it had risen to almost 70. The death rate had fallen twice as rapidly between 1938 and 1950 as between 1921 and 1937. Infants, children, and young adults had benefitted most. The death rate from childhood diseases had tumbled 90 per cent. Almost as dramatic were declines in the death rates for influenza-

[5] *Ibid.*, 24; Robert A. Hardt, "A Pharmaceutical Manufacturer Looks at the Food and Drug Administration," *Antibiotics and Chemotherapy*, 6 (May 1956), 316-18; George P. Larrick, "Can We Rely on Modern Medicines?," mimeographed text of Mar. 15, 1957, address; Smith cited in *FDC Reports*, Dec. 19, 1960.

[6] Larrick, "Can We Rely on Modern Medicines?"; Richards, "A Clinician's View of Advances in Therapeutics," in Paul Talalay, ed., *Drugs in Our Society* (Baltimore, 1964), 31.

pneumonia and for infectious diseases. "How much value can we place on 3.2 million American lives?" asked Austin Smith rhetorically in 1959. "These are the lives that can be attributed in large part to the chemical revolution in medicine."[7]

Drugs discovered during this revolution dominated the market. Ninety per cent of the prescriptions written by doctors, noted the FDA Annual Report in 1956, called for drugs not commercially available when the new drug safety clearance required by the 1938 law went into effect. And the new drugs prescribed were curative "high-powered bullets" unlike the "old-fashioned shotgun medication to alleviate symptoms" which had dominated the prerevolutionary era. Of the thousands of drugs marketed in earlier times, only about a hundred, asserted a pharmacologist in 1928, were "by common consent deemed essential for treating the sick." Other authorities thought the basic list should be much more limited than that. In the new day, pharmaceutical manufacturers accelerated a trend already started, curtailing production of botanical medicines, to concentrate on the new and potent chemical agents. One firm, Smith Kline & French, for example, had marketed some 15,000 products during the 1920's; by the late 1950's their line contained fewer than 60.[8]

If drug entities were fewer, the total market was vastly expanded. The tendency toward therapeutic nihilism was reversed. With truly effective drugs, doctors prescribed—in time overprescribed—and pharmaceutical production boomed. In the early 1930's Americans spent less than $200,000,000 for prescription medication; by 1957 the sum had reached $2,000,-000,000. Problems would arise in time to cast some shadows over the new miracle of prescription drugs, problems of prices and profits and promotion, problems of unexpected side effects and adverse reactions, problems of bacterial strains

[7] Bureau of the Census, *Historical Statistics of the United States, Colonial Times to 1957* (Wash., 1960), 25; Public Health Service, *Vital Statistics of the United States, 1950,* i (Wash., 1954), 145; Smith cited in *Newsweek,* 54 (Dec. 7, 1959), 88.

[8] *1953 Annual Report of the U. S. Department of Health, Education, and Welfare* (FDA), 200; Stieglitz, *Chemistry in Medicine,* 496; R. T. Stormont, "From Alchemy to Antibiotics," *FDC Law Jnl.,* 11 (Feb. 1956), 98-99; Frank H. Wiley, "The Analysis of Drugs," *ibid.,* 16 (Dec. 1961), 733-34; Mahoney, *The Merchants of Life,* 33, 35-36.

developing a resistance to drug action. But the chemotherapeutic revolution, with its unquestioned benefits for public health, had ushered in a new and irreversible age.[9]

The double pressure of this revolution and the new and stricter law posed for proprietary manufacturers many crucial problems. Major proprietors, under constant urging from Proprietary Association officials, made such haste to bring their labeling within the bounds of legal rectitude that they won commendation from Food and Drug officials. Of 284 actions taken by FDA against proprietaries for human use in one seven-year span, only four belonged to Proprietary Association members. Commissioner Crawford, addressing the Association, was willing to grant that most violations "by honest and well-intentioned manufacturers" arose "from inadvertence, accident, or thoughtlessness." Relations were so friendly that FDA officials helped the Proprietary Association prepare an industrial film on the proper uses of self-medication.[10]

But many proprietary formulas in wide use when the new law came into effect relied heavily on the same botanicals that were dropping from the pages of official pharmacopeial volumes and becoming outmoded in prescription medication as the drug revolution surged on. Nor did important segments of the proprietary industry expand research facilities to the same extent, in order to establish the efficacy of products on the market and to find new ones, that pharmaceutical manufacturers did. Prior to 1938, Frederick Cullen, the Proprietary Association's medical consultant, said, "true research was extremely spotty." The Association sought to encourage research, and conditions improved. But two decades later Cullen thought not all investigation was as thorough as might be, some of it.

[9] Mary Ross, "Potions and Pills, The High Cost of Mystery," *Survey*, 67 (Jan. 1, 1932), 372; George Larrick before a House Committee, cited in *FDC Law Jnl.*, 13 (Apr. 1958), 230. For information on some of the problems that arose, see the essays in Talalay, *Drugs in Our Society*, and see below, ch. 19.

[10] *FDC Reports*, Nov. 18, 1957, 6; Charles W. Crawford, "Problems of Compliance and Enforcement under the Drug Law," mimeographed text of May 18, 1947, address; *PI*, 226 (Feb. 25, 1949); 227 (Apr. 22, 1949), 15. See ch. 9 for the early reaction of major proprietors to the 1938 law.

aimed primarily at discovering data that might be used to counter criticism of therapeutic claims should this arise. The ratio of research cost to sales for drug products sold direct to consumers was only a third that for prescription pharmaceuticals. Critics outside the industry also were somewhat skeptical. Dr. Albert B. Holland, Jr., head of FDA's Division of Medicine, addressing the Association in 1958, posed for proprietors the frank question, "How many proprietary products are actually supported by good, sound scientific data?" His answer was not reassuring. Too many proprietaries, he judged, were still "not acceptable for advertising in first-rate medical journals." Too few "good papers on proprietaries" appeared in the medical literature. Holland urged an expansion of solid research, not the "all-too-common 'cookbook' paper for promotional purposes only."[11]

Thus there was some threat to traditional proprietaries because of inadequate scientific undergirding for their efficacy. Sometimes the threat was countered by changing the formula, while retaining the trade name, introducing new ingredients developed through research. Often, as in the early days of the new law, label claims were sharply restricted to avoid the "false and misleading" charge.

Traditional proprietaries confronted other pressures during the chemotherapeutic revolution. Pharmaceutical manufacturers themselves began to enter the self-medication field. Not all of the new discoveries in their ever-expanding laboratories turned out to be drugs requiring the prescription legend. The 1938 law was "ambiguous" regarding the line between prescription and self-medication drugs. Food and Drug Administration policies restricted most medicines cleared through the "new drug" procedures—like the sulfonamide successors of sulfanilamide—to the doctor's prescription pad. But the FDA also insisted that, if a drug could be used safely by laymen when labeled with adequate directions, that drug should be released

[11] Proprietary Association *Executive News-Letter* 482 (June 7, 1959); James F. Hoge, "Government Interest in the Drug Business," mimeographed address distributed with *ibid.*, no. 59-21, May 29, 1959; *FDC Reports*, Apr. 14, 1945, white 6-7; *Drug Trade News*, 36 (Dec. 25, 1961), 27, 37; Holland, "Who Will Be First?," *FDC Law Jnl.*, 13 (July 1958), 471-72.

for self-medication sale. Many pharmaceutical companies marketed "over-the-counter" drugs, sometimes restricting their promotion to doctors and druggists, but increasingly advertising them, through the press, magazines, radio, and television, direct to the lay public.[12]

Indeed, the distinction that had once existed between ethical drugs and proprietaries began to break down, both on scientific and corporate grounds. Prescription drugs as well as self-medication items could be "brand name specialties"— and hence proprietary articles, each the exclusive property of a single manufacturer: by 1959, of the 409 drugs most prescribed in the nation 83 per cent were brand-name specialties and only 17 per cent generic-name drugs. For reasons both of the best utilization of research and of economic stability, large corporate complexes that marketed both prescription and self-medication drugs developed. A drug trade attorney sought to explain this trend.[13]

"There was a time," James F. Hoge asserted, "when proprietary manufacturing was separated completely from the pharmaceutical; when one was east and the other west and when ne'er the twain would meet. Now the time has apparently come when manufacturing interests look to proprietary products for stability, for balance. Pharmaceutical products are, by their nature and in the circumstances of their use, more dramatic and spectacular. But likewise they are more liable to obsolescence; are more susceptible to new, quick and sensational discoveries; to revolutionary research developments." During years when pharmaceuticals "leveled off" in sales, the steady sale of proprietaries proved a decided financial asset. "The time is at hand," Hoge said, "when there is more than a meeting of the twain. There is actual merging. . . ."[14]

There were two avenues that merged to reach the same goal.

[12] Larrick, "Pharmacy at the Crossroads," mimeographed text of Aug. 24, 1959, address; Robert L. Swain, "Our Self-Defeating Pharmacy Laws," *FDC Law Jnl.*, 14 (Apr. 1959), 263-66; *FDC Reports*, Sep. 19, 1955, 13-41; Aug. 21, 1959, 18.
[13] *Ibid.*, July 4, 1960, 17-18; Mahoney, 26.
[14] Hoge, "Government Interest in the Drug Business."

Pharmaceutical companies launched proprietary remedies and acquired control of established proprietary firms. Proprietary companies began marketing prescription drugs and purchased pharmaceutical concerns. The result was the appearance of large and growing diversified firms, making and marketing drug products of all types—as well as cosmetics, toilet articles, egg dyes, and what not. Nor did merging stop at this point. Manufacturers whose major products had been razors, chemicals, liquor, petroleum, soap, sundries entered the drug field. A significant share of proprietary medicine sales, as time went on, fell to the lot of a handful of the large diversified producers. By 1956 five companies controlled over two-fifths of the American proprietary market.[15]

This market was large, surpassing a billion dollars before the end of the 1950's. But proprietaries were not maintaining their proportionate share of the total drug market. Early in the century proprietaries outsold prescription drugs by over two to one, and by the eve of World War II sales of the two types were roughly even. After two decades of the chemotherapeutic revolution, however, the prescription drug market had become three times as large as that for proprietary drugs. Furthermore, over-the-counter pharmaceuticals were gaining business at a more rapid rate than were the old-line proprietaries. And proprietary sales were not keeping pace with increases in population or in consumer spending.[16]

The role of legitimate self-medication had shrunk with the 1938 law. The bulk of the business was confined to the treatment of minor ailments. By 1954, as any peruser of newspaper ads or viewer of television commercials might have surmised, analgesics, mainly aspirin and compounds containing aspirin, led the proprietary market. Following in order, according to the Census of Manufactures, were laxatives, vitamins, cold

[15] *JAMA*, 112 (June 3, 1939), 2276-78; *Drug Trade News*, 33 (Mar. 10, 1958), 30; *FDC Reports*, Feb. 6, 1954, white 12; Jan. 2, 1956, 15; Aug. 12, 1957, 3; Aug. 26, 1957, 3, 17; Nov. 11, 1957, 22; Feb. 3, 1958, 20; Apr. 27, 1958, 24; June 16, 1958, 13; Aug. 18, 1958, 20; Sep. 15, 1958, 18; Mar. 2, 1959, 7; Aug. 17, 1959, 17; May 23, 1960, 9-10.
[16] *Newsweek*, 51 (June 16, 1958), 62; Hoge, "Government Interest in the Drug Business"; *FDC Reports*, Apr. 29, 1957, 1-8.

and cough preparations, antacids and stomach remedies, antiseptics, liniments, and tonics.[17]

Not that all was smooth sailing even here. Common symptoms, like headache, coughing, constipation, in some cases properly treatable with home medication, might also herald serious disease. An Atlanta chest specialist, checking medical textbooks, found 137 different causes for coughing. How was the ordinary citizen to know if his cough denoted a minor irritation or tuberculosis? Expert opinion was by no means unanimous as to just how much self-medication might be safe. Some medical specialists thought the zone should be drastically restricted; proprietors generally wanted it enlarged. The Food and Drug Administration came to insist that even the commonest remedies must bear label warnings against possible hazards. If pain persisted or recurred frequently, the consumer should consult a doctor. Laxatives should not be taken when abdominal pain was present, possibly indicating appendicitis. Antihistamines might cause drowsiness, and the user should avoid driving a car or operating machinery. Aspirin should be kept out of the reach of children.[18]

Furthermore, even the most used and safest self-medication drugs might, through their promotion, become dangerous and illegal. To find the border between legitimate proprietaries and quackery was as hard at one extreme as to find the border between ethical drugs and proprietaries at the other. Proprietary Association spokesmen recognized the need "to draw lines between good and not-so-good self-medication products." "Part of our program," asserted the organization's executive vice-president, "should be . . . to make clear that intelligent, directed self-medication, with reliable products, made by reputable manufacturers, is in the public interest, whereas uncontrolled, unsound self-medication with quack

[17] Bureau of the Census, *United States Census of Manufactures: 1954*, II, *Industry Statistics*, Part 1, *General Survey and Major Groups 20 to 28* (Wash., 1957), 28C-10 through 28C-12.

[18] Andrew Sparks, "How Good Are Physical Checkups?," *Atlanta Jnl. and Constitution Mag.*, Apr. 15, 1956, 26; N. E. Cook, "Our Mutual Problems," mimeographed text of Aug. 26, 1957, address; *FDC Reports*, Aug. 14, 1954, pink 2-3; FDA "Labeling Recommendations in the Interest of Children's Health," Mar. 18, 1957; FDA news release on label warnings, Mar. 25, 1960.

THE CHEMOTHERAPEUTIC REVOLUTION

products made by quack manufacturers is not." To draw this line, he readily admitted, would be "difficult."[19]

Fundamentally, quackery is what quackery does. Kenneth L. Milstead, a Food and Drug official, employed this concept in seeking to mark the border beyond which quackery lay.[20]

"When," said Dr. Milstead, "an untrue or misleading health claim is deliberately, fraudulently or pretentiously made for a food, drug, device or cosmetic, this is quackery. . . .

"It matters not whether the quackery is practiced by the witch doctor or the licensed medical practitioner; the Indian medicine man or the pharmacist; the proprietary drug manufacturer or the prescription drug manufacturer; the health food manufacturer or the clerk in the health food store; the health lecturer, the self-styled nutritionist, the doorstep diagnostician, the fly-by-night operator or some of our most respected food, drug, device and cosmetic manufacturers—it is still quackery.

"It matters not which mask it wears—ignorance, superstition, fear, gullibility, folklore, myth, half-truth, or falsehood —it is still quackery.

"And, it matters not whether the article is harmless or whether it gives some psychosomatic relief; whether it is cheap or whether it has value for other purposes; whether it is produced by an obscure firm or whether it is produced by a 'reputable' firm—the promotion of it is still quackery."

The speech in which Dr. Milstead formulated this eloquent definition was delivered before a conference of pharmacists. During World War II, a few of the thousands of American pharmacists had engaged in shady practices—"quackery" as Milstead defined it—that eventually led to a revision in the 1938 law making it easier than it had been to draw the line between prescription and self-medication drugs. Word reached the Food and Drug Administration from a Navy base in Maine that the venereal disease program was encountering difficulty because some sailors were attempting to treat their gonorrhea by dosing themselves with sulfathiazole. One sailor in particular, buying the prescription drug easily at a waterfront phar-

19 Howard A. Prentice, cited in *FDC Reports*, May 22, 1961, 15.
20 Milstead, "Enforcement of Antiquackery Laws," 458.

macy, had continued taking small amounts of sulfathiazole until his ailment had become sulfa-fast. Complications developed which put the sailor in the hospital for a long stretch of time. The drugstore, the FDA found, was doing a land-office business in the illegal sale of sulfathiazole at a dime a tablet. Investigation revealed similar breaches of the law by druggists near military bases elsewhere in the country.[21]

Suspicious that such sales were being made by Sullivan's Pharmacy in Columbus, Georgia, two Food and Drug inspec-. tors, on separate occasions, posed as would-be customers and, without prescriptions, sought to buy sulfathiazole. They were successful. The druggist in each case took a dozen tablets from a bottle, put them into a small box, and handed them to the inspector in exchange for his money. All that was written on the box was the name of the drug—and it was misspelled— "SULFOTHIAZAL." When the district attorney hailed the druggist into court, Sullivan denied that he had broken the law. Both his buying of the drug, from an Atlanta branch of the manufacturer, and his selling of the drug, he argued, had been solely intrastate.[22]

The district judge agreed with the government's contention that, though the transactions did take place within the state of Georgia, nonetheless the 1938 law applied. Congress had meant to preserve the integrity of labeling until it reached the ultimate consumer, else much of the protective power of the law might be denied. And sulfathiazole was too dangerous a drug for consumers to use to treat themselves. The bottle from which the druggist had taken the tablets bore not only the caution that the drug was for use "only by or on the prescription of a physician," but also the further warning that physicians "should familiarize themselves with the use of" sulfathiazole before administering it, because in some people the drug might

[21] Larrick, "The Federal Food, Drug, and Cosmetic Act and Pharmacy," mimeographed text of June 13, 1950, address; *1944 Report of the Food and Drug Administration*, 27-28.

[22] United States v. Sullivan, an Individual, Trading as Sullivan's Pharmacy, 67 Fed. Supp. 192 (1946), in Kleinfeld and Dunn, *Federal Food, Drug, and Cosmetic Act, 1938-1949*, 319-27; Jordan James Sullivan, Trading as Sullivan's Pharmacy v. United States, 161 Fed. (2d) 629 (1947), in *ibid.*, 334-37; United States v. Sullivan, Trading as Sullivan's Pharmacy, 332 U. S. 689 (1948), in *ibid.*, 350-58.

cause "severe toxic reactions." Daily blood and urine examinations were suggested to check on dangerous abnormalities that might develop—anemia, for example.

Sullivan appealed his case to the circuit court, and there the judges, taking a less flexible constitutional position, supported him. The law was not "plain enough," they ruled, "to make criminals of retail grocers and druggists" who had bought their wares within their state. Thus, pending a final verdict from the Supreme Court, the FDA's efforts to restrict over-the-counter sale of dangerous drugs lay in jeopardy. In January 1948, however, the Supreme Court, in a divided opinion, reversed the circuit court, ruling that action against Sullivan for his sale of sulfathiazole was within the law and constitutional. Even though the sale was intrastate, it came within the law's provision forbidding "the doing of any . . . act with respect to, a . . . drug . . . if such act is done while such article is being held for sale after such shipment in interstate commerce and results in such article being misbranded." The language of the law was broad and sweeping. It mattered not "how long after the [interstate] shipment the misbranding occurred" or "how many intrastate sales had intervened." The ultimate consumer must be protected.

Thus reassured by the highest tribunal in the land, the Food and Drug Administration accelerated its campaign against the sale of hazardous drugs without prescriptions. Other medicaments besides the sulfas fell into this category—thyroid extract, benzedrine sulfate, and various barbiturates among them.[23]

But sales without prescriptions were not the only problem. In their investigations, Food and Drug inspectors had discovered another way in which prescription drugs were being abused. This was the indiscriminate, unauthorized refilling of prescriptions. Checking on drugstores suspected of illegal sales, inspectors were often told that, while this drug or that could not be sold without a prescription, once the pharmacist had a prescription on file, he could supply virtually an unlim-

[23] *1948 Report of the Food and Drug Administration*, 556; *1949 Report*, 25-26; Larrick, "Indiscriminate Sale of Dangerous and Habit-Forming Drugs," *FDC Law Jnl.*, 5 (May 1950), 251-57.

ited quantity of the drug in question. This happened most often with barbiturates.[24]

These drugs, a product of the German chemical industry, had appeared on the market early in the century. Depressants of the central nervous system, they provided doctors with valuable therapeutic tools, useful for treating epilepsy, certain nervous conditions, and for bringing sleep to the distraught. But their potential for harm was also great. The 1938 law had placed them in the list of dangerous drugs and had required labeling their habit-forming potentialities. War and postwar stresses increased both their use and their misuse. Medical scientists took note of an increasing rate of barbiturate addiction, which in some ways was worse than narcotic addiction. Deaths from accidental overdosage and from suicide were rising. In 1948 drug manufacturers produced 24 sleeping pills for every man, woman, and child in the nation, a quantity far above legitimate needs. FDA inspectors, in their rounds, discovered tragic case histories. While most pharmacists practiced their profession responsibly, in some instances the source of the drug leading to tragedy was a prescription endlessly refilled.[25]

A woman in a town in the Midwest, the mother of three children, was discovered, upon admission to a hospital, to be a barbiturate addict. A check on her source of supply revealed that she had had a prescription for 30 capsules refilled 16 times within three months. Another woman, who had been mildly afflicted with high blood pressure, was found dead in her bed. Investigation at the pharmacy named on her prescription showed that she had secured 23 refills for 20 barbiturate capsules during the preceding six months.[26]

In Kansas City a woman's neighbors, noting accumulating milk bottles and newspapers, summoned the police. Breaking into the house, they found the woman's body on the floor,

[24] N. E. Cook, untitled text of mimeographed address given before District of Columbia Pharmaceutical Association, Nov. 15, 1950.

[25] Leonard P. Prusak, "Barbiturate Control by Legislation," *FDC Law Jnl.*, 5 (Sep. 1950), 598-603; Stieglitz, 485-86, 491; *Literary Digest*, 97 (June 16, 1928), 65-66; *PI*, 164 (July 1933), 21; *N.Y. Times*, Dec. 16, 1951; *1949 Report of the Food and Drug Administration*, 25-26.

[26] Cook, Nov. 15, 1950, address.

mutilated by rats. She had been dead about three days. Her estranged husband told the authorities she had become addicted to barbiturates. From smudges of finger marks knee-high on the wallpaper, it appeared that a great deal of the time she had been too heavily drugged to walk. The husband gave police the name of the California drugstore near their former home from which his wife had been buying her drugs. The mailbox contained a package notice, but so much time had elapsed the package had been returned to the sender. A Food and Drug inspector got the husband's sister to write the drugstore, saying the woman could not pick up the package and asking that it be mailed again. Shortly two bottles arrived, each containing 500 barbiturate capsules. Investigation revealed that five years previously the woman had secured a prescription for 15 capsules. The druggist had refilled the prescription 43 times for a total of 7,000 capsules. The doctor who had written the prescription was never consulted about refilling it.[27]

As such disheartening instances mounted, the Food and Drug Administration decided to take action. A number of states had no laws regulating prescription refills, and in some of the states that did, enforcement was woefully inadequate. After the Sullivan decision, which was followed by an amendment to the 1938 law covering its main point, the FDA could move against illegal sales on the retail level with a greater feeling of security. In October 1948, speaking before the National Association of Retail Druggists, Commissioner Dunbar announced a new FDA policy. All prescription refills, he said, would henceforth be considered as illegal unless they had been specifically authorized by a physician. The question FDA officials had posed for themselves, agency spokesmen told various groups of pharmacists, was, "Is a prescription once filled still a bona fide prescription when presented for refilling without the doctor's knowledge and approval?" The answer they had come to, after consulting the laws of various states and foreign nations, as well as scholarly works on prescription writing, was "No." An unauthorized refill meant that

[27] Crawford, "The Federal Drug Law and the Druggist," mimeographed text of Oct. 18, 1950, address.

the pharmacist, not the physician, was doing the prescribing. This amounted to over-the-counter selling of prescription legend drugs.[28]

While recognizing the hazards in unauthorized refills, organized pharmacy objected strenuously to the FDA's method of attacking the problem. Most prescription refills, pharmacy spokesmen argued, dealt with safe drugs, and refilling amounted to 40 per cent of the total prescription business. Legal control of pharmacy was traditionally a state instead of a national concern. To have the Food and Drug Administration enter so massively into the sacred physician-pharmacist-patient relationship seemed ominous. The answer to the unscrupulous minority should not be federal intervention, but more effective state laws and better education. So disturbed were pharmacists at the FDA's position, and legal actions initiated under it, that they sponsored a proposed law, introduced by a pharmacist member of the House of Representatives, which would exempt from the jurisdiction of the Food and Drug Administration all products dispensed upon prescription or prescription refill. The FDA naturally opposed this measure.[29]

In the wake of this action, leaders of the National Association of Retail Druggists and FDA officials engaged in conversations looking toward a compromise. If a new law could ban only unsafe refilling, then the major part of the prescription business would continue unhampered by possible federal intrusion. But what was unsafe? The draft eventually presented to the Congress by Congressman Carl Durham and Senator Hubert Humphrey, pharmacists both, specified three categories of drug prescriptions which could not be refilled by pharmacists without specific authorization of the physician: drugs, like the barbiturates, which were habit-forming; new drugs released for marketing by the FDA with the stipulation they be limited to prescription sale; and other drugs to be designated by the FDA, after a hearing, which could be

[28] Crawford, "The Federal Drug Law and the Druggist," *FDC Law Jnl.*, 5 (Dec. 1950), 812-22; Walton M. Wheeler, Jr., "Prescription Refills," *ibid.*, 5 (Nov. 1950), 746-54. The Miller Amendment became law June 24, 1948.

[29] *Ibid.* The Durham Bill was introduced into Congress Apr. 12, 1949.

employed safely and effectively only under the supervision of a doctor.[30]

The third category seemed of signal importance to Food and Drug officials, for, with respect to all drug products, it would permit the drawing of a sharp line between prescription and self-medication items. This line the 1938 law had not drawn, and regulatory efforts to mark it had not had much success. A "broad twilight zone" continued to exist. The problem was not only the over-the-counter sale of hazardous drugs. Drugs safe for use by laymen, even sodium bicarbonate, were being marketed as prescription items so that their vendors could avoid labeling them with adequate directions for lay use, counting on advertising claims to impress the consumer mind.[31]

Food and Drug officials also were pleased to have the standard of effectiveness written into the draft law. They recognized that consumer safety lay not alone in a drug's inherent lack of toxicity. The circumstances under which a drug was used played a central role in safety. A non-toxic diuretic, used by a layman to reduce swelling in his ankles, might be extremely hazardous if the swelling was caused by heart or kidney disease. Such a diuretic, FDA's George Larrick told a Congressional committee, should not be permitted on the market for self-dosage. "We submit," Larrick asserted, "that it is just as important that a drug be effective in the hands of the person who acts as his own physician as that it be safe in the sense that it will not poison him."[32]

[30] *Ibid.* The history of the Durham-Humphrey Act is traced in Richard J. Hopkins, "Medical Prescriptions and the Law: A Study of the Enactment of the Durham-Humphrey Amendment to the Federal Food, Drug, and Cosmetic Act" (Emory University: unpublished Master of Arts thesis, 1965).

[31] Testimony of Federal Security Administrator Oscar R. Ewing, *Federal Food, Drug, and Cosmetic Act: Hearings before the Committee on Interstate and Foreign Commerce, House of Representatives, . . . on H. R. 3298* (82 Cong., 1 ses., 1951), 20. A Senate subcommittee also held hearings: *To Amend Section 503 (b) of the Federal Food, Drug, and Cosmetic Act of 1938, As Amended: Hearings before the Subcommittee on Health of the Committee on Labor and Public Welfare, U. S. Senate, . . . on S. 1186 and H. R. 3298* (82 Cong., 1 ses., 1951). House Report 700 and Senate Report 946 issued from these hearings.

[32] Larrick, House Hearings, 94.

To many pharmacists, physicians, and drug makers, however, this section of the Durham-Humphrey bill seemed even more threatening than recent FDA administrative policies. These groups did not trust the Food and Drug Administration to draw the line. James Hoge and Charles Wesley Dunn explained the opposition of proprietary and pharmaceutical manufacturers. To give the FDA administrative authority to separate self-medication from prescription drugs, wrote Hoge, "introduced a plan for the regulation of the drug industry to an extent never heretofore proposed or contemplated." The administrative hearings, he thought, would prove to be "snares and delusions." The whole concept was Tugwellian and, if enacted, would "increasingly restrict the right of self-medication," something that Congress in 1938 had "stated was not to be restricted but made safe." An ominous clue had been forthcoming at the Congressional hearings. The Federal Security Administrator, while testifying, had been asked if there was any possibility that a prescription refill might be required for aspirin. He had said no, not as of the moment, although a future Administrator might put the issue up for hearing. Dunn likewise thought the proposed law portended "governmental control of the drug business and the medical profession, which can be used to socialize them in the most invidious sense; and it amounts to life-or-death control over non-prescription drugs."[33]

So Congress, yielding to these sentiments, removed from the bill the FDA's authority to decide, after administrative hearings, which were prescription and which non-prescription drugs. Instead, the Durham-Humphrey Act, passed in October 1951, contained an objective definition of prescription drugs. Included in this category was any drug intended for human use which "because of its toxicity or other potentiality for harmful effect, or the method of its use, or the collateral measures necessary to its use, is not safe for use except

[33] Hoge, "The Durham-Humphrey Bill," *FDC Law Jnl.*, 6 (Feb. 1951), 135-41; Hoge, "Major Drug Law Problems," *ibid.*, 6 (Dec. 1951), 933-35; Dunn, "The Durham-Humphrey Bill," *ibid.*, 5 (Dec. 1950), 854-65; and their similar testimony at the hearings: House Hearings, 75-87 (Dunn), 191-206 (Hoge); Senate Hearings, 103-19 (Hoge); 148-52 (Hoge written statement); Ewing on aspirin, House Hearings, 38.

under the supervision of a practitioner licensed by law to administer such drug." Gone from the earlier bill was the word "effective," though something of its flavor lingered on. Dangerous drugs as so defined, as well as habit-forming drugs and new drugs clearing FDA procedures as prescription items, must bear the prescription legend and not be refilled by pharmacists without the specific authorization of physicians. The FDA might issue advisory lists, but the initiative still rested with manufacturers to decide whether or not their therapeutic wares fit the Durham-Humphrey definition. If disagreement arose between a manufacturer and the FDA, the issue could be settled in the courts.[34]

Enforcing the Durham-Humphrey Act, in fact, did not prove placid. In seeking to apply the new statutory definition, the FDA, as always, moved in the midst of conflicting scientific opinions and divergent economic interests. In the main, the agency continued to act within its interpretation of the 1938 law: to provide as much self-medication as might be safe. But safety, as a result of the new amendment to the law, was a more sophisticated standard than before. Some drugs once thought safe for self-medication, experience had shown, proved not to be—sulfa in salves, for example—and the FDA returned them to the prescription legend. Demanding requirements were set for moving prescription drugs to over-the-counter status: thorough data on the length and extent of use, the nature of any side reactions encountered, evidence on differences in response to the medicine with respect to sex and age, acute and chronic toxicity studies, and much else. When ten pharmaceutical manufacturers petitioned to exempt hydrocortisone ointment from the prescription dispensing requirement, doctors and pharmacists opposed the move. Too much of this powerful drug, dermatologists testified, might get into the user's system, especially if he neglected to heed the label warnings and overused the ointment. Evidence was presented, through a public opinion study run for the American College of Apothecaries, that this indeed might happen. Two-thirds of

[34] 65 Stat. 648. Analysis of the law appears in Dunn, "The New Prescription Drug Law," *FDC Law Jnl.*, 6 (Dec. 1951), 951-69, and in *F&D Rev.*, 35 (1951), 227.

the consumers interviewed showed lack of familiarity with label warnings on a dozen nationally advertised proprietaries. Persuaded by such evidence, the FDA forbade the change.[35]

The Proprietary Association objected to the hydrocortisone ointment decision. "It seems," said Dr. Cullen, "the effect of this hearing is an attempt to present again at the federal level the issue of self-medication as it has not been raised since the enactment" of the 1938 law. If switches from prescription to over-the-counter status became increasingly difficult, noted a drug trade journal, the proprietary industry would "face a dubious future insofar as really new products, containing modern therapeutic ingredients" were concerned.[36]

Some pharmacists sided with the Proprietary Association, seeing greater profits in a high volume of over-the-counter sales. But the majority of pharmacists favored releasing drugs from prescription status only slowly. The issue became involved in a long-standing dispute between pharmacists and proprietary manufacturers, the restrictive sales controversy. Arguing that many proprietary products posed hazards if used unwisely, pharmacists sought to confine their sale to drugstores. In this way the pharmacist, knowing his customers, could point to label warnings, caution against excessive purchases, and generally exercise some supervision over self-medication in the interests of public health. The proprietary industry, on the other hand, charged that the pharmacists' alleged solicitude for public health was specious and their desire to restrict sales to drugstores "simply a matter of private profit." Changes in marketing patterns were indeed increasing proprietary sales in groceries and supermarkets and decreasing sales in drugstores. Whatever the motivation, pharmacy groups undertook to change state pharmacy laws to stem this tide. The Proprietary Association, aided by drug wholesalers, grocery associations, and some pharmaceutical manufacturers, fought to defeat such laws and, where laws

[35] Cook, "Over-the-Counter Sales and the Pharmacist," *Antibiotics and Chemotherapy*, 6 (May 1956), 315-16; *FDC Reports*, May 29, 1954, pink 2; Aug. 7, 1954, white 14; Aug. 14, 1954, pink 2-3; Nov. 13, 1954, 13-15; Sep. 10, 1956, 8; Dec. 17, 1956, 8-10; May 13, 1957, 11-14; FDA press release, Jan. 17, 1957.
[36] *FDC Reports*, Oct. 15, 1956, 9-10.

existed, to have them interpreted in the courts to their advantage. One concession the Proprietary Association was willing to make: to limit sales of medicines by non-drug outlets to those proprietaries promoted to the lay public, thus excluding over-the-counter pharmaceuticals promoted only to the health professions. But pharmacy organizations would not accept this compromise and fought state bills, sponsored by the Proprietary Association, that sought to enact this definition into law. Pharmacists hoped to ban from non-drug outlets all home medications that required warning labels under the law, and all medications listed in the *Pharmacopeia* or other official compendiums—including milk of magnesia and aspirin. The battle raged on, on the whole inconclusively, although with varying fortunes on various fronts. Nor has it ended. In place of the two-class division in medication set forth in the Durham-Humphrey Act, the American Pharmaceutical Association has recently been campaigning for a four-class structure, one group to consist of proprietaries needing such caution in their self-use that only a pharmacist personally should sell them.[37]

The abuse which started events moving toward the Durham-Humphrey Act, the unauthorized refilling by some pharmacists of prescriptions for dangerous drugs, was quite satisfactorily resolved by that statute. But this did not end the illegal usage of barbiturates. Thrill-seekers and addicts sought these powerful hypnotics through other channels, and the bootleg black market boomed. Enough sleeping pills were produced in the year the Durham-Humphrey bill was passed,

[37] William F. Weigel, "State Legislation Restricting the Sale of Drugs," *FDC Law Jnl.*, 13 (Jan. 1958), 48-56; Sol A. Herzog, "The Advantages to the Public of Restricting the Sale of Drugs and Medicines to the Retail Drug Store under the Supervision of Registered Pharmacists," *Amer. Jnl. Pharm.*, 126 (May 1954), 177-84; *Drug Trade News*, 29 (Oct. 25, 1954), 1; *FDC Reports*, Feb. 17, 1945, white 5; Mar. 13, 1954, white 14-15; Sep. 25, 1954, pink 1, 4, white 2; Nov. 20, 1954, 11; May 30, 1955, 3; May 14, 1956, 16; Dec. 10, 1956, 9-10; May 18, 1959, 16-18; William S. Apple, "The Pharmacist and the Public Health," *Emory University Qtly.*, 21 (Summer 1965), 118-21; Apple, "APhA Statement before House Subcommittee on Intergovernmental Relations," *Jnl. Amer. Pharmaceutical Assoc.*, ns 4 (May 1964), 212-16, 219; Carl L. Vitalie, "Reclassification of Drugs: A New Look at a New Idea," *Pharm USC* (June 1965), 7, 36-37.

a doctor said, to put every person in the United States to sleep for 20 years. Half the capsules, he estimated, were used for non-medical purposes. A similar diversion from legitimate purposes occurred with the amphetamines, used by truck drivers, for example, to disguise tiredness. The misuse of these drugs, indeed, expanded into one of the nation's most serious social problems. An ever larger portion of the Food and Drug Administration's limited resources went into tracking down illegal sources of "bennies" and "goof balls." The work was not only time-consuming for FDA inspectors, but hazardous as well.[38]

Greatly preoccupied by this emerging form of "quackery," the FDA could not devote so much attention to medical quackery of more traditional forms. Nor was traditional quackery in a moribund state, safely to be neglected. Quite the reverse: despite the more potent, really curative medicines available to doctors, quackery, with its false medicines, was growing. Indeed, paradox though it might be, the very success of the chemotherapeutic revolution contributed greatly to quackery's reinvigoration. Never before the exciting age of miracle drugs had so many people met so much publicity in such varied media about the field of health. In 1936, for example, the *Saturday Evening Post* had run two medical articles and had not mentioned a drug in its editorial columns during the whole year; in 1956 the *Post* published 36 articles on health, referring to 72 different drugs a total of 330 times. Each new therapeutic wonder, real or would-be, received full and exciting coverage in the press and magazines, on radio and television. "Readers are not just more medically conscious," a drug trade journal stated, "but more drug conscious too." Health was something that could be bought. As always, the average citizen had difficulty in analyzing the credentials of competing vendors.[39]

[38] Larrick, "The Food and Drug Administration's Battle against Unlicensed Merchandisers of Bootleg Drugs," mimeographed text of Oct. 19, 1955, address; Dr. Donald Dukelow, cited in *Atlanta Journal*, Mar. 20, 1953. Much more thorough legislative controls over such dangerous drugs were passed by the Congress in 1965 and given to the FDA to administer.

[39] *FDC Reports*, Dec. 16, 1957, 7-10; Herbert Ratner, "Are Ameri-

"More and more," the FDA's director of public information said, "people believe in miracles, not only the real miracles of scientific achievement but also the fake miracles of promoters and charlatans." "Americans have come to believe," stated a president of the American Medical Association, "that science is capable of almost everything. Any glib salesman who has a white coat and calls himself a doctor can take a black box, a powder, a pill, or a liquid and set out to capitalize on it."[40]

So science and pseudo-science advanced hand in hand.

---

cans Overmedicated?," *Saturday Rev.*, 45 (May 26, 1962), 8; Russell S. Boles, "When Medicine Makes the Headlines," *ibid.*, 34 (May 19, 1951), 7; Wallace F. Janssen, "Quackery and the News," *Public Health Reports*, 74 (July 1959), 635-38.

[40] *Ibid.*, 636; Dr. Louis M. Orr cited in *Newsweek*, 52 (July 7, 1958), 48-49.

# 13

## MAIL-ORDER "HEALTH"

*"No other country in the world begins to approach
our national use of direct selling by mail. The public
has amazing confidence in products so advertised. . . .
The quacks with their nostrums, the miracle makers
who can bring new sexual vigor to old men, grow hair
or make it 'permanently' vanish, develop the bust, cure
every ill from cancer to hemorrhoids, produce pills to
make skinny people fat or fat people skinny, persist in
their efforts, but we believe we have made the going
considerably tougher. . . . The promoters of these
schemes always think up a new wrinkle when we put
them out of business, and it is amazing the diversity
and the novelty of the schemes that are involved."*

—ABE M. GOFF, GENERAL COUNSEL, POST OFFICE DEPARTMENT,
1957[1]

WHILE the chemotherapeutic revolution brought an increasing array of new and effective drugs to treat the ailments
of mankind, quackery's ineffective nostrums still flourished.
The most outlandish and unscrupulous of therapeutic claims
reached would-be customers through the comparative privacy
of direct mail advertising. In the Post Office Department, a
yeoman's guard of inspectors and lawyers sought to stem this
vicious tide.

In 1938, the year of the new food and drug law, broad-
gauge cure-alls led the list of actions initiated by the Department. Some 28 purported panaceas, with curative promises
running through the whole range of human disease, were
entered on the solicitor's docket. Next in order of frequency

[1] *False and Misleading Advertising (Weight-Reducing Preparations),
Hearings before a Subcommittee of the Committee on Government Operations, House of Representatives* (85 Cong., 1 ses., 1957), 67.

[ 282 ]

came male-weakness remedies, heirs as it were of Man Medicine, which had engaged the Department's attention a quarter of a century before. Some 25 of these alleged rejuvenators were docketed in 1938. Cures for obesity, baldness, cancer, diabetes, tuberculosis, piles, and a score of other ailments and conditions required attention.[2]

A decade later the pattern remained much the same. Panaceas still sought to cure all ills. Diseases like cancer and diabetes, promoters said, could still be eradicated with recipes sent by mail. Busts could be built up, virility quickened. In the never-never land of direct mail promotion, anything was possible. Regardless of changes in medical science, in legal regulation, in educational expansion, the same old utopian assurances, reminiscent of quackery's most ancient days, continued to gull the credulous and enrich the unconscionable.[3]

In fighting medical mail frauds, the Post Office Department continued to use its time-tested procedures. Clues as to suspicious promotions came from various sources: from surveys of magazine advertising; from come-on letters sent to inspectors whose earlier test letters had gotten their names on new mailing lists; from consumer complaints; from suggestions made by other regulatory agencies, the American Medical Association, the National Better Business Bureau. Assuming the role of customer, under fictitious names, inspectors received the full range of promotional build-up and bought the product. Under the long liaison with the Food and Drug Administration, the Department secured analyses of drugs and expert scientific counsel in comparing real therapeutic value, if any, of drugs and devices with claims made in the advertising. When the data were all assembled, a Post Office lawyer wrote the promoter a pre-citation letter, explaining precisely what was wrong with his advertising. If the scheme seemed obviously fraudulent, the letter requested a voluntary abandonment of the whole enterprise. The Department might ask in response merely a letter saying the scheme had been given up—and later an inspector would check to make sure. Or the

[2] Calendar year 1938, Fraud and Lottery Docket, vol. 11, Office of the Solicitor for the Post Office Dept., Records of the Post Office Dept., RG 28, NA.

[3] Calendar year 1948, *ibid.*, vols. 16 and 17.

Department might require the promoter to sign an affidavit of discontinuance. The affidavit pledged the promoter to return money received in response to objectionable advertising and to abandon further use of such advertising. Should the promoter disobey, the document stated, postal officials could issue a fraud order immediately. In cases not wholly disreputable, the pre-citation letter suggested what particular advertising claims struck the Department as wrong. Post Office officials might accept an affidavit that was less than 100 per cent desirable in order to get quick action on stopping the worst claims, realizing how long the proprietor could continue these claims to the detriment of the public welfare if he chose to fight the Department through the protracted machinery of formal action. Some 60 to 70 per cent of cases initiated were settled by compromise.[4]

Formal action began with a fraud complaint served on the proprietor. This document was resorted to immediately to launch a case against a perennial offender or one engaged in a scheme so large or hazardous as to make it a matter of serious public concern. The complaint listed specifically alleged violations of the law and usually summoned the promoter to a hearing. Before 1951 the same procedures were followed as in the Man Medicine case: the same lawyer might assemble the evidence, conduct the hearing, and make recommendation for action to the Postmaster General. In that year, however, the Supreme Court ruled that the Post Office Department must follow the provisions of the Administrative Procedure Act, passed by Congress in 1946 to ensure fair treatment of those brought to the bar of quasi-judicial proceedings by administrative agencies. This led to the creation in the Department of hearing examiners, impartial "judges" selected by the Civil Service Commission and insulated from the Department lawyers who prepared and presented the Department's case. Following prescribed procedures, the examiner conducted a hearing based on the complaint, taking

---

[4] Interview with Abraham Levine, attorney in the Office of the General Counsel, Apr. 5, 1961; *Procedures of the Post Office Department, Rules of Practice in Proceedings Relative to Fraud and Obscenity Orders . . . Amended Effective February 24, 1960*; Hearings before House Subcommittee, 73.

testimony from witnesses appearing for both the Department and the remedy promoter and then rendering an initial decision, which became final unless either party decided to appeal. The Department's chief legal officer acted for the Postmaster General in rendering a decision on the appeal. Loopholes in the Department's organizational structure, found by ingenious counsel for defendants and made the basis of successful court action, led to the creation of a Judicial Officer, separate from the General Counsel, to act as the Department's appellate judge. Thus in 1958 the prosecuting and judicial functions were clearly separated. From the Judicial Officer's decision, the Department had no further appeal. A proprietor, if not satisfied that justice had been done, could carry his case on into the federal courts.[5]

In the days of Man Medicine, proceedings had been more summary. The new procedures, while protecting the promoter's rights, gave him enhanced opportunities for stalling tactics. "When you get one of these fellows who is really in the business," the General Counsel stated at a Congressional hearing in 1957, "he delays the proceeding and files all kinds of motions and objections because he can continue to operate until we issue a final order." Clever proprietors, Post Office attorneys were convinced, planned a campaign with an eye on the calendar. Knowing they could push their advertising and maintain their selling while the administrative and court proceedings went their deliberate ways, promoters manufactured just enough of their "health" product to last until the final word was in. And their sales price was inflated to encompass the cost of lawyers' and court fees and possible fines in case of criminal conviction, which they tended to regard as a standard expense of doing business. If the final word was a

[5] *Ibid.*, 89; Levine interview; Cates v. Haderlein, 342 U.S. 804 (1951); Reilly, Postmaster, v. Pinkus, trading as American Health Aids Co., 338 U.S. 269; Pinkus v. Reilly, 157 Fed. Supp. 548 (1957); Columbia Research Corporation and Allerton Pharmacal Corporation v. Schaffer, 256 Fed. (2d) 677 (1958); Vibra Brush Corp. v. Schaffer, 256 Fed. (2d) 681 (1958); *FDC Reports*, Jan. 20, 1958, 17; Sep. 22, 1958, 7-8; *Procedures of the Post Office Department . . . Relative to Fraud and Obscenity Orders*, 1960. Prior to 1951 hearings in fraud cases were considered optional with the Department.

fraud order, their stock of merchandise was exhausted anyway. And new promotions beckoned.[6]

Indeed, since settlement by compromise was possible at any point during the administrative process, promoters often hung on until the midnight hour, reaping profits from sales, then agreed to an affidavit of discontinuance, thus avoiding even the stigma of a fraud order. Not infrequently they had begun a new venture even while the old was still in litigation.[7]

Despite the dilatory tactics of besieged proprietors and despite the Department's small staff of inspectors and lawyers devoted to medical mail fraud work, their pace of action was creditable. "The Post Office Department," concluded the Blatnik subcommittee of the House after its 1957 hearings on the advertising of obesity remedies, "has a reasonably laudable overall record in expeditiously handling fraud cases." Still, the elapsed time from the receipt of a complaint to a final decision within the Department—with court appeal still possibly to come—averaged nearly 200 days.[8]

For some years the Postmaster General had held the view that he posssessed the authority, when the public interest was great enough, to issue a temporary impounding order. This prevented a concern from receiving its mail until a fraud proceeding should be established against him. This power was very rarely used, and scarcely at all in medical fraud cases. Its legal basis was vague, and in 1959 a circuit court decided that the postal laws did not permit it. The next year Congress sought to remedy this weakness. In cases involving serious public interest, the new law authorized the Department to go to a district court and plead for an injunction. This would temporarily tie up a promoter's incoming mail until the question of fraud could be settled by the more time-consuming regular procedures. The Department, anxious that its first test case under the law be a solid one, moved warily. Up to 1966, no effort to secure an injunction had been brought in court.[9]

[6] Hearings before House Subcommittee, 42, 66; Levine interview.
[7] Hearings before House Subcommittee, 42.
[8] *False and Misleading Advertising (Weight-Reducing Remedies)*, House Report 2553 (85 Cong., 2 ses., 1958), 15.
[9] Frederick M. Hart, "The Postal Fraud Statutes: Their Use and

Just as court decisions forced the Post Office Department to institute more elaborate judicial proceedings, so too did a crucial Supreme Court decision place upon the Department a more difficult burden of proof in securing a fraud order against a promoter of medical wares. The Department had recognized that, when it asked the Department of Justice to launch a criminal case against a proprietor, clear-cut evidence of fraudulent intent must be established. But, from early in the century into the 1940's, in Departmental proceedings aimed at fraud orders, less demanding standards were set. If therapeutic claims for a drug or device could be shown to be false, fraud was presumed. Fraud orders issued on the basis of such logic were not questioned by the courts. In 1949, however, Justice Hugo Black, speaking for the nation's highest tribunal in a case without dissent, changed all that. Barring the receipt of a person's mail, he indicated, was a harsh penalty. In order to warrant this severe step, Black ruled, "proof of fraudulent purposes is essential—an 'actual intent to deceive.'" Proof that an incorrect statement had been made as part of the promotion was not sufficient.[10]

"That's the case that killed us," a Post Office attorney noted later. For proving the fraudulent state of a promoter's mind in the 1950's was as difficult a task for the Post Office Department as the same burden had been in the 1920's for the Food and Drug Administration. The circumstances led to the pre-built alibi. Before launching a promotion, the proprietor would seek scientific counsel from doctors of questionable reputation, and, being assured that a given ingredient possessed therapeutic merit, he would initiate his scheme. When hailed to a Departmental hearing, he could assume the role of injured innocence. If his claims were false, he had made them in all good faith, relying on his "experts."[11]

---

Abuse," *FDC Law Jnl.*, 11 (May 1956), 248-53; Greene v. Kern, 269 Fed. (2d) 344 (1959); Levine interview; interview with Ralph B. Manherz, attorney in the Office of the General Counsel, July 26, 1962; Levine to author, Jan. 20, 1966. The act providing the authority to appeal for an injunction, 74 U.S. Stat. 553, became law July 14, 1960.

[10] Hearings before House Subcommittee, 71-72; Reilly v. Pinkus, 338 U.S. 269.

[11] Levine interview; Hearings before House Subcommittee, 79. Efforts

Justice Black, in the Reilly v. Pinkus decision, did enunciate one method by which it would be possible to establish fraud from the facts presented in a case. "An intent to deceive might be inferred," he suggested, "from the universality of scientific belief that advertising representations are wholly unsupportable." This ruling provided a further clarification of the significant McAnnulty decision that had influenced all governmental efforts to combat quackery since 1902. The McAnnulty rule did not bar a finding of fraud, Black stated, "whenever there is the least conflict of opinion as to the curative efforts of a remedy," but, in such a case, the promoter's fraudulent intent must be established. When medical knowledge became "crystallized in the crucible of experience," however, and that knowledge denied that a given drug could benefit a given ailment, then one who sold that drug to treat that ailment perpetrated a fraud.[12]

Black's lesson for the shrewd promoter was plain: avoid remedies purporting to cure cancer, diabetes, tuberculosis, concerning which knowledge had "crystallized in the crucible." Seek out instead the grey zone, in which, even though medical opinion leaned heavily in one direction, a minority position might at least be vigorously argued and honest intent asserted. Then postal authorities must prove state of mind.

That promoters learned this lesson well, the trend in fraud cases demonstrated. Surging to the top in almost equal numbers were three types of grey zone schemes: arthritis remedies; vitamins and other nutritional promotions—often a new vehicle for conveying ancient sexual prowess claims; and drugs and devices offered for weight reduction.[13]

It had been an obesity treatment that lay behind the Su-

---

in Congress to eliminate the obligation upon the Department to prove fraudulent intent on the part of a promoter in order to issue a fraud order have so far failed, most recently in 1966, when the House unanimously passed H.R. 16706 but the Senate did not bring the measure to a vote. *Wash. Post*, Aug. 16, 1966; Levine interview, Nov. 1, 1966; *False or Misleading Mail Matter: Hearings before the* [House] *Subcommittee on Postal Operations* (89 Cong., 2 ses., 1966).

[12] Reilly v. Pinkus, 338 U.S. 269; Edgar R. Carver, Jr., "The Rule in the McAnnulty Case," *FDC Law Jnl.*, 5 (Aug. 1950), 508-12.

[13] Levine interview, Apr. 5, 1961.

preme Court's ruling in Reilly v. Pinkus. "I'm the only man," Joseph J. Pinkus later told a reporter, "who ever beat the Post Office in the Supreme Court of the U.S. by a unanimous decision." And he conveyed the impression to the reporter that his victory had been won on grounds of medical efficacy. Such was certainly not the case. The Pinkus triumph was procedural. In the Post Office hearing, his attorney had not been permitted to cross-examine physicians who testified for the Department concerning statements in other medical works than the volumes they had referred to. As to the value of Pinkus' product, Justice Black asserted, the evidence was sufficient to support the Postmaster General in finding that advertising claims misrepresented its power to take off weight. But proving fraud required something more.[14]

The case had begun five years before. Pinkus, through his American Health Aids Company, vended a product known as Kelpidine, along with counsel on reducing sent with the drug to customers. Extensive advertising in magazines and on the radio offered an easy road to loss of weight. Picturing a shapely young woman in a bathing suit, one advertisement promised:

# REDUCE SAFELY

## NO EXERCISE
## NO REDUCING DRUGS
## ABSOLUTELY HARMLESS
### LOSE 3 to 5 lbs. a WEEK yet eat plenty!

### Follow the KELPIDINE REDUCING PLAN
Simply take a half teaspoonful of KELPIDINE with any meal (preferably at breakfast).
EAT AS YOU USUALLY DO. DON'T CUT OUT fatty, starchy foods, just CUT DOWN on them. That's all there is to it![15]

[14] *Advertising Age*, 23 (Nov. 3, 1952), 66; Reilly v. Pinkus, 338 U.S. 269.
[15] Fraud Order Jacket 7343, Records of the Post Office Dept., RG 28, NA; Fraud and Lottery Docket 14/303 and State and District Court Docket 1/36, *ibid.*; Fraud Order 27,936, May 7, 1945.

Kelpidine was dried seaweed from the Pacific Ocean. The prescribed diet offered to customers cut down their eating to between 800 and 1,200 calories a day. No matter what the advertising promised, nothing in the labeling of Kelpidine referred to it as a reducing agent or as an adjunct to a reducing diet. It was, the label said, a "nutritional supplement for increasing daily intake of iodine from ocean vegetation." Ocean kelp and any iodine it contained, two physicians testified at the hearing, possessed no value in treating obesity. A doctor appearing for Pinkus asserted that the iodine in kelp was an "anti-fat for reducing," but he admitted that he had never prescribed it for that purpose nor knew of any other doctor who did. The only test he ever had made of kelp, he said, was putting some in his mouth and swallowing it with water. Nor, said the Post Office medical witnesses, could kelp "reduce the feeling of hunger" by adding "bulk" to a diet low in calories, as some of Pinkus' advertising claimed. A daily diet of 1,000 calories, these witnesses testified, was "rigid" and "severe," and Pinkus' physician agreed. Even this diet, if it could be followed, would not ordinarily take off as much weight as three pounds a week. Loss of weight at this rate, in any case, might well prove harmful, especially to patients with heart and kidney disease. None of the advertising, however, conveyed to the would-be customer that he would be buying advice to curtail his eating so drastically. The regimen would certainly not let him "eat plenty" or eat as he "usually does," as the American Health Aids advertising promised. So a fraud order was issued in 1945.

What Pinkus wanted to have read into evidence to question the Department's medical witnesses about were certain old medical works and dictionaries in which kelp had been suggested as having some value in reducing. Being denied this privilege by the hearing examiner, Pinkus sued for an injunction to prevent the fraud order from being put into effect. He won his point in the district court and, when the government appealed, in the circuit court and finally in the Supreme Court.[16]

[16] *Ibid.*; Pinkus v. Walker, 61 Fed. Supp. 610 (1945); Pinkus v. Reilly, 71 Fed. Supp. 993 (1947); Pinkus v. Reilly, 170 Fed. (2d) 786 (1948); Reilly v. Pinkus, 338 U.S. 269 (1949).

Kelpidine was by no means the only drug of contention between Joseph Pinkus and postal authorities. A peripatetic scholar, Pinkus had attended a college of osteopathy in Missouri, Montclair State Teachers College in New Jersey, New York University, Harvard, Columbia (where Teachers College awarded him the Master of Arts degree). Teaching for a time at both high school and college levels, Pinkus found his true métier as mail-order promoter. "He seems to direct all of the tremendous amount of nervous energy stored in his wiry frame," noted a trade press reporter, "into new ideas for his business." And Pinkus was remarkably fecund. Like an expert juggler, he skillfully kept many items going simultaneously. His range of interest was broad—perfumes, guns, dolls, gems, hit tunes, lingerie, reproductions of Confederate currency. Health items, however, led to his main controversies with the Post Office Department.[17]

Postal authorities got Pinkus to sign affidavits, either to stop his business or tone down his claims, for such promotions as Stop Smoke Chewing Gum; Hairgon Exolator, a device for the removal of excess hair; and T-M-X tablets, which were lauded in advertising for their quick restoration of "vim, vigor and vitality" and their power to enable any user "to start enjoying life to the full again." Pinkus lost a court challenge when he sought an injunction to stop a fraud order leveled against his Spot Reducer, a vibrating gadget. His misrepresentations, the judge ruled, must be intentionally false because for one of his earlier obesity remedies, the drug Fucine, Pinkus had represented to the public that a vibrating device could not reduce weight. Within this defeat, however, Pinkus won a sort of victory. Post Office attorneys at the hearing had sought to present evidence that Pinkus' device could neither reduce total weight nor, as he claimed, take pounds and inches away safely from "most any part of your body where it is loose and flabby." The departmental decision, however, ruled that the spot-reducing claims were not at issue, only the matter of total weight. So promoters were given a green light

[17] *Advertising Age*, 23 (Nov. 3, 1952), 66-68; Hearings in [later] American Healthaids Co., Solicitor's Docket, 1/319; Spot Reducer Co., Solicitor's Docket, 1/63; *NBBB Service Bull.*, Periodical No. 1652, Nov. 24, 1958.

on selling devices promising to massage ugly dimensions down to graceful size.[18]

A more significant Pinkus triumph involved a proposition offered to the public not for making the fat slender but for making the skinny put on pounds. It was in the More-Wate case that Pinkus' lawyer found the loopholes in Post Office Department organization after the methods of operation had been changed to fit the Administrative Procedure Act. Because investigatory and judicial functions were not properly separated, and because the changed structure had not been published in the *Federal Register*, he argued, the legal requirements of the act had not been met. A judge agreed. Other cases were lost on these same grounds, and promoters with fraud orders lined up at the Department to have the orders rescinded. So a great deal of effort went for nought. In due course, after the Department had remedied these faults, a new case was initiated against More-Wate, and Pinkus signed an affidavit agreeing to modify his claims.[19]

Pinkus' promotions brought millions of dollars to his post office box in Newark. And other mail-order promoters, through their frequent contact with Post Office lawyers, became almost as familiar faces as the postal inspectors on-the floors below. Maye Russ, then director of the Food, Drug, and Cosmetic Division of the National Better Business Bureau, chronicled for the Blatnik subcommittee the complicated careers of several of these perennial litigants. "Sometimes," she said, "the names of relatives of a person whose activities have been curbed by postal-fraud actions, appear as principals of new companies which engage in similar practices. Such techniques permit multiple offenses without the appearance of the promoter's name in a succession of violations, thus encumbering effective prosecution of the undisclosed principal."[20]

[18] Stop Smoke Co., Solicitor's Docket 7/33 (1955); Hairgon Exolator, General Counsel's Docket 1005 (1960); T-M-X Co., General Counsel's Docket 1524, Post Office Dept. Docket 2/30 (1961); Spot Reducer Co., Solicitor's Docket 1/63 (1951-60); Pinkus v. Reilly, 178 Fed. Supp. 399 (1959).

[19] Pinkus v. Reilly, 157 Fed. Supp. 548 (1957); *FDC Reports*, Jan. 20, 1958, 17 and Sep. 22, 1958, 7-8; More-Wate Co., General Counsel's Docket 1155 (1960).

[20] Spot Reducer Co., Solicitor's Docket 1/63; Hearings before House Subcommittee, 43-45.

Promotions did not necessarily end with the securing of fraud orders. If a promoter forsook direct mail solicitation and marketed his wares through retail drugstores, his product could sell on. Indeed, he could continue to get grudging help from the postal service. For a fraud order did not permit the Post Office Department to restrict a proprietor's mailing of third-class handbills and brochures. So advertising containing the very claims condemned in a fraud order could be delivered by mailmen to the mail boxes of the citizenry announcing the worthless drug or device for over-the-counter sale at a local store.[21]

Nor did the citizen into whose box such a circular was delivered have much chance of knowing that the product had been tested by postal authorities and found wanting. "What publicity," Congressman Blatnik asked the inspector in charge of mail fraud investigations, "is given to these mail fraud orders and to affidavits of discontinuance?"[22]

"Frankly," Inspector William Callahan replied, "not as much as I would like to see given them." They were published in the *Postal Bulletin,* sent to all postmasters, and a public record was made available to members of the press. But newspapers were not much interested in publishing news of this kind. Such indifference had led to the discontinuance of press releases, which the Department had issued some years before. Shortly after the Blatnik hearing, a press release service was resumed. Newspaper reporting of fraud orders, however, remained minimal. While, even with their frustrations and their failures, the Department saved the public millions of dollars by stopping shady promotions, the public remained largely ignorant of this measure of protection.[23]

The American people learned little about either the grey-zone repeaters or the imaginative individualists, whose amazing therapeutic doctrines found their way into postal archives —like those, for example, of "Saint George," whose gospel of health went forth from "Faith Farm." Although he had received no training in either theology or medicine, Saint

[21] House Report 2553 (85 Cong., 2 ses., 1958), 22.
[22] Hearings before House Subcommittee, 81-82.
[23] *Ibid.* The Post Office Department Information Service issues frequent releases entitled "Enforcement Action: Fraud and Mailability."

George, alias Morris Katzen, claimed to have had a vision from God while in a trance aboard a ship in the Persian Gulf. The vision instructed him that Jesus Christ, the all-powerful healer, was not a person but a mythical personification of the sexual fluid within the body. "The best natural healing," Saint George wrote, "is accomplished by retaining the sexual fluid; by retaining the wind; and by not being too hasty with bowel movements." Such a regimen would purify the blood, vanquish common ailments, banish nervous disorders, and provide the best chance for curing cancer. Katzen's direct mail advertising summarized his basic doctrines and offered for sale books he had written, *Keys to Life* and *The Elixir of Life*, in which the theories were more fully elaborated so that, he said, they could be practiced by the purchaser to his everlasting benefit. Katzen fought a fraud order on constitutional grounds, asserting that the order would violate the first amendment's prohibition against governmental establishment of religion. But the Post Office Judicial Officer did not agree, citing an earlier court decision: "A religious ingredient is no better defense to a charge of fraud than to a charge of murder."[24]

It is understandable that Post Office inspectors and attorneys, while proud of their successes, should sometimes fall prey to the feeling that they were ploughing the sea. The main business of the Department, after all, was to deliver the mail. Fighting fraud was an incidental, if significant, sideline. Postal inspectors had some 250 different types of investigations for which they were responsible, medical mail fraud being only one. Procedures were more complicated and legally demanding than they once had been. Hard-won victories did not seem to diminish the number of potential foes. The repeaters kept repeating, learning from their experience, so new cases were often more difficult to develop than earlier ones. New promoters entered the medical mail-order game day by day. Criminal action, sometimes resorted to, proved not to be a compelling deterrent. In many jurisdictions, indictments were difficult to obtain. Cases were always time-consuming. Fines, when imposed, amounted to only a small percentage of the profits from the ventures. Jail sentences were infrequent and usually

[24] Post Office Dept. Docket 2/73; Fraud Order 62-258 (1962).

short. The hardened promoter sometimes continued to carry on his operations from his cell.[25]

The Postmaster General, in 1957, announced that the use of the mails to promote medical quackery was at the highest level in history. Medical mail frauds, he asserted, were more lucrative than any other criminal activity. Facing such a challenge, the Blatnik committee learned, the Department had three inspectors devoting their full-time energies to medical mail fraud work. Other inspectors helped with individual cases, and a handful of lawyers sought to carry the heavy legal load. Despite some enlargement of the medical mail fraud staff, the contest continued woefully uneven.[26]

"Because of the widespread plying of the fake medicine trade," another Postmaster General stated in 1961, "it is imperative that we use our limited resources wisely. . . . For this reason, our inspectors have been instructed to concentrate their efforts on the more serious perpetrations, which affect the most people in the worst way, rather than to be diverted by 'fringe' cases, which might consume more time and labor than their investigation and prosecution justify." Of all types of fraud, he indicated, the sale of specious drugs and devices was the most difficult to prosecute. "The peddling of fake medical cures," despite the dedicated efforts of the Department's small staff, continues to be "the most prominent fraudulent activity conducted through the U.S. mails today."[27]

[25] Levine interview, Apr. 5, 1961; Miriam Ottenberg, *The Federal Investigators* (Englewood Cliffs, N.J., 1962), 310.

[26] Postmaster General Arthur E. Summerfield cited in Post Office Dept. release, May 12, 1957, reproduced in Hearings before House Subcommittee, 170-71; *ibid.*, 80.

[27] Postmaster General J. Edward Day, mimeographed text of Oct. 6, 1961, address.

# 14

## PROPRIETARY ADVERTISING
## AND THE WHEELER-LEA ACT

*"Something is very wrong when an advertising campaign, redolent with deception, can run its merry course across the country until it dies of exhaustion and is buried by its sponsors. Small wonder that sensible people shake their heads in wonderment when the Federal Trade Commission digs it out of its grave and orders it reinterred with solemn legality. Now, this may be racked up as a statistic of law enforcement, but in my judgment it has failed in its two essentials—protection of the consumer and protection of the law-abiding competitors of the false advertiser. I say that the Commission had better concentrate on halting false advertising while it is still claiming victims, rather than wagging a wise finger at the misdeeds of yesteryear. . . . We're going to serve injured business and consumers with a squad car instead of a hearse."*
—FTC CHAIRMAN PAUL RAND DIXON, 1961[1]

TWENTY-FIVE years after the publication of *Your Money's Worth*, the editors of *Consumer Reports* asked Stuart Chase to take a retrospective look at what had happened to advertising since he and F. J. Schlink had loosed their devastating blast. "The advertising of . . . patent medicines," Chase wrote, "was perfectly terrible in 1927, and it is terrible today."[2]

When Chase rendered this gloomy progress report in 1954, the Wheeler-Lea Act, intended to strengthen the Federal

[1] Dixon, "False Advertising Is No Minor Matter," mimeographed text of Apr. 17, 1961, address.

[2] Chase, " 'Your Money's Worth' Twenty-Five Years Later," *Consumer Reports*, 19 (Feb. 1954), 93.

Trade Commission's policing powers over advertising, had been on the statute books for almost 16 years. That law, designed in part by members of the House of Representatives to prevent the Food and Drug Administration from gaining control of advertising, had indeed expanded the FTC's scope of coverage and increased the sanctions at the Commission's disposal. No longer were only the "unfair methods of competition" of the 1914 law illegal; illegal also by the 1938 amendment were "unfair or deceptive acts or practices in commerce." Thus, consumers could be protected explicitly and not merely as a by-product of protecting business competitors. New sections were also added aimed directly at false advertising of food, drugs, devices, and cosmetics. In determining falsity, not only were "representations made or suggested" to be taken into account. The law barred the failure of advertisers to make affirmative disclosures necessary for consumer protection. In weighing advertising, the Commission must consider "the extent to which the advertisement fails to reveal facts material in the light of . . . representations or material [presented in an advertisement] with respect to consequences which may result from the use of the commodity . . . under the conditions prescribed in said advertisement, or under such conditions as are customary or usual."[3]

The Wheeler-Lea Act tightened procedures to speed up the date on which cease and desist orders of the Commission would become final and effective. A civil penalty was added for violation of an order, a fine of up to $5,000 for each violation upon conviction of the offender in federal district court. When orders had been carried to a circuit court and there affirmed, violators could be checked by contempt proceedings. With respect to foods, drugs, devices, and cosmetics, the Commission was authorized to apply to a district court for an injunction to stop advertising under way or planned, pending a resolution of the legality of the advertising through the Commission's usual procedures. For two types of advertising

[3] 52 U. S. Stat. 111. Charles Wesley Dunn, in *Wheeler-Lea Act, A Statement of Its Legislative Record*, has brought together texts of the various drafts of this bill, committee reports, selections from hearings, and pertinent passages from the *Congressional Record*.

in the food, drug, device, and cosmetic field, criminal action was made possible by the new law. If the Commission believed that the commodity advertised might be "injurious to health," or that the advertiser intended "to defraud or mislead," the agency could turn the facts over to the Department of Justice. Upon conviction in court for such a violation, a maximum sentence of $5,000 fine, six months' imprisonment, or both, might be imposed. For second offenders these maximums were doubled.

These broadened definitions and increased penalties, as Congressman Lea saw his handiwork, would protect the consumer and check the unscrupulous advertiser without converting the FTC law "into a criminal statute" to harry the respectable businessman. But even before the law was passed critics wondered if it could do much good. The bill "is absolutely without teeth," charged Congressman Kenney during the House debate, and he and other opponents in the House and Senate sought to point out the weaknesses of the supposed strengthening amendments. No sanction could be levied, they said, until after a cease and desist order had been secured, a long and tedious process during which the advertiser could keep on until he had virtually milked his market through his false claims. Even securing an injunction would take much time. "The injunction may say 'Stop,'" Kenney asserted, ". . . but the disseminator has already stopped. His false advertising for the year has been done." The next year would bring a new kind of false appeal or a new product. Nor would the criminal provision really aid the consumer. Few nostrums posed actual physical danger to the user, and the Wheeler-Lea definition did not cover the kind of danger that came from using innocuous medications for serious ailments and thus delaying recourse to proper medical advice. As to deliberate fraud, FDA experience had shown the well-nigh insuperable difficulties of proving fraud in court. For these reasons, Congressman Chapman predicted, the criminal clause would see rare use. In short, the bill made "no substantial change" in advertising controls that had been in force for 20 years. Patent medicine racketeers would not be deterred. The citizen, falsely thinking he was being given enhanced protection, would be deceived. If the bill should pass, the worried Copeland told the Senate, "the consumers of this country will be raped."[4]

Part of this alarm was prompted by the desire of Copeland and other members of Congress to keep the regulation of advertising in the not-yet-enacted Food, Drug, and Cosmetic law. Their gloomy predictions nonetheless contained much truth. The Wheeler-Lea Act has not permitted the FTC to control the advertising of self-medication drugs with the rigor which the FDA, under its 1938 law, has regulated labeling. Stuart Chase has been by no means the only observer who, upon looking backward, has not seen as much improvement in patent medicine advertising as he could have wished.

Questionable advertising campaigns, as Congressmen forecast, have run their course while FTC procedures have slowly unwound, from complaint, to initial hearing before an examiner, to hearing before the full Commission; from testing the Commission's cease and desist order in a circuit court to final judgment on appeal in the Supreme Court. (In one celebrated case, it took the Commission 16 years to remove the "liver" from Carter's Little Liver Pills.)[5] When an order was finally confirmed in court, no penalty—save bad publicity—accrued to the offender if he stopped using the advertising complained about. By then he very often had changed to a new approach in any case, so FTC orders, as a Commissioner acknowledged, attacked "the misdeeds of yesteryear" instead of current distorted promises "still claiming victims."[6]

[4] The main House debate took place Jan. 12, 1938, *Cong. Record* (75 Cong., 3 ses.), 391-424; both proponents and opponents had expressed their views in *Extension of Federal Trade Commission Authority over Unfair Acts and Practices and False Advertising of Food, Drugs, Devices, and Cosmetics*, House Report 1613 (75 Cong., 1 ses.). Copeland in Senate, Mar. 14, 1938, *Cong. Record* (75 Cong., 3 ses.), 3289.

[5] The case ran from the complaint in 1943 to the Supreme Court's denial of certiorari in 1959 on Carter's appeal from a 9th Circuit Court opinion. Complaint, In the Matter of Carter Products, Inc., FTC Docket 4970; Carter's Products, Inc., v. FTC, 268 Fed. (2d) 461; 36 U.S. 884. Some 11,000 pages of testimony and 750 exhibits were involved in this case. Sigurd Anderson, "Consumer Fraud: The Role of the Federal Trade Commission," mimeographed text of Mar. 11, 1960, address.

[6] For a summary of some of the lengthy FTC cases, see James Cook, *Remedies and Rackets: The Truth about Patent Medicines Today* (N.Y., 1958), 56-61, 186-87. David H. Vernon, "Labyrinthine Ways: The Handling of Food, Drug, Device and Cosmetic Cases by the Federal

Nor did the injunction and criminal provisions of the Wheeler-Lea Act prove of outstanding significance in halting exaggerated therapeutic promises. Immediately after the law's enactment, the injunction did serve to stop a number of egregious nostrum advertisers, but then its use fell off. Only some 40 injunctions were secured during the decade and a half following 1938. Congressman Chapman's prediction concerning the rare use of the criminal clause proved sound: through 1960 criminal prosecutions brought under the law had numbered only two. These two potential weapons, as a Commissioner suggested, became "rusty through disuse."[7]

Like the FDA, the FTC has had an enormous task to perform with woefully inadequate resources and staff. Responsible for anti-monopoly policing across the whole complex span of the nation's economic life, charged with combatting unfair competitive methods and deceptive acts in every field of commerce, the FTC could devote only a small portion of its attention to the false advertising of proprietary remedies. Nor has Congress been generous in its financial support. In 1962 the Commission had only a quarter more employees than it had had two decades earlier.[8]

Policy continuity with respect to false advertising has been a more difficult problem at the FTC than has policy continuity regarding labeling at the FDA. Food and Drug Commissioners until 1966 rose through the ranks, acquiring experience and attitudes toward problems confronting the agency which they served as administrative heads of policy. Few Commissioners at FTC have been elevated from the permanent staff. Appointed from divergent backgrounds and reflecting differing perspectives, the Commissioners cannot provide the same type of continuing cohesive policy. Serving the FTC not only as a multi-member head but also as a sort of court,

Trade Commission Since 1938," *FDC Law Jnl.*, 8 (June 1953), 367-93; "The Regulation of Advertising," *Columbia Law Rev.*, 56 (Nov. 1956), 1035-36; Dixon, "False Advertising Is No Minor Matter."

[7] Vernon, "Labyrinthine Ways," 370; interview with Frederick W. Irish, chief, FTC Division of Scientific Opinions, Mar. 28, 1961; Dixon, "Some Obligations of Your Consumer Franchise—a F.T.C. Point of View," mimeographed text of May 15, 1961, address.

[8] Dixon, "Let's Get Rid of Uncertainty," mimeographed text of Apr. 28, 1962, address.

the Commissioners stand somewhat aloof from their career aides. In the 1920's and since that time a change in the Commission majority has sometimes brought a sudden shift in policy lines.

The two 1938 laws posed different standards for labeling and advertising, the latter much less severe. Whereas the FDA could attack labeling "false or misleading in any particular," the FTC could only combat advertising "misleading in a material respect." Thus a broad, grey border zone continued in which exaggerated advertising assertions retained legality. The Wheeler-Lea Act had not been intended to circumscribe puffery. Senator Wheeler had made that clear during the debate. The FTC's chief examiner reiterated the point soon after the law went into effect. This assurance was seldom absent from addresses given by Commissioners before trade association conventions.[9]

Despite all the handicaps, the Commission made earnest efforts during the first few years under its new law to fight the most obvious evils. Since "advertising in the field of proprietary medicines," as Commissioner Robert Freer told the Proprietary Association, was "in large measure responsible for consumer and Congressional demand for stricter regulation," this category received major attention. Observers gave the FTC staff high marks for their diligence and zeal. Increased surveillance of advertising was launched, with attention for the first time to the foreign language press and increased emphasis on radio commercials—by this time the medium receiving the largest single share of advertising dollars. Campaigns attacked abuses in the promotion of alleged cures for obesity, arthritis, cancer, ulcers, and headaches. There was continued great reliance on use of the Commission's informal procedures, warning advertisers of their errors before launching official actions, settling cases by stipulations, thus avoiding the effort and expense of preparing cases for presentation before trial examiners. Indeed, large manufacturers sometimes complained that small manufacturers of similar products bar-

[9] Wheeler in *Cong. Record* (74 Cong., 2 ses.), 6592; James A. Horton in *Twenty-Ninth Annual Meeting, American Drug Manufacturers Association* (Baltimore, 1940); Robert M. Dyer, "False and Misleading Advertising," *FDC Law Jnl.*, 5 (Sep. 1950), 570-89.

gained therapeutic claims away by stipulation that might well have been retained had a proper fight been made. A batch of injunctions was secured against advertisers who failed to reveal harmful potentialities in their abortifacients, aphrodisiacs, and so-called cures for obesity and dipsomania. Disreputable device advertising also felt the pressure of action by the FTC. Although most of the actions launched aimed at the most disreputable fringe of proprietary advertisers, big names were not neglected. Listerine and Alka-Seltzer, for example, showed up in FTC complaints.[10]

A key driving force in this campaign against proprietary advertising was J. J. Durrett, FTC chief of medical opinions. While with the FDA, Durrett had earned the antagonism of proprietors by his forthright skepticism about the value of their wares. He had sought FTC cooperation in clamping down on manufacturers who promoted their salves and analgesics as preventives for the flu. Later disagreeing with his FDA colleagues over such issues as how vigorously to assail acetanilid-bromide pain-killers, Durrett left the agency, migrating to the FTC. He brought his strong opinions with him. Durrett's judgment, in the early Wheeler-Lea days, played a major role in determining which cases the FTC would launch in the health field and what strategy of attack the Commission would employ.[11]

Durrett's presence at FTC, perhaps, as well as lingering resentments from the bitter jurisdictional battle for control of

[10] Freer, "The Wheeler-Lea Act," mimeographed text of May 17, 1938, address; T. Swann Harding, "Has Truth in Advertising Been Achieved At Last?," *Amer. Jnl. Pharm.*, 192 (Aug. 1940), 325-26; "The Consumer and Federal Regulation of Advertising," *Harvard Law Rev.*, 53 (1940), 828-42; *FDC Reports*, Feb. 11, 1939, pink 3, white 1-2; Feb. 18, 1939, 3; Nov. 10, 1945, white 1-3; *Advertising As a Factor in Distribution*, part 5 of *Report of the Federal Trade Commission on Distribution Methods and Costs* (Wash., 1944), ix; Ewin Davis, "Federal Trade Commission Procedure—with Particular Reference to Advertising of Medicinal and Cosmetic Preparations," mimeographed text of Sep. 30, 1940, address; Robert E. Freer, "Recent Activities of the Federal Trade Commission," mimeographed text of Sep. 27, 1939, address; *JAMA*, 113 (Aug. 12, 1939), 596-97. *Annual Reports* of the FTC have been used *passim*.

[11] *FDC Reports*, Nov. 17, 1945, white 1, 2; Oct. 17, 1950, 11; Mar. 24, 1951, 5-8; *PI*, 210 (Mar. 16, 1945), 11; interview with John J. McCann, Mar. 15, 1961; see ch. 5 above.

advertising, led to a coolness between the Commission and the Food and Drug Administration that lasted for a decade and a half. Commission lawyers tried drug cases unaware of FDA's regulatory position on the questions at issue. For some proprietary products, like acetanilid-bromide mixtures and antihistamines, the FTC sought more rigorous advertising restrictions than the FDA required for labeling. For other products, like arthritis-rheumatism remedies, the reverse was true. Not until the Eisenhower administration did the agencies negotiate a peace treaty that restored harmony and established a measure of liaison on policies in overlapping areas.[12]

One of Durrett's prime objectives was to give the "affirmative disclosure" provision of the Wheeler-Lea Act meaning in practice. Proprietors thought Durrett much too extreme in insisting that their advertising warn the public of injuries that might occur and advise the public of benefits they must not expect from taking medicines. Both the Commission and the courts curtailed Durrett's eagerness. In 1947 a shift in the voting majority on the Commission brought a decision that warnings about possible hazards from the use of certain laxatives, headache remedies, and other self-medication drugs need no longer appear in advertising, at least until scientific data became clearer that substantial injury was possible. Three years later the Supreme Court refused to hear a circuit court judgment that also circumscribed the affirmative disclosure principle. The case involved a blood tonic, Oxorin Tablets, made by a manufacturer named Alberty. In this instance, the Commission had gone along with Durrett, ordering Alberty to limit claims for the tablets to conditions due to simple iron deficiency anemia, and then to add "that the condition of lassitude is caused less frequently by simple iron deficiency anemia than by other causes and that in such cases this preparation will not be effective in relieving or correcting it." Giving the Wheeler-Lea Act a narrow construction, the circuit court

[12] F&D Rev., 29 (Oct. 1945), 214-17; FDC Reports, Apr. 10, 1954, 13-14; June 12, 1954, pink 2-3; Oct. 2, 1954, white 5-6; "Working Agreement between FTC and FDA," FTC press release, June 9, 1954, containing text of agreement signed by Oveta Culp Hobby, Secretary of the Department of Health, Education, and Welfare, and FTC Chairman Edward F. Howrey.

held that the Commission had not proved the need for this warning in order to prevent consumer deception. "There is a limit to the Commission's power," the judges ruled. "It is not given a general charter to police the expenditure of the public's money or generally to do whatever is considered by it to be good and beneficial."[13]

The FTC staff also encountered troubles regarding the nature of their evidence. Many early Wheeler-Lea cases had been won before the five-member board when the staff presented medical experts as witnesses who, though never having tested the products at issue, could assert from their pharmacological knowledge that the ingredients in the nostrums could not possibly possess the therapeutic effects claimed for them in advertising. But the Commission came to give less credence to such experts and greater weight to the opinions of satisfied users who asserted that, whatever the experts said, they had indeed been cured. Manufacturers also began to defend themselves at hearings by presenting the results of clinical trials. Doctors on the Commission staff might be persuaded that this scientific evidence was "inadequate, preliminary and inconclusive," but it sounded impressive and could not easily be countered by the statements of medical experts who themselves had not tested the drugs in clinical trials. The small scientific staff of the Commission had neither the time nor money for many such efforts, and it was hard to persuade reputable outside scientists to devote their energies to proving by tedious research the falsity of claims which, to them, seemed prima facie ridiculous. So cases were lost. In the Cystex case, for example, medical experts asserted that the drug possessed no value in treating kidney and bladder disorders. But the company presented medical witnesses who had run clinical tests which, they testified, had demonstrated some merit in the product. The Commission, in denying an order, told its staff that allegations must be supported with a preponderance of evidence. It was "carefully-designed, extensively-used advertising," Durrett wrote, that presented "the real problem confronting the Commission.

[13] *FDC Law Qtly.*, 2 (Sep. 1947), 334; *PI*, 220 (Sep. 12, 1947), 15; Alberty v. FTC, 182 Fed. (2d) 36, certiorari denied, 340 U.S. 818; Jack Graeme Clark on Alberty case in *Cornell Law Qtly.*, 36 (Spring 1951), 534-41.

... Such claims involved practically the entire range of knowledge developed by the medical sciences."[14]

These defeats were symptomatic of a general slackening of the earlier vigor with which the Commission had responded to the Wheeler-Lea Act. The reformist New Deal days were gone, and the nation was enjoying postwar prosperity. President Truman's appointees to the five-member board were business-oriented. One of them, Albert Carretta, addressing the Proprietary Association, suggested his perspective in his title: "The F.T.C.—When Will It Assume the Role of the 'Friendly' Policeman?" In the past, Carretta believed, the Commission had leaned too far toward "abstract justice, untempered by the equities of fact and circumstance." In the friendlier atmosphere which Carretta desired, the number of medical advertising cases shrank. After 1950 no new campaigns were launched. The effort in that year, aimed at antihistamines promoted as cold cures, proved not a complete success: the Commission sought to attack the safety of these drugs for self-medication after the FDA had already authorized their use. Another sign of slackness in the Commission was evident: little effort was made to check on whether or not the more than 4,000 cease and desist orders outstanding were being obeyed. President Eisenhower's first appointee, Edward Howrey, who came as chairman, did seek to remedy this oversight. But being more interested in the anti-monopoly than the advertising phases of FTC's authority, Howrey restricted advertising surveillance and refrained from pressing new advertising cases. In 1954 the Commission did not issue a single new complaint in the drug field.[15]

[14] Irish interview; Irish, "The Control of False Advertising by the Federal Trade Commission," Proprietary Association *Executive Newsletter* 59-23 (June 12, 1959); *Drug Trade News*, 29 (Oct. 11, 1954), 9; 30 (Mar. 14, 1955), 8; 32 (Sep. 23, 1957), 29; *FDC Reports*, May 1, 1954, white 10. Cases revealing the Commission's changing view of evidence involved Cystex, 51 FTC 206, and Lipan, 51 FTC 616. An example of the staff's response, in developing clinical evidence, is the case against the Brotherhood of Good Samaritans for Victims of Arthritis, 53 FTC 470. Durrett, "Our Health and the Federal Trade Commission," *Jnl. Med. Assoc. of Alabama*, 13 (Mar. 1943), 158.

[15] Carretta, "The F.T.C.—When Will It Assume the Role of the 'Friendly' Policeman?," mimeographed text of June 9, 1953, address;

During these days, a drug trade reporter later noted, the FTC was "a headless, drifting agency which acted desultorily and seldom hurt anybody very much." The Commission had done "little more than play around with a situation which affects the pocketbooks, and sometimes the health, of a large proportion of the U.S. population." Frustrated staffmen in the agency did not believe the law had been given a "real tryout."[16]

In such a regulatory atmosphere, quackery was emboldened and customarily cautious advertisers were severely tempted. As in the depression, competitive pressures led to a progressive inflation of therapeutic claims. When one promoter in a given product line, taking a chance that the FTC might remain passive, promised greater benefits, other promoters had to follow or risk losing their share of the market.[17]

Even in the period before the FTC's relaxed enforcement, proprietary advertisers had developed ways of expanding their persuasiveness with little legal hazard. They sought to keep their exaggerations minor instead of "material." "The careless and false advertisers," an early critic noted, "may tell as many little fibs as they please just so they do not put in a big whopping misstatement of a material fact." They talked about "the irrelevant as if it were pertinent," made "factual statements" that did "not apply to the product or the situation described," and especially used "weasel words in small print." Qualifying phrases proliferated, which might protect the advertiser if hailed in by the FTC but still escape a would-be customer's attention, statements like "In the absence of organic trouble, this will build your blood back to normal" and "Perhaps your kidneys are to blame." Ads might ask in large type, "What do doctors prescribe for headache?," and then print in even larger letters the name of the proprietary. The link forged in the consumer's mind could well survive the more revealing story given in small type below these headlines.[18]

FDC Reports, May 22, 1954, white 9-14; Jan. 2, 1956, 6-8; Apr. 2, 1956, 3-5; Sep. 9, 1957, 5.

[16] Stephens Rippey, "Lines from Washington," Drug Trade News, 32 (Sep. 23, 1957), 29; 33 (Feb. 24, 1958), 28.

[17] FDC Reports, Sep. 9, 1957, 5.

[18] Harding, "Has Truth in Advertising Been Achieved At Last?,"

Radio offered still more opportunities for evading the spirit while abiding by the letter of the law. "The spoken word," a critic noted, "can be made to say one thing and mean another." He asked his readers to listen for "the sly formula of implication and innuendo" which radio commercials exhibited, including precautionary statements which the "Federal Trade Commission has obviously requested the advertiser to insert and the advertiser has obviously instructed the announcer to 'kill' by inflection."[19]

And then came television, bringing, as a Commissioner said, "the pitchman off the street into our parlors." Beginning in the late 1940's, TV advertising became by 1955 a billion-dollar business. To the hard-sell spoken word was added visual impression, and proprietary manufacturers became inveterate users of the medium. Reaching back into the ancient days of patent medicine promotion, they revived symbols of evil from the devil's dark domain, and now the fiendish creatures wiggled. Spectators peered inside the body, watched limp intestines undulate with vigor when plied with laxatives, observed the exciting race of pain-relievers from stomach to brain, harkened to white-coated actors impersonating doctors. And TV advertising paid off: one "relaxant capsule," an agency executive said, had gotten sales results within a few weeks that in pre-TV years would have taken ten years to achieve. Grumbling about the ubiquity of television advertising began to be heard in many quarters, and some of its specious therapeutic counsel, one pharmacologist said, was "as potentially dangerous as a loaded gun."[20]

All American advertising had boomed mightily since the depression days, when the basic utility of this form of economic enterprise had been seriously questioned by Chase and

---

325-34; "Patent Medicine Shows," *JAMA*, 119 (June 27, 1942), 714; "Advertising for Home Remedies," *ibid.*, 145 (Mar. 31, 1951), 986-87.

[19] R. M. Cunningham, Jr., "Medicine Men of the Air," *New Republic*, 111 (Oct. 23, 1944), 515-17.

[20] Commissioner Sigurd Anderson, "Modern Advertising—Uses and Abuses," mimeographed text of Sep. 27, 1956, address; David Seligman, "The Amazing Advertising Business," *Fortune*, 54 (Sep. 1956), 107-109; *FDC Law Jnl.*, 13 (Oct. 1958), 664; *FDC Reports*, Sep. 2, 1957, 15; Sep. 9, 1957, 17; Oct. 7, 1958, 22; *Drug Trade News*, 33 (Jan. 27, 1958), 2; (June 2, 1958), 2.

Kallet and Schlink. In the postwar decade alone—while FTC
resources were inching up—the total volume of advertising
had trebled, reaching an annual expenditure of ten billion
dollars. A new storm of protest was rising, but little of the
critique would strike at the fundamental usefulness of this
social institution as the "guinea pig" muckrakers had done.
Few commentators would blast all advertising as "economic
waste." "As capitalism itself has grown more productive (and
popular) in the U.S.," a writer in *Fortune* asserted, "it has
come to be more generally accepted that advertising has a
good deal to do with the rising U.S. standard of living."
Even Stuart Chase had mellowed. "Advertising has an important task," he acknowledged, "in a high energy economy."
Except for several product categories, advertising was "less
lethal" than when he and Schlink had written *Your Money's
Worth*. Radicals had stopped attacking it "with loud rebel
yells." Advertising, in short, had won its war with its severest
critics, by making some concessions, by counterpropaganda,
and especially by continuing to develop "weapons of persuasion" in the technique of appealing to customers which were
more effective in selling without being so assailable on rational grounds as violations of the "truth."[21]

While under heavy fire during the depression, the advertising industry constantly augmented the sums it spent on psychological research, becoming by 1940 one of the largest customers for studies of human behavior. Copywriters continually
improved ways of making claims which, if they had been
explicit, would have violated the Wheeler-Lea Act, but, being
implicit, escaped official censure. Their goal was to endow
their ads with "psychological techniques of persuasion so emotionally powerful and subtle that they could induce a determined opponent of advertising to buy the product even if he
disbelieved the claims advertised for it." This goal was best
achieved by presenting their appeals through "stereotyped
images and unequivocal symbols," often pictorial, rooted in
fundamental emotional drives. Ads presented vicarious experiences, implying they might be actualized by using the prod-

---

[21] Seligman, "The Amazing Advertising Business," 107, 110; Chase,
" 'Your Money's Worth' Twenty-Five Years Later," 93-95.

uct, playing on basic cravings for security, status, prestige, companionship, love, sexual fulfillment.[22]

During World War II, as during World War I, the advertising profession employed its most effective weapons in behalf of the national interest. And in the postwar decade, with the advent of television, psychological probing of the consumer expanded so markedly "as to render the findings of the prewar era almost elementary by contrast." Over 80 firms engaged in and sold what came to be called "Motivation Research." This alliance between "Freud and the Hucksters" prospered because, when tested by the yardstick of expanding sales, it yielded excellent results.[23]

In the mid-1950's, when the Federal Trade Commission's regulatory efforts were at low ebb, sporadic criticisms of advertising began to coalesce into a major movement. It was not the existence of advertising that came to be condemned but its excesses: the noisiness and abominable taste of television and radio commercials, the cynicism of some of the craft's grey-suited practitioners, the unethical alliances summed up in the word "payola." Critics worried too about advertising's very potent social role: the unnerving effect of its constant prodding of emulative anxieties, the depreciation of more basic values through glorifying of materialistic satisfactions. Advertising's amazing success at motivating conduct in the marketplace through appeal to irrational drives—through "hidden persuaders"—brought increasing uneasiness to many thoughtful citizens. In various ways these cumulating concerns acted to re-energize the FTC.

Amid the wide range of advertising's vulnerabilities, proprietary advertising was a most conspicuous target. The American Medical Association grew increasingly concerned about the white-coated pseudo-doctors who lauded "new" drugs—

[22] A probing discussion of these trends appears in Otis Pease, *The Responsibilities of American Advertising: Private Control and Public Influence, 1920-1940*, 167-203.

[23] *Ibid.*, 202-203. The literature on "Motivation Research" is vast. See Perrin Stryker, "Motivation Research," *Fortune*, 53 (June 1956), 144ff.; Ralph Goodman, "Freud and the Hucksters," *Nation*, 176 (Feb. 14, 1953), 143-45; "Consumer Motivation," *Consumer Report*, 22 (June 1957), 299-301. The work that most aroused the public was Vance Packard, *The Hidden Persuaders* (N.Y., 1957).

like the bioflavonoids and chlorophyll—without adequate scientific proof. Sensitive common citizens grew ever more irritated at drug commercials, objecting to learning about their "potential intestinal difficulties between Beethoven and Mozart." The Commission "can regulate medicine claims," commented a newspaperman, "about as well as a gardener can regulate autumn leaves in a high wind." What spurred the FTC most directly, however, was the reflection of these pressures on Congressional committees. Appropriation committees in both Houses raised probing questions about the FTC's policy on proprietary advertising. In 1957 a subcommittee of the House Committee on Government Operations, chaired by Congressman John A. Blatnik, held hearings on misleading advertising in the weight-reducing field. From this examination the FTC emerged with very poor marks indeed. Physicians and a representative of the Better Business Bureau spoke out most critically about abuses in obesity-cure promotion. FTC defense of its policies did not impress committeemen as adequate. The fact of a court defeat in 1946—in a case the Commission admitted had not been well presented—was no excuse for the ensuing "12-year paralysis." "In this [obesity] field," Blatnik's final report charged, "the attitude of the Commission has been one of indifference and apathy," and as to false and misleading advertising generally, "the Commission's record has been one of incredible delay and procrastination." As a result, with respect to slenderizing wares alone, "the American consumer" was "being bilked out of approximately $100 million" expended annually on these preparations.[24] In 1959, probing the quiz show scandals, the House Legislative Oversight Subcommittee found that one of the major programs involved had been sponsored by a proprietary manufacturer.[25]

Responding to successive waves of pressure, the FTC

[24] *FDC Reports*, May 30, 1955, 18; Apr. 2, 1956, 3; May 26, 1958, 17-18; *Drug Trade News*, 31 (Jan. 16, 1956), 1, 33; letter to editor, *Harper's Mag.*, 202 (Apr. 1951), 20; Cook, *Remedies and Rackets*, 65; *False and Misleading Advertising (Weight-Reducing Preparations): Hearings before a Subcommittee of the Committee on Government Operations* (85 Cong., 1 ses., 1957); *False and Misleading Advertising (Weight Reducing Remedies)*, House Report 2553 (85 Cong., 2 ses., 1958).

[25] *FDC Reports*, Oct. 12, 1959, 21.

brought greater and greater pressure to bear on proprietary advertisers. In 1955 21 complaints were issued in the drug and cosmetic field. Late in the year, Chairman Howrey, resigning under fire from the House Small Business Subcommittee, was replaced by John Gwynne, who was more interested in policing advertising. In the first year of Gwynne's chairmanship, more complaints and orders were issued than in any year since World War II. Monitoring was once again improved by the creation of a special radio-TV "task force," which put attorneys in Washington and in FTC field offices to work listening and watching to catch the tone of voice and note the facial expression of advertising pitchmen: previous monitors had merely read the scripts. "Quite a few" of the misleading claims picked up by this method, Gwynne told the Senate Appropriations Committee, would "have to do with drugs." New complaints began to issue: against a series of arthritis-rheumatism remedies with such nationally known names as Mentholatum, Infra Rub, and Heet; against the shampoo Lanolin Plus; against Rolaids, which sought to boost its antacid qualities by showing television viewers—falsely, the FTC charged—that concentrated stomach acid could burn a hole in a cloth napkin. The FTC also resurrected the affirmative disclosure principle, dead since the Alberty case, applying it first to a series of hair treatment salons which were failing to tell readers of their advertising that most cases of baldness were impervious to their methods. Stronger liaison was established with the Federal Communications Commission, which henceforth received copies of FTC documents relating to actions against radio and television advertising. After the Blatnik hearings, but before the subcommittee issued its blistering report, the FTC started a campaign against weight-reducing remedies.[26]

[26] 1956 FTC Annual Report, 2, 38-39; 1957 Annual Report, 3, 37; 1958 Annual Report, 41; 1959 Annual Report, 6, 48; *FDC Reports,* Aug. 15, 1955, 3-9; Jan. 2, 1956, 6-8; Jan. 21, 1957, 5; May 20, 1957, 4; July 15, 1957, 8-10; July 22, 1957, 4; July 21, 1958, 10; *Drug Trade News,* 30 (Aug. 15, 1955), 4; 32 (Mar. 25, 1957), 27; (Apr. 22, 1957), 1; 33 (Sep. 22, 1958), 14; *Business Week,* Apr. 6, 1957, 73; FCC Order 57-172, "Liaison between Federal Communications Commission and Federal Trade Commission," *Federal Register,* Apr. 6, 1957.

The quiz scandals made big headlines and increased consumer complaints about commercials tenfold in the FTC's mail. This too intensified the Commission's campaign. "If the creative ability of those who develop advertising gambits—and who are, I understand, rather handsomely remunerated for it—is of the genius variety we are led to believe, they should have no difficulty in reconciling their imaginative fantasy with legality of phraseology." Such was the sarcastic judgment of the Commission's new chairman, Earl Kintner, who had been elevated to that position from within the agency, which he had served as general counsel. Expanding monitoring around the clock, the FTC challenged TV commercials that seemed to show one thing while actually showing another, complaining, for example, about the "protective shield" claim for Gardol in Colgate's toothpaste. The Commission also began to include in its actions, along with the manufacturer, the advertising agency that had prepared the copy. This publicity was unwelcome. "What disturbs Madison Avenue," a business periodical noted, "is that the government seems intent on turning advertising's own tools of communication against it."[27]

While adding "a few lead weights" to "the enforcement club," Kintner at the same time sought to persuade industry and the media to take giant steps toward self-reform. He and his Commission colleagues made many addresses in which pleading and warning were intertwined. The warning flag, of course, had long been out, but too few advertisers had seemed to see it. After the Blatnik hearings, Dr. Cullen had counselled Proprietary Association members to recheck their advertising and make changes, if necessary, "to stem the tide."[28]

Self-regulation machinery at the highest echelons of advertising was tightened up, with full support from the American Medical Association. Some physicians desired a forthright anti-self-medication stand, but the AMA's House of Delegates

[27] *FDC Reports,* Nov. 23, 1959, 14; Jan. 11, 1960, 15; Apr. 25, 1960, 23-24; *Business Week,* Dec. 19, 1959, 73-74, 76; Jan. 23, 1960, 34; *FDC Law Jnl.,* 15 (Feb. 1960), 95; 1960 FTC Annual Report, 53-54.

[28] *FDC Reports,* June 13, 1960, 13-15; Kintner, "The Current State of Advertising," mimeographed text of June 15, 1960, address; Proprietary Association *Executive News-Letter* 492 (Aug. 16, 1957).

directed an augmentation of liaison with the radio-television industry to raise advertising levels voluntarily. After an informal conference, attended by representatives of the AMA, the National Better Business Bureau, the proprietary industry, and advertising agencies and media, the AMA became a sustaining member of the NBBB, thinking it "the most practical coordinating agency." This new "mechanism" of coordination, a committee reported to the 1958 AMA convention, would produce good results. The House of Delegates did enact a resolution condemning advertising that urged self-treatment for indigestion, constipation, and anemia, although a committee report complimented the proprietary industry generally on its diligent efforts at self-policing. The specter of "socialized" medicine doubtless played a role in the AMA's efforts to wrestle with an admittedly serious problem in a wholly voluntaristic way. Indeed, a committee resolution calling for stricter governmental controls on advertising was pigeonholed.[29]

The National Association of Broadcasters, as a token of the new cooperative efforts, amended its code to ban actors in drug commercials from wearing white coats. "Dramatized advertising involving statements or purported statements by physicians, dentists or nurses," the new rule said, "must be presented by accredited members of such professions." A special committee of the Television Code Review Board was appointed to survey commercials and draft some "common-sense guideposts" for those preparing them. With respect to laxatives, for example, the subcommittee suggested the avoidance of "techniques which over-dramatize the discomfort of one requiring a laxative, which emphasize the speed or efficiency of the laxative, [and] which duplicate the mechanics of elimination by charts or props." Barred completely from showing by stations which wished to display the Code Board's seal of approval were commercials promoting feminine hygiene products and hemorrhoid remedies.[30]

[29] *FDC Reports,* May 26, 1958, 17-18; June 30, 1958, 9-11; *Drug Trade News,* 33 (July 14, 1958), 1, 27; *JAMA,* 167 (July 19, 1958), 1508.
[30] *Drug Trade News,* 33 (June 30, 1958), 1; 34 (Oct. 5, 1959), 1, 14; excerpts from NAB "Television Code Review Board Special Sub-Committee Report on Personal Product Advertising," in Proprietary As-

This last taboo revealed some of the difficulties inherent in self-regulation. One of the giants of the proprietary industry, AMHO-Whitehall, marketed a profitable treatment for piles called Preparation H. The Code Review Board warned television stations that they would lose their seal of approval if they continued showing Preparation H commercials. Over a score of stations preferred the advertising revenue to the seal. In any case, many stations were not members of the National Association of Broadcasters and of those that were, some were not subscribers to the code. AMHO-Whitehall increased its dollar outlay for television advertising in behalf of Preparation H.[51]

Certainly, by the early 1960's, neither renewed efforts at self-regulation nor reinvigorated regulation by the Federal Trade Commission had solved the problem of either taste or "truth" in proprietary advertising. Of all the complaints reaching the National Better Business Bureau, those in the health field headed the list. In a poll conducted by the National Audience Board, deodorant commercials struck consumers as most obnoxious. "All TV commercials for deodorants stink," wrote one spokesman for the public, Brooks Atkinson of the *New York Times.* "Many of the others are harrowing in one way or another. The trip hammer that pounds on the nerves, the bolts of lightning that split the head of the junior executive, the flaming stomach walls, the liver acid that burns holes in a cloth, the pockets of rotting food between teeth—portray the American body as one of nature's abominations."[32]

Uneasiness continued within the industry. "When you sit," said the vice-president of a major proprietary concern, "as I have so often in these past months, with Government officials or with advertising men from other industries and discuss the problems facing advertising today, we in the drug business are most frequently considered to be the bad boys. We are the ones who are called the rotten apples in the barrel." And an advertising agency official, speaking to his fellows, was equally

---

sociation *Executive News-Letter* 59-44 (Oct. 23, 1959); *FDC Reports,* Aug. 26, 1957, 17.
[31] *Ibid.,* May 11, 1959, 16; June 22, 1959, 13.
[32] *Wash. Post,* July 8, 1960; Aug. 1, 1961; *N.Y. Times,* June 16, 1961.

disturbed. "Some of the advertising now on the air for deodorants, laxatives, corn removers, 'sick headache' remedies, cold and sinus inhalants, and girdles and brassieres needs to be thrown off and kept off the air. For if there is nothing more beautiful to the maker of nose spray than a map of the nasal passages, at least he mustn't insist upon showing it in parlor projection."[33]

"To say that the Government's enforcement of the truth-in-advertising law has been ineffectual," adjudged a *Consumer Reports* editorial, "is to put a good face on the matter. It has been close to a farce." Still another FTC chairman, Paul Rand Dixon, surveying the Commission's past from the vantage of 1961, was forced to assess that record gloomily. The agency had not yet found a way to stop false advertising while it was "still claiming victims."[34]

Abuses with respect to prescription drug advertising, exposed in the celebrated hearings conducted by Senator Estes Kefauver, led to the enactment of legislation in 1962 which placed control of such advertising within the authority of the Food and Drug Administration.[35] By the mid-1960's no similar major confrontation and resolution of the questionable techniques in drug advertising to consumers had yet occurred.

[33] Donald S. Frost, a Bristol-Myers vice-president, Proprietary Association *Executive News-Letter* 14-60 (Apr. 8, 1960); Fairfax Cone of Foote, Cone & Belding, *Business Week*, Apr. 30, 1960, 86, 88.
[34] "The FTC's Squad Car," *Consumer Reports*, 26 (July 1961), 425-26; Dixon, "False Advertising Is No Minor Matter."
[35] Kefauver-Harris Drug Amendments of 1962, 76 U.S. Stat. 780. See ch. 19 below.

# 15

## MEDICINE SHOW IMPRESARIO

---

*"What's Hadacol? Well, basically, it's a patent medicine—a little honey, a little of this and that, and a stiff shot of alcohol hyped up with vitamin B. Actually it's a great deal more. It's a craze. It's a culture. It's a political movement."*

—NEWSWEEK, 1951[1]

---

ONE of the Federal Trade Commission's "customers" during the summer of 1950 was a Louisiana state senator named Dudley J. LeBlanc. Pausing briefly to sign a stipulation which promised to tone down his advertising claims, LeBlanc quickly turned his amazing energies to promoting the gaudiest comet to flash across the nostrum sky in the 20th century. Hadacol was, as Morris Fishbein said, the "apotheosis of nostrums."[2]

LeBlanc, during the heyday of his fame, was fond of telling inquiring reporters how it had all begun. In 1943, he said, he got a bad pain in his right big toe. The pain spread to his knees, his arms, his neck. Three different doctors gave him three different diagnoses—gout, arthritis, beriberi. Each treated him without success. While in a New Orleans hospital, he overheard his wife say: "He really is sick. I never saw Dudley so bad. I just don't know if I'll ever see him alive again."[3]

---

[1] 37 (Apr. 16, 1951), 32.

[2] In the Matter Of The LeBlanc Corporation, a corporation, and Dudley J. LeBlanc, an individual, Stipulation 8034, Aug. 17, 1950, FTC; Fishbein, "Hadacol—Apotheosis of Nostrums," *Postgraduate Medicine*, 9 (Feb. 1951), 175-77.

[3] The story exists in a number of versions containing some contradictions in details. This account is a composite taken from Norma Lee Browning's *Chicago Tribune* series, Feb. 18, 19, 20, 1951; *Newsweek*, 37 (Apr. 16, 1951), 32-33; Maynard Stitt, "Cousin Dud's Hadacol," *Amer. Mercury*, 73 (Sep. 1951), 7-15.

LeBlanc sought to escape from the hospital. As he hobbled out he met an old friend, another doctor, who told him he looked like "walking death." Hearing LeBlanc's symptoms, the doctor offered to cure them. So LeBlanc went with him to his office for an injection. Like magic the medication began to cure his condition. Each shot brought further improvement. LeBlanc was naturally curious. So he asked: "Doc, whazzat stuff you got in dat l'il ole bottle?"

"Dude, you crazy?" the doctor answered. "You think I give away my secrets to a man in the patent medicine business?"

Several days later the doctor was busy and told his nurse to give LeBlanc his shot.

"She wasn't so smart as him," LeBlanc later reminisced. "Nor so careful either. She left the bottle on the table. When she finished I gave her that old Southern Chivalry, you know, 'after you, Gertrude.' As soon as she turned her back I shoved the bottle in my pocket."

Taking the bottle to his hotel, LeBlanc read the label, then got some books to find out what the label meant. His injections, he found, were mostly B vitamins. "Then I figured to myself," LeBlanc said, "this is it."

*It*—as he shortly worked things out—proved to be an elixir of 12 per cent alcohol, plus some of the B complex vitamins, iron, calcium, and phosphorus, dilute hydrochloric acid, and honey. LeBlanc mixed the first batches in big barrels behind his Abbeville, Louisiana, barn, nearby farmers' daughters stirring it with boat oars. Everybody sampled it, and the ailing felt improved. LeBlanc put his product on the market. It took hold fast.[4]

"They came in to buy Hadacol," recalled a Lafayette pharmacist, "when they didn't have money to buy food. They had holes in their shoes and they paid $3.50 for a bottle of Hadacol."[5]

"From Down on the Delta"—so ran a later advertisement—"Came the Thrilling News! First to try HADACOL . . . first to see with their own eyes how this unknown new health formula marches into the battle against the pain and suffering of disease

[4] Hadacol bottle label; *Chicago Tribune*, Feb. 18, 1951.
[5] Clayton Kirkpatrick in *ibid.*, Nov. 5, 1951.

. . . were the plain-living hard-to-convince families of Louisiana's romantic delta land, direct descendants of the famed Acadians who settled there 200 years ago. The wonderful news of HADACOL traveled fast. Along the fantastically twisted shores of the lonely bayous . . . across the sweltering sugar plantations into the tangled backwoods . . . in the picturesque settlements of Labadieville, Bayou Goula, Lafourche and Grand Conteau the French-speaking natives passed the word until the whole delta country knew about HADACOL."[6]

LeBlanc himself was a Cajun who traced his ancestry back nine generations to Acadia and France. Indeed, he was a professional Acadian, once penning a booklet about the great 18th-century migration from Nova Scotia to Louisiana, once escorting a group of Cajun girls dressed like Evangeline back to Grand Pré, stopping off at the White House to say hello to President Hoover. Born in 1895, the son of a blacksmith, LeBlanc spoke only the Cajun patois until he was almost ten. Poor but ambitious, he paid for some schooling by organizing a pants-pressing service. He served a while in World War I, then went on the road as salesman for shoes, tobacco, patent medicines. LeBlanc also launched a burial insurance company. And, playing up his Cajun heritage, he entered politics.[7]

In 1926 LeBlanc beat a Huey Long–backed candidate for the post of public service commissioner for southern Louisiana, and soon he was representing two Cajun parishes in the state senate. In 1932 LeBlanc made his first race for governor, opposing a candidate hand-picked by the Kingfish from his Senate seat in Washington. (Huey, incidentally, had once served part of his apprenticeship as traveling salesman for Wine of Cardui.) The race was bitter. LeBlanc tried to outdo Long's social welfare promises, offering a $30-a-month pension to all Louisiana citizens over 60. And charges of disloyalty to

[6] *New Orleans Item*, Oct. 14, 1948.

[7] LeBlanc, *The True Story of the Acadians* (n.p., 1932); on p. 90 is a photograph of the Louisiana party and President and Mrs. Hoover. Biographical data in souvenir program for 1951 Hadacol Caravan Show; *Chicago Tribune*, Feb. 18, 19, 20, 1951; Stitt, "Cousin Dud's Hadacol," 7-15; David Nevin, "The Brass-Band Pitchman and His Million-Dollar Elixir," *True*, Mar. 1962, 16-28, 114.

the white race flew thick and fast. Huey termed Dudley's Thibodeaux Benevolent Association "a nigger burial lodge and shroud and coffin club," accusing its promoter of putting dead Negroes in expensive coffins and later transferring them to pine boxes for burial. Long also circulated pictures of LeBlanc and his Negro associates in the burial association. LeBlanc responded with pictures of Long distributing tax-bought textbooks to Negro children. At the end of this mudslinging campaign, Long's candidate beat LeBlanc handily in the primary.[8]

Selling out his burial association, LeBlanc began to manufacture patent medicines: Dixie Dew Cough Syrup and Happy Day Headache Powders. Three factors brought this venture to an end. First, competition was keen and profits not suitably rewarding. Second, in 1941, the Food and Drug Administration seized some of the Powders. The mixture of aspirin, acetanilid, caffeine, milk sugar, and the laxative phenolphthalein, the libel said, was dangerous to health when used according to directions and certainly not efficacious for the long list of ailments listed in the labeling. No claimant appearing in court, the Powders were condemned and destroyed. And third, LeBlanc built a better mousetrap. As a result of his big-toe crisis, he formulated Hadacol. The name was a contraction of Happy Day Company plus the "L" for LeBlanc's own initial.[9]

The senator boosted sales for his own product throughout the Cajun country by reading testimonials in French over a radio station. Shortly he expanded to printing testimonials in both French and English newspaper advertising. And what testimonials they were! "I no longer suffer from asthma," wrote a man from Iowa, Louisiana. "Crippling rheumatism for 10 years long . . . now I walk again," wrote a woman from St. Martinsville. "Was suffering terribly from disease of the blood . . . now back to work," wrote a man from New Orleans. "I do not have heart trouble any more," wrote a woman from Port Arthur, Texas. "This is to certify," wrote a man from Arnauds-

[8] Allan P. Sindler, *Huey Long's Louisiana: State Politics, 1920-1952* (Baltimore, 1956), 51, 76-78; Huey Long as salesman, *Standard Remedies,* 21 (July 1935), 14.

[9] *Chicago Tribune,* Feb. 18, 1951; *Newsweek,* 37 (Apr. 16, 1951), 33; DDNJ 434 (the seizure took place Mar. 21, 1941).

ville, "that I . . . was suffering from ulcers of the stomach. . . .
One doctor told me that I was suffering from cancer. . . . I
decided to be operated on and my wife persuaded me to take
HADACOL. . . . I can now eat almost everything . . . even pork.
In fact, I feel perfectly well. I work hard in the field with no
ill effect." In 1948 LeBlanc gathered up his glowing crop
of testimonials and reprinted them in a pamphlet called *Good
Health Life's Greatest Blessing*—replete with pictures of the
testimonial givers. In sections on anemia, arthritis, asthma,
diabetes, epilepsy, heart trouble, high and low blood pressure,
gallstones, paralytic stroke, tuberculosis, and ulcers, LeBlanc
cited his grateful customers who praised Hadacol for curing
them of these serious ailments.[10]

The Hadacol bubble began to expand enormously, growing out from the romantic delta land to cover the broader
South. Lafayette became a boom town, as LeBlanc tore down
houses and a school to enlarge his plant. Experts at promotion
were hired from major proprietary concerns in the East. And
as sales grew fast, LeBlanc's advertising campaign grew faster.
Toward the end of 1949, he found he owed a tremendous tax
bill which he did not have the ready cash to pay. So LeBlanc
told his advertising manager to wipe out the bill by plunging
the whole sum in new advertising. During the last two months
of the year over $300,000 carried the Hadacol message far
and wide.[11]

In entering the Atlanta market, for example, LeBlanc blan-
keted the area with newspaper ads and radio spots before he
shipped any of his tonic to the city. He ran a radio contest,
which required the listener to identify "Dixie," and winners
were sent coupons good for a bottle of Hadacol. Going from
drugstore to drugstore, recipients found no Hadacol in stock.
Then LeBlanc sent in trailer trucks loaded with the medicine.
His salesmen, however, would let each drugstore operator
have only a single case, saying that Hadacol was in short

[10] Interview with Wallace F. Janssen of FDA, June 19, 1956; *New
Orleans Item*, Oct. 14, 1948; *Atlanta Constitution*, Sep. 21, 1948; *Baton
Rouge Advocate*, Apr. 11, 1945; the Hadacol folder in the AMA's Dept.
of Investigation contains a copy of *Good Health Life's Greatest Blessing*.
[11] *Chicago Tribune*, Nov. 5, 1951; *FDC Reports*, Oct. 6, 1951; Stitt,
"Cousin Dud's Hadacol," 7-15.

supply, but would be available through wholesalers. Some druggists ordered from every wholesaler. In two days the Hadacol trucks were empty.[12]

In 1950 Hadacol grossed at least $20 million within its sales area of 22 states, by far the largest sum spent for any proprietary in the world. And both sales and advertising were still expanding. Toward the close of the year, LeBlanc's advertising bill ran to a million dollars a month, taking in about 700 daily papers and 4,700 weeklies and 528 radio stations. For various reasons, the style of his ads became, if not less subdued than earlier in the bayous, at least more circumspect. For one thing, LeBlanc was aware that the Food and Drug Administration was observing his operations with suspicious interest. Whereas the Hadacol package labeling made no undue claims, FDA inspectors had noted what might be construed as misleading promises painted on LeBlanc's fleet of white trucks. Chief Inspector George Larrick, indeed, had notified the FDA office in New Orleans to trail a truck laden with Hadacol and, when it crossed a state line, to seize the cargo, alleging the truck slogans as mislabeling. Somehow LeBlanc became aware his truck was being followed. He phoned Larrick in Washington to report that all trucks were being repainted. For another thing, there was the FTC stipulation which LeBlanc had signed. Although the trade press commented on the mildness of this restraint, the senator had promised to stop saying that Hadacol would "restore youthful feeling and appearance," that it would ensure "good health," indeed, that it possessed any therapeutic value other than that resulting from a dietary deficiency of the ingredients it contained. So gone from LeBlanc's advertising were any references to asthma and to cancer. As far as promises went, Hadacol was now good for what ailed you, if what ailed you was what Hadacol was good for.[13]

This message was, of course, more subtly phrased. One ad depicted a man laboriously climbing from a swamp over almost insurmountable boulders atop which shone a glorious sun. The

[12] Nevin, "The Brass-Band Pitchman," 24.

[13] *Business Week*, Jan. 6, 1951, 72; *PI*, 232 (Sep. 1, 1950), 77; interview with George Larrick, Aug. 4, 1965; FTC stipulation 8034. *Drug Trade News*, 29 (Aug. 30, 1956), 6, gave Hadacol's 1950 gross as $24,000,000.

boulders bore labels—fatigue, vague aches and pains, nervousness, tiredness, stomach bloat. Who among the readers had not suffered from one or another of these assorted ailments? And who would not yearn to escape such a "'rocky road' through life?" Yet, in deference to the FTC, LeBlanc added to each boulder, in addition to the big-print name of its malady, a small legend reading: "When due to lack of Vitamins $B_1$, $B_2$, Niacin and Iron."[14]

If heart trouble and epilepsy were gone from printed testimonials, tributes of gratitude involving lesser ailments still formed the backbone of Hadacol advertising. Hundreds of men, women, and children lauded the tonic from the pages of the press and over the airwaves. A septuagenarian minister who could neither eat with comfort nor sleep with ease noted "a wonderful change" before he had taken half a bottle. A lad of 13 who lacked energy even to ride his bicycle took Hadacol and became center on his football team. A rundown housewife who couldn't keep up with her housework began with the first bottle to regain her pep, and 15 bottles later was going strong. Names and addresses and photographs of these satisfied customers—most of them smiling buoyantly—accompanied their testimony. LeBlanc had aides who went out to follow up the letters that came pouring in. These letters came not from men and women of distinction, but from America's millions whose names seldom appeared in newspaper headlines. They worked on railroads, in retail stores, in pottery factories. Some were veterans of military service. Now and then a writer held local governmental responsibility, like the post of chairman of a county parole board. The reader who perused the testimonials found them penned by humble people like his neighbors and himself. If he was of religious bent, he might be pleased to note the devout praise of Hadacol from a clergyman. If he was awed by the health professions, he might find persuasive commendations from an apprenticed pharmacist and a nurse. If he held education in esteem, the happy Hadacol experience of college students might seem impressive.[15]

14 *Atlanta Journal*, Apr. 12, 1951.
15 *Ibid.*, Mar. 13 and Apr. 24, 1951; *Emory* (Univ.) *Wheel*, Mar. 27,

As he refurbished the testimonial, so too did LeBlanc exploit other stock techniques of the old-time nostrum vendor. He boastfully cited for all to read the statistics of Hadacol sales. Twenty million bottles in ten months. Twenty-seven million bottles in a year. Three great new factories. An endless caravan of white Hadacol-distributing trucks, each emblazoned "For a Better Tomorrow." Admitting his own amazement at a success outreaching his "wildest dreams," LeBlanc let his reader draw the inevitable conclusion: so many millions can't be wrong. But should a potential customer still remain skeptical, LeBlanc was willing to let him be the final judge. "You have to be satisfied," his ads assured; if you should find that Hadacol fails to help, take comfort in the fact that LeBlanc *will gladly send back your money.*" So had promised the maker of Dr. William Judkin's Patent Specific Ointment in 1826.[16]

LeBlanc also resurrected the old-time medicine show and built it to gargantuan proportions. In the summer of 1950 a caravan of 130 vehicles, including steam calliopes, toured 3,800 miles through the South, LeBlanc's medicine troupe playing one-night stands in 18 cities. Heavy advertising heralded the show's approach, and each night, on the average, 10,000 fans brought their Hadacol box tops as admission fees to hear a Dixieland band play "Hadacol Boogie" and "Who Put the Pep in Grandma?," to watch Chicago chorus girls illustrate the history of the female bathing suit, and to observe the antics of such big-name performers as Connie Boswell, Carmen Miranda, Roy Acuff, Minnie Pearl, Mickey Rooney, Chico Marx, George Burns, and Gracie Allen. LeBlanc himself served as master of ceremonies, posing with his show girls, joshing with his customers, and lauding in stentorian tones the virtues of the South.[17]

"I spent a cool half million for talent and stuff on this tour,"

---

1951; *Chicago Tribune*, Mar. 13, 1951; Nevin, "The Brass-Band Pitchman," 26.

[16] *Atlanta Journal*, Nov. 11, 1950, Mar. 13, 1951.

[17] *Time*, 55 (June 19, 1950), 81-82; R. Raynolds and T. G. Harris, "Yahoo Hadacol!," *Life*, 29 (Sep. 18, 1950), 23-24 *passim*; Joseph Roddy, "Million-Dollar Medicine Man," *Look*, 14 (Dec. 5, 1950), 34-43.

LeBlanc boasted, "but I sold more than three million bucks' worth of Hadacol along the way." He also showed to tens of thousands of his fellow Southerners the brash, earthy, self-confident extrovert who made the Hadacol they paid for. A short, round man, wearing rimless glasses, a Texas hat, and black-and-white shoes, LeBlanc's bragging and chuckling and gaudy showmanship turned him into a celebrity, and this sold medicine. Those who saw the shows and read of LeBlanc's antics in the press knew him to be a man of humble origin, like themselves, who, in the great American tradition, had climbed the ladder of financial success by the exercise of native shrewdness.[18]

The senator followed up his Southern tour with an assault on the West Coast citadel of show business. Bolstered by Groucho Marx and Judy Garland, LeBlanc wound up his gigantic carnival with a month's stand in Los Angeles. All this was calculated to open up the Western market.[19]

The next summer LeBlanc began again with an even bigger show, traveling in a 17-car special train. Clowns kept the assembling crowds happy, taking long drinks from bottles of Hadacol, which lit up their false eyes and noses. Cesar Romero ran the performers through their paces, and there was something for almost everyone—a beauty contest for hometown talent, pony and bicycle prizes for the kids, both a sweet band and Dixieland, dancing girls, tumblers, comedians, songs from Carmen Miranda and Minnie Pearl, a midget and a man over nine feet tall ("before" and "after" taking Hadacol). Even Jack Dempsey took the stage, making a pitch for war bonds.[20]

What the youngsters, hoping to win a pony, thought of the Hadacol jokes that kept cropping up would be hard to guess. These tall and raw tales all aimed in one therapeutic direction —to imply that Hadacol possessed great merits as an aphrodisiac and as a sustainer and restorer of both male and female potency. Even before the shows, this legend had begun to

[18] *Ibid.*

[19] *Time,* 57 (Jan. 22, 1951), 60, 62; *Newsweek,* 37 (Apr. 16, 1951), 32-33; *Los Angeles Times,* Jan. 16, 1951.

[20] *Atlanta Journal,* Aug. 12, 1951; *Atlanta Constitution,* Aug. 24, 1951; Hadacol Caravan Show souvenir program. The author attended the Atlanta show, Aug. 23, 1951.

[ 324 ]

spread across the South. Any and all old jokes, decent and indecent, which related to sexual prowess were dug up and revamped with the Hadacol label. The senator told them himself. It was reported that he had hired gagsters to accelerate the process. At any rate, Hadacol humor became a national sensation, approaching the epidemic proportions of jokes about the Model T or WPA. This triumph of folk culture, whatever his role in creating it, LeBlanc could not but welcome. In none of his printed advertising could Hadacol's claims rival its miraculous properties as circulated by word of mouth. And the FTC could not interfere. Potency appeal may well have provided a bigger market for Hadacol than the dread diseases of the abandoned testimonials.[21]

Another kind of "potency" concerning Hadacol also became the subject of widespread talk. Could the popularity of the tonic be due in some measure to the 12 per cent of alcohol that it contained? Was Hadacol a descendant of the long line of "boozers" and "bracers" with which patent medicine history was replete? LeBlanc laughingly brushed this possibility aside. Himself a devotee of Old Forester, he could not see anyone's using Hadacol as a drink. It was just about as alcoholic as wine, and any drugstore had on its shelves a number of patent tonics of higher proof. Hadacol's label asserted that the alcohol was present "as a Preservative." It was hard to imagine a customer feeling the slightest titillation if he used Hadacol according to directions, spreading an ounce of alcohol over 16 doses taken during a period of four days.[22]

Nonetheless there was evidence that upon occasion the label directions were honored in the breach. In some areas of the South, dry by local option, druggists sold Hadacol by the shot. In certain Midwestern communities, where minors were forbidden to purchase liquor, Hadacol flowed freely at parties of the high school set. "Teen-agers," the executive of an Illinois village asserted, "can get plastered on Hadacol."[23]

[21] *Ibid.*; Stitt, "Cousin Dud's Hadacol," 13; Nevin, "The Brass-Band Pitchman," 26; Herbert Halpert, "Hadacol Stories," *Kentucky Folklore Record*, 2 (Jan.-Mar. 1956), 13-14.
[22] *Chicago Tribune*, Mar. 28, 1951; Stitt, "Cousin Dud's Hadacol," 12-13; *Newsweek*, 37 (Apr. 16, 1951), 32.
[23] *Ibid.*; *Chicago Tribune*, Mar. 15 and 28, 1951.

Insofar as it was used as a beverage, Hadacol must have been a drink of desperation. It was not cheap: depending on whether one bought the eight-ounce $1.25 bottle or the 24-ounce $3.50 "family economy size" jug, the "recommended adult daily intake" cost 31 or 29 cents, and the faithful disciple would spend over $100 a year. Wine, as LeBlanc was fond of pointing out, cost less. And Hadacol was not palatable in any usual sense. LeBlanc, who knew that the common citizen expected his medicine to taste somewhat nasty, thought Hadacol tasted like "dirt." "It contained vitamins," he explained, "and they come from dirt and that's how it tasted." Other samplers variously described the flavor as "musty," "metallic," "fishy," as similar to "weak iodine," "bilge water," "emasculated wine." The odor of the murky brown brew called forth remembrance of liniments and horse medicine. Indeed, one would suppose after a gingerly experimental sip, that inveterate users conditioned themselves to the flavor not for the sake of pleasure but from the sternest sense of duty.[24]

Despite LeBlanc's disclaimer and the handicaps of price and flavor, some steps were taken to treat the tonic as a liquor. The suburban village of Northbrook, near Chicago, banned the sale of Hadacol by any retail outlets except licensed liquor stores. An ordinance to the same effect, proposed in the Atlanta city council, brought Roland LeBlanc, Hadacol's chief chemist, to oppose the resolution. The committee, according to the minutes, "assured Mr. LeBlanc that the co-authors of the proposed resolution were not serious in their intent when they presented the ordinance." It did not become law, of course. More in earnest was the House of the Illinois General Assembly, which did pass a resolution entreating LeBlanc, in view of the alcohol in his product, to stop using testimonials of children. Citation of letters like that from the mother asserting that her daughters, aged two and three, "indulge in an occasional nip for their stomach's sake," the legislators decided, was advertising "of doubtful propriety."[25]

[24] Nevin, "The Brass-Band Pitchman," 26; friends of the author are responsible for the descriptions.
[25] *Chicago Tribune*, Mar. 28, 1951; Police Committee of Atlanta Council minutes, Apr. 11, 1951, cited in letter to author from H. T.

If some governmental figures regarded Hadacol with skepticism, the same was more markedly true of members of the medical profession. This must have disappointed LeBlanc, for he strove diligently to win the approval of doctors just as he sought in his advertising to convey the impression that Hadacol possessed the sanction of orthodox medicine. The phrase kept reappearing, "HADACOL is recommended by many doctors." LeBlanc explained that all efforts at "improving" his tonic were undertaken under the control of a medical director, Dr. L. A. Willey, who supervised the "clinical" activity of "20 other medical experts throughout the country."[26]

By means of letters bearing Willey's facsimile signature, LeBlanc appealed to physicians in many areas to give consideration to Hadacol as an "ethical proprietary." He would gladly send samples. "We cordially invite you," his research director wrote, "to conduct clinical tests, among a group of your own patients, with HADACOL . . . on a fee basis per patient."[27]

If LeBlanc won any recruits from the ranks of physicians by his stratagem, the doctors enlisted against the counsel of the American Medical Association. "It is to be hoped," reported the AMA's Bureau of Investigation in the pages of the *Journal*, "that no doctors of medicine will be uncritical enough to join in the promotion of Hadacol as an ethical preparation. It is difficult to imagine how one could do himself or his profession greater harm, from the standpoint of the abuse of the trust of a patient suffering from any condition. Hadacol is not specific medication. It is not even a specific preventive measure. It could not be eligible for serious consideration by the Council on Pharmacy and Chemistry."[28]

The Bureau of Investigation had other stern things to say. The only L. A. Willey for whom a record could be found was a man who had been convicted in California of calling himself a doctor though he had no medical degree and of practicing

Jenkins, Chief of Police, May 11, 1951; *Chicago Tribune*, Mar. 14, 1951; *JAMA*, 146 (June 9, 1951), 566; *Atlanta Journal*, Mar. 29, 1951.
[26] *New Orleans Item*, Dec. 17, 1950; "Hadacol—the Ethical(?) Proprietary," *JAMA*, 145 (Jan. 13, 1951), 107-108.
[27] *Ibid.*; copy of Willey letter, Nov. 6, 1950, in Hadacol folder in the AMA's Dept. of Investigation.
[28] *JAMA*, 145 (Jan. 13, 1951), 107-108.

medicine though he had no license. As to the dangers of Hadacol, the Bureau had in its files a letter from an Arkansas doctor,
telling of a diabetic patient who gave up insulin to treat herself
with Hadacol; she immediately went into a diabetic coma and
almost died. As to Hadacol's therapeutic merits, the Bureau
made the significant statement, "Although Hadacol has been
advertised to the laity as being a more assimilable form of
administration for the vitamins, neither the U.S. *Pharmacopeia*
nor the Council [on Pharmacy and Chemistry] recognizes alcoholic elixirs containing these substances as a dosage form."

What then was Hadacol good for? One answer was that
which occurred to LeBlanc himself when the question was put
to him by Groucho Marx on television. Hadacol, replied its
maker smilingly, "was good for five and a half million for me
last year."[29]

So, into 1951, the Hadacol bandwagon rolled on. There
seemed no bottom to LeBlanc's promotional bag of tricks. He
circulated Captain Hadacol comic books loaded with advertising. He lured children into salesmanship with such prizes as
luminescent T-shirts. He sponsored theater parties, admission
by box top. He installed in railroad terminals three-dimensional
displays of healthy, well-molded maidens beside the familiar
Hadacol package. He let it be widely known he was looking
for a parrot who could repeat clearly and often "Polly wants
Hadacol." When found, Polly would travel about the country
to drugstores and sales conventions in a limousine bearing her
name in gold.[30]

As sales mounted and LeBlanc's fame spread, the senator
looked covetously again at the Louisiana governorship. Some
of his advertising, perhaps, had been subtly aimed in that
direction all along. Once again following in the tradition of
his predecessors, LeBlanc presented himself to the nation as
a great humanitarian. In his advertising ventures, he exploited
both his own colorful personality and his political career. Le-
Blanc the man, LeBlanc the humanitarian, and LeBlanc the
statesman stood before the public as a mighty three-in-one.

[29] Martin Gardner, *In the Name of Science*, 229.
[30] *Business Week*, Jan. 6, 1951, 76; *Chicago Tribune*, Oct. 1, 1950,
Feb. 19, 1951; the railroad station display was seen in Cincinnati.

"Senator" was invariably prefixed to LeBlanc's name in Hadacol promotion. His legislative achievements were included in the advertising record to validate his claim to the title "Humanitarian Statesman, and Great Friend of the People." He had "always championed the cause of the oppressed, the poor and the underprivileged." He was, he said, "the first candidate for governor to advocate Old Age Pensions." He claimed credit for the $50 monthly pension then being paid to "the deserving senior citizens of Louisiana." He was a proponent of legislation for veterans and "successfully enacted into law a measure providing for the selection of a service commissioner" to ensure justice for Louisiana veterans from the state and national governments. Moreover, "during his entire political career, he . . . never cast a ballot or vote against a man or woman who must toil to earn his or her livelihood."[31]

How was LeBlanc's humanitarian statesmanship related to Hadacol? It was "because his heart has always beat in sympathy with the cause of the oppressed, the infirm, the lame and the sickly, [that] through endless effort and study he has developed today's great HADACOL, one more addition to his long record of service to humanity."[32]

Other incidents reveal LeBlanc's shrewdness in associating with his remedy the forces of political power and prestige. When General Douglas MacArthur was called home from Korea and his name was dominating headlines, LeBlanc reaped headlines of his own by offering MacArthur a Hadacol vice-presidency. Earlier LeBlanc, even though a Southerner, reached back into history and came up with Abraham Lincoln. A large ad presented the faces of both Lincoln and LeBlanc, with quotations from them both. The Lincoln citation, it happens, was a garbled version of the statement which historians have not been able to establish that Lincoln ever made, the one about fooling the people. After the quotation there followed this line: " 'You were right, Mr. Lincoln,' says Senator Dudley J. LeBlanc."[33]

[31] *Atlanta Journal*, Mar. 13, 1951.     [32] *Ibid.*
[33] *Chicago Tribune*, Apr. 16, 1951; *Atlanta Journal*, Nov. 11, 1950. The same fooling-the-people quotation had been used 50 years before to promote Hale's Honey of Horehound and Tar for the Cure of Coughs and Colds. *Amer. Messenger*, 58 (Mar. 1900), 47.

LeBlanc forged yet one more link between patent medicine and politics. On his grand excursions through the South, he had himself photographed in animated conversation with other political figures. An issue of *Look* carried pictures of the Louisiana state senator conferring separately with the mayor of Baton Rouge, the mayor of New Orleans, and the governor of Alabama. "Senator," Governor "Kissin' Jim" Folsom was saying, "that sure is some medicine business you got."[34]

To LeBlanc, then, politics and patent medicines were a reversible reaction. He used his political career to promote Hadacol; he also used Hadacol to promote his political career. Defeated twice for the Louisiana governorship by Long machines, LeBlanc looked toward another try against another Long machine in 1952. The senator's friends worked hard at building up draft-Dudley sentiment, and after some pretense of coyness LeBlanc yielded. Spreading the gospel through his advertising that he was "the best friend the poor people ever had," LeBlanc also insisted he would be good for business. The state's greatest need, he said, was a sure-fire promoter to persuade the outside world, skeptical of Longism, that Louisiana was a pretty fine place for industrial investment. And what better promoter than the millionaire state senator? LeBlanc, a shrewd observer noted, was "widely respected as a money maker, a man who built something out of nothing," and at the same time was regarded as "a slightly comic figure, which doesn't hurt him here." Commentators began to predict that LeBlanc had a chance to win. The Longs got worried. They determined to fight fire with fire. They started a patent medicine of their own.[35]

It's a pity, in a way, that the campaign could not have been fought out in this pseudo-medical atmosphere, between Hadacol and Vita-Long, up to the day of the voting. But in midstream LeBlanc sold his horse. The senator had claimed shortly

[34] Roddy, "Million-Dollar Medicine Man," 34-43.
[35] Sindler, *Huey Long's Louisiana*, 186, 234-35; Perry H. Howard, *Political Tendencies in Louisiana, 1812-1952* (Baton Rouge, 1957), 163; T. Harry Williams to author, May 6, 1951. The Food and Drug Administration eventually brought a seizure action against Vita-Long, which was uncontested. DDNJ 3811.

before that Hadacol sales might reach $75 million for 1951. He was in the midst of his second fabulous summer medicine show tour. So his announcement, in August, that he had let Hadacol go took the nation by surprise. It soon became known that the price was $8 million, of which a quarter million was in cash, the rest to be paid from profits through the years, and LeBlanc was to stay on as sales manager at an annual salary of $100,000. The buyer was the Tobey-Maltz Foundation of New York, organized for cancer research by a plastic surgeon, which quickly leased the tonic to a syndicate of Northern businessmen.[36]

Within a very short time the Yankee purchasers let it be known they had been stung. Hadacol's books were not what they had seemed to be to the New York accountants who had examined them before the sale. LeBlanc, the new owners charged, had concealed two million dollars in unpaid bills, and more than another two million, listed as assets under "accounts receivable," was really Hadacol out on consignment, a great deal of which was flowing back. The whole enterprise had become vastly overextended. Even while the senator had continued his flamboyant drumbeating, the market had passed the saturation point. The new owners went into bankruptcy; the creditors organized. LeBlanc had shrewdly wriggled out just in the nick of time. "If you sell a cow," he told the press, "and the cow dies, you can't do anything to a man for that."[37]

But the senator had other troubles. The FTC, believing his latter-day advertising had violated his earlier stipulation, issued a complaint. The Bureau of Internal Revenue charged him with owing some $650,000 in income taxes. And, despite the glee Louisiana voters took in the trick he had pulled on Yankee city slickers, the bursting Hadacol bubble killed his gubernatorial hopes. LeBlanc sought to secure the post of lieutenant-governor on the ticket of several of his rivals and,

[36] *Business Week*, Jan. 6, 1951, 72, 74; *N.Y. Times*, Aug. 28 and 31, 1951.

[37] *Chicago Tribune*, Sep. 21 and Nov. 5, 1951; *N.Y. Times*, Sep. 27 and Oct. 4, 1951; *FDC Reports*, Oct. 6, 1951. The financial aftermath of the Hadacol crash dragged on for nearly a decade. *Chicago Daily News*, May 6, 1960; *Chicago Tribune*, May 7, 1960.

failing, campaigned manfully for governor until the end. When the votes were counted, Cousin Dud wound up in seventh place.[38]

The Hadacol trade name lived on but never recouped an iota of its erstwhile fame. LeBlanc himself sought to carry on. After a time, indeed, he launched a new tonic, and Kary-On was its name. But it did not carry the senator either to his former fortunes or to the governorship.[39]

Hadacol in its heyday, however, and its colorful promoter, penetrated Southern folklore, and the myth of both is still widely remembered with a certain amused fondness. The millions needlessly expended, or spent for Hadacol instead of proper medical care, tend to be forgotten.

[38] Complaint, Sep. 28, 1951, in FTC Docket 5925 (this was eventually dismissed on the grounds that LeBlanc no longer had a voice in the control of the business, *50 FTC Decisions* 1028); *N.Y. Times,* Sep. 21, 1951; Sindler, *Huey Long's Louisiana,* 234-35, 238.

[39] Several efforts were made to revive Hadacol sales. FTC Docket 5925; *PI,* 248 (Nov. 19, 1954), 108; *FDC Reports,* Dec. 24, 1962; *Drug Trade News,* Aug. 15, 1966. On Kary-On: *FDC Reports,* Feb. 20, 1954; May 23 and July 18, 1955; Jan. 23, 1956; 52 *FTC Decisions* 607; *Newsweek,* 55 (Feb. 22, 1960), 84.

# 16

## "YOU ARE WHAT YOU EAT"

*"After studying the eating habits of the American people for a number of years, I found thirty distinct Disease Conditions: vitamin-deficient, mineral-starved, cooked food-enervated, sun-cheated, clothes-insulated, coffee-soaked, spice-irritated, tobacco-poisoned, constipation-befouled, oxygen-deprived, sugar-acidified, meat-polluted, starch-clogged, salt-ified, mustard-plastered, pepperized, jelly-bowled, pop-bloated, vinegar-jagged, chocolate-coated, mashed and creamed, toasted and roasted, ice-cubed, tea-tannined, sauce-jaded, night-hawks, morning-deadheads, heat-treated, sex-depleted, and gravy-saturated. That's the average human being today."*

—ADOLPHUS HOHENSEE, LECTURE IN DENVER, 1952[1]

"HADACOL was a very, very meritorious product," insisted its inventor, Dudley J. LeBlanc, in talking with a reporter a decade after the B-vitamin tonic boom had collapsed. "Who is to say that those people weren't helped for those ailments? The doctors? Who can believe them? No, my friend, there's still much that's not known about nutrition."[2]

About one thing, at least, LeBlanc was right. Nutrition, as a science, was as yet incomplete. Because of what was not yet known and the complexity of what *was* known, nutrition, during the 20th century, has provided a happy hunting ground for those who would beguile the American public into buying their questionable wares.

[1] FDA file on Hohensee, Interstate Sample No. 14-497L, FDA Records, Washington.
[2] David Nevin, "The Brass-Band Pitchman and His Million-Dollar Elixir," *True*, March 1962, 26.

"In 1900," one of the nutrition pioneers has written, "we were almost blind to the relations of food to health." Six years later, the year the first Pure Food and Drugs Act became law, a research scientist spoke of protein, carbohydrates, and fats as "still the nutritional trinity." In that same year, however, a number of significant papers were published proving the trinity by no means adequate. Other food factors, as yet not clearly recognized, must be included in the diet if good health was to be maintained. A growing wave of research by food chemists confirmed this view, and a decade later pathologists, hitherto preoccupied with the aftermath of the germ theory, joined forces with the chemists in nutritional research. In 1911 a Polish chemist, Casimir Funk, working at the Lister Institute in London, coined the word "vitamine" for these needed food factors. The next year Funk published a paper suggesting the theory that various diseases—beriberi, scurvy, pellagra, rickets —resulted from the lack of vitamins in the diet. Empirical observations in the past had pointed in this direction. Now controlled research began to establish such surmises as demonstrated fact. At the University of Wisconsin in 1913 Elmer McCollum identified the need in animal diets for a fat-soluble nutrient which, adopting Funk's nomenclature, he christened Vitamin A. By 1926 two components in vitamin B, as well as vitamins C, D, and E, had also been found as necessary to health. During the 1930's, while Congress struggled to enact a stronger food and drug law, scientists in their laboratories identified the chemical structures of the vitamins and, in some cases, created them by synthesis. Nor were vitamins the only indispensable nutrients. Research confirmed or discovered the need for amino acids and minerals, even though in the most minute amounts. Successive scientific studies revealed the ever greater complexity of nutrition. Nonetheless, in McCollum's view, 1940 marked a plateau, the successful achievement of the primary goals of nutritional science, to discover what chemical substances were required for an adequate diet in domestic animals and man. More than 40 such nutrients had, by then, been proved necessary.[3]

[3] Elmer V. McCollum, *A History of Nutrition* (Boston, 1957), vi, 153, 201, 217-18, 224, 229-416 *passim*, 420-21; Elizabeth N. Todhunter,

Since the days of the pyramids, food and health had been inextricably intertwined in folklore, and food faddism ran rampant in 19th-century America. Relics of ancient myths, indeed, still cherished in the popular mind, made the task of 20th-century nutritional proprietors much easier. Commercial exploitation of food folklore began at least as early as the origin of the packaged cereal industry. Religion, health, and business enterprise converged in Battle Creek. Corn Flakes began as Elijah's Manna, and one of the early therapeutic uses suggested for Grape Nuts was as a preventive for appendicitis.[4]

Popular interest in the nascent nutritional revolution, coupled with popular concern about food shortages during World War I, opened the way for an upsurge of food promotion with health overtones. Since advertising techniques had just reached the stage to make the most of such an opportunity, Americans, during the prosperity decade, were constantly besought to buy physical well-being and to banish ailments by eating cheese, bread, and cereals, by imbibing milk and carbonated drinks. Yeast and chocolate bars vaunted their vitamin content. Vitamin pills, like Mastin's Vitamon Tablets— "Give You That Firm Flesh Pep"—received a big play. And cod liver oil, long a staple in the proprietary field, enjoyed a new vogue with the discovery that it was a source of vitamin D. So-called extracts of this oil were promoted with claims that the vitamin value was retained while the fishy taste was banished.[5]

The Food and Drug Administration discovered otherwise. Beginning to assay these products in 1926, the agency found therapeutic claims exaggerated and vitamin content low or

"The Story of Nutrition," in *Food: The Yearbook of Agriculture 1959* (Washington, 1959), 12-18.

[4] Ronald M. Deutsch, *The Nuts among the Berries* (N.Y., 1961), 13-65; Gerald Carson, *Cornflake Crusade* (N.Y., 1957), *passim*, Elijah's Manna at 183, Grape Nuts and appendicitis at 162.

[5] Deutsch, 145; Pease, *The Responsibilities of American Advertising*, 94; *Printers' Ink: Fifty Years, 1888-1938*, 318; Harrison Graves, "Marketing a Proprietary," *Standard Remedies*, 8 (Oct. 1922), 20; Mastin's ad in Medicine-Remedies folder, General Corres. of Office of Sec. of Agric., 1921, RG 16, NA; George P. Larrick, "The Pure Food Law," in *Food: The Yearbook of Agriculture 1959*, 446.

missing. Combining persuasion with legal action, the FDA succeeded in eliminating from the labeling of many "extracts" any reference to cod liver oil. Moreover, the whole broad front of "health foods" increasingly troubled the agency. In 1929, through a press release, Walter Campbell issued a warning to the American people. "The use of the word ['health']," Campbell said, "implies that these products have health-giving or curative properties, when, in general, they merely possess some of the nutritive qualities to be expected in any wholesome food product. The label claims on these products are such that the consumer is led to believe that our ordinary diet is sorely deficient in such vital substances as vitamins and minerals, and that these so-called 'health foods' are absolutely necessary to conserve life and health." Such misrepresentation, Campbell promised, the FDA would "combat."[6]

The next year Campbell's aide, Paul Dunbar, speaking before trade associations of canners and wholesale grocers, scolded the sinners in their ranks. Nutrition news, he said, had "appealed immensely to the popular fancy. . . . In its ignorance of the present limitations of scientific knowledge it has been disposed to accept without reservation the most extreme, and in some cases ridiculous claims for the wholesomeness and health-giving qualities of various products. Unfortunately, a certain element of the advertising profession proceeds upon the theory that a market may be obtained for almost any product if its imaginary virtues are exploited in impressive scientific terms, and unfortunately this theory appears to be correct. A glowing statement to the effect that Jones' carrot bread or Smith's turnip breakfast food contains all the known vitamins, will restore the elasticity of youth to the bones and muscles of the aged, and will ward off all known diseases is likely to be seized upon with avidity, especially by those who are in need of the very rejuvenating effects they are promised by the enthusiastic advertiser. The magic words 'health giving' are today the most overworked and loosely applied in the advertising lexicon."[7]

[6] *Ibid.*; *1928 Report of Food, Drug, and Insecticide Administration*, 4-5; FDA Press Notice, May 22, 1929, Press Notice file, FDA, Washington.
[7] *F&D Rev.*, 14 (Feb. 1930), 41-44.

"Do you want the consuming public to get the idea," Dunbar asked the processors, "that they should turn to this particular delicacy only when in unsound physical condition? Don't you want your product to appeal to the well rather than to the invalid class?"

The Food and Drug Administration began taking actions in a modest way against unwarranted nutritional claims. Breakfast food factories across the country were inspected for labels of doubtful propriety. A small unit was created, which in 1935 became the Division of Vitamins, to study the some 400 products—foods and drugs—being promoted with general or specific claims of vitamin efficiency. In Chicago, 23,365 packages of Congoin were seized—the product was really yerba maté, the Latin American "tea." "Absolutely alone," Congoin's advertising had promised, "it will support life for weeks on end." Cases were won against a new and growing type of racket, the multi-vitamin cure-all. The product might be, like Catalyn, milk sugar, wheat starch and bran, and epinephrine, but its label boasted—falsely—potency in all vitamins from A through G, and promised to cure high and low blood pressure, Bright's disease, dropsy, and goiter.[8]

If FDA activity might induce caution in the multi-vitamin promoter, other trends in the 1930's spurred him on. While scientists insisted that all needed nutrients could be secured through a varied and well-balanced diet, careful surveys of depression America revealed that one-third of the nation's families consumed a diet that had to be regarded as poor.[9] Widespread publicity given to such surveys worried even the well fed, and the grimmest quotations torn from the context of such scientific reports appeared promptly—and remained for years—in the pamphlets penned by purveyors of nutrition nonsense.

As the second World War loomed, the National Academy of Sciences and the National Research Council appointed a

[8] *Ibid.*, 15 (May 1931), 139; 19 (Aug. 1935), 173-76, and (Oct. 1935), 221; *1932 Report of Food and Drug Administration*, 10-11; *1936 Report*, 15; *1939 Report*, 24-25; United States v. Lee, 107 Fed. (2d) 522. The Vitamin Division became the Division of Nutrition in 1949.

[9] Hazel K. Stiebeling, "Food in Our Lives," in *Food: The Yearbook of Agriculture*, 5.

Food and Nutrition Board to develop a table of "Recommended Daily Allowances for Specific Nutrients." In 1941 the first list was issued, indicating the number of calories and the quantities of nine nutrients needed for good nutrition by most persons with higher than average requirements. The Board recognized that people sick or suffering from malnutrition might need more. They acknowledged that 11 other nutrients were essential for health, but, because of inadequate data or because deficiencies were not likely to occur, desirable quantities of these could not be specified. The Board recommended, in view of diet inadequacies discovered in the surveys, that some foods be "enriched" with vitamins that had by then been synthesized by chemists. This concept was not entirely new. Iodine had been added to salt as early as 1924 to help prevent the development of goiter. Vitamin D had later been added to milk and vitamin A to margarine. The Food and Nutrition Board proposed enriching bread and other grain products with several vitamins and iron. So as the war came, with the hazard of new food shortages, the staple diet of Americans was more adequate in nutrients than it had ever been before.[10]

By this time too, the Food and Drug Administration had been given by Congress new and more effective authority over health food claims. The 1938 law declared as misbranded a food promoted for "special dietary purposes" which failed to label information about "its vitamin, mineral, and other dietary properties" which the FDA deemed "necessary in order fully to inform purchasers as to its value for such uses." Under this provision the agency set forth not "recommended" but "minimum daily requirements" of the key known nutrients and required manufacturers to label their products in terms of these requirements.[11] Under the law, too, a "food" was also a "drug" if therapeutic claims were made for it, and the FDA's burden of proving a drug misbranded was less demanding than under the earlier law. Thus new weapons lay at

[10] Ruth M. Leverton, "Recommended Allowances," in *ibid.*, 227-30; Todhunter, "The Story of Nutrition," 17, 20-21.
[11] Sec. 403 (j) of the law; FDA press release, Nov. 22, 1941.

hand to combat inflated nutritional claims. Fortunate this was, for the battle threatened to loom large indeed.

Many factors favored the nutritional promoter. The war years did bring a drab diet to civilians, as well as an increase in emotional strain. To treat ailments, real or imaginary, physicians in private practice were in short supply. As a consequence, self-diagnosis and self-treatment expanded. Wartime and postwar prosperity made it easier for the common citizen to pay the high prices charged by nutritional salesmen for their wares. The continuing concern by reputable nutritionists to safeguard and improve the American diet aided the disreputable, who asserted that their supplements would do just that. After the war, better eating habits plus the "enrichment" program improved the nation's nutritional level. The millennium, however, was not yet reached. Postwar surveys continued to show inadequacies. A comprehensive study in 1955, for example, revealed that about one-tenth of America's families consumed a diet that was nutritionally poor, and nearly half the families fell below the Food and Nutrition Board's recommended level with respect to one or more essential nutrient.[12] The proper solution, nutritional experts stated, lay in wiser food selection, not in expensive commercial supplements. But those with vitamins to sell made the most of the surveys. Even large manufacturing concerns of great prestige, medical scientists asserted, oversold the value of their vitamins.[13] Promoters less scrupulous sought to frighten the nation into the conviction that America faced widespread starvation.

The initial successes of the FDA, employing the weapons of the 1938 law, in circumscribing patent medicine quackery tended to push fringe promoters toward the greener pastures of nutrition. Vaguer claims seemed legally safer. Vitamins and minerals were seldom sold blatantly as cancer or diabetes cures. The supplements and tonics, rather, promised to "increase vigor" or "prevent wearing out" because of nutritional deficiency. Often such promises were accompanied by "adroit

---

[12] Corinne Le Bovit and Faith Clark, "Are We Well Fed?," in *Food: The Yearbook of Agriculture*, 620; Janet Murray and Ennis Blake, "What Do We Eat?," in *ibid.*, 609-19.

[13] "Shotgun Vitamins Rampant," *JAMA*, 117 (Oct. 25, 1941), 1,447.

references to disturbances of the digestive, circulatory, and nervous systems." In all this carefully worded doctrine, the would-be customer might well read or hear the idea of "cure." But because of the sly phrasing, and the complicated nature of nutritional science, the Food and Drug Administration faced a formidable regulatory task.[14]

Policing the claims of nutritional promoters became a heavy burden for the FDA also because increasingly salesmen in the realm of food faddism relied on oral speech. This reduced the risk of detection. It also put the pitchman in direct contact with his potential customer. Thus was revived the face-to-face persuasiveness of the old-time patent medicine barker. The Nutrilite network of door-to-door salesmen proved to be a prototype for other similar ventures, like Abundavita and Nutri-Bio. Nutrilite officers, under the terms of the 1951 injunction, promised not only to limit their claims drastically but also to inform their salesmen what they could and could not say about this vitamin-mineral-alfalfa-parsley-watercress mix. In the privacy of residential living rooms, FDA inspectors, posing as customers, sometimes discovered that salesmen failed to exercise the agreed-upon restraint. But legal action against isolated vendors did not hamper Nutrilite's growth. Five years after the injunction, when the Federal Trade Commission looked into Nutrilite's sales practices, the force had expanded by a third and totaled 20,000 doorbell-ringing women and men. Sales in 1956 amounted to $26,000,000.[15]

Another forum for nutritional pitchmen who possessed hortatorical skill was the lecture platform. Gayelord Hauser, a suave and talented performer, revived in the 1930's the ancient art of the popular health lecture course. Heralded by advertising, the course began with a free lecture or so, continued for a fee. Hauser, a man on cordial terms with American movie stars and English nobility, lauded five "wonder" foods—skim milk, brewer's yeast, wheat germ, yogurt, and blackstrap molasses—and touted his own writings on nutrition. His appeal

[14] *1944 Report of Food and Drug Administration*, 28-29; *1945 Report*, 43.

[15] On the Nutrilite injunction, see ch. 9. *F&D Rev.*, 39 (Nov. 1955), 169; 41 (July 1957), 115, and (Dec. 1957), 212; 42 (Mar. 1958), 38; *FDC Reports*, Dec. 16, 1957, 15-16.

was amazing. When *Look Younger, Live Longer* was published in 1950, the book stayed on best seller lists for over a year and during that time sold a third of a million copies.[16]

Of the two score and more lecturers who entered upon the nutritional lyceum circuit, not all were as smooth and polished as Gaylord Hauser. One of the rougher breed was Adolphus Hohensee. In 1943 the Better Business Bureau of St. Louis sent a telegraphed inquiry to the American Medical Association: Who was Hohensee? The AMA did not yet know. As the months passed, the AMA took increasing interest in this recruit to the ranks of nutrition spielers. So did the FDA.[17]

Hohensee, diligent inquiry revealed, had set forth from Chevy Chase, near Washington, shortly before, promoting his line of Vita Health Foods. Nothing in his background seemed to qualify him as a nutrition expert. To be sure, he had been born in Poland, the same country as Casimir Funk. But Hohensee had had no formal training in vitamin research. He had come to America early in the century as a young boy. So far as the FDA could learn, Hohensee's schooling ended in 1918 with a single semester of high school level work, taken at the Washington Missionary College in Takoma Park. For this he received four hours of credit. Hohensee worked for a time as a soda jerk. His whereabouts during the 1920's could not be discovered. In 1933 Hohensee operated a real estate scheme in Galveston. He collected fees from owners who wished to sell their property, but he expended little effort at making sales. Charged with mail fraud, Hohensee pleaded guilty, spent a month in jail, with five years of probation to follow. He returned to Washington and entered the sightseeing tour business with his wife's car. Within three years he had acquired 140 cabs and some gas stations. During these years Hohensee's life was rugged. He was arrested for various misdemeanors, including the passing of bad checks. Four charges of assault were brought against him, but none was prosecuted. In

[16] Deutsch, 158-70; *JAMA*, 108 (Apr. 17, 1937), 1359-60; *Newsweek*, 37 (Mar. 26, 1951), 58-59; U.S. v. 8 Cartons . . . Blackstrap Molasses, 97 Fed. Supp. 313; U.S. v. 8 Cartons . . . Blackstrap Molasses, 103 Fed. Supp. 626.

[17] List of health lecturers drawn up in 1948 by FDA, in personal file, J. J. McCann Jr., FDA; Adolphus Hohensee folder, Dept. of Investigation, AMA.

the early 1940's, for reasons of his own, Hohensee shifted from transportation to nutrition. Soon after launching his travels as lecturer, he also shifted his home base, moving from the Washington suburbs to a farm near Scranton, which he named El Rancho Adolphus.[18]

Hohensee was 42 in 1943, a tall, broad-shouldered man, stocky and robust, weighing over 200 pounds. His neck was thick, his face fat, his head round and balding. He sported a small black mustache which he kept waxed and pointed. His eyes were dark and piercing. Hohensee's physical stamina seemed never to wane. He could lecture night after night for two to three hours without tiring. His sharp, loud, and commanding voice, a voice devoid of jollity but skilled at expressing sarcasm and scorn, never weakened during his lectures. It was a powerful and flexible instrument, ranging from "whispering confidentiality to shouting hate" through all the variations in between. Hohensee dressed with some elegance, although his strenuous antics during an evening of lecturing often left him rumpled.[19]

Billing himself as an M.D. in his early forays, Hohensee quickly met challenge. So he sought to acquire whatever kinds of health degrees he could. He secured in 1943 an Honorary Degree of Doctor of Medicine from the Kansas City University of Physicians and Surgeons, an institution that had been listed as unaccredited by the AMA for 15 years and that was closed in 1944 by the Missouri State Board of Medical Examiners. Hohensee added Doctor of Naturopathy degrees, without attendance, from schools in Oklahoma and Indiana. And in 1946 he passed an examination and was granted a chiropractic license by the state of Nevada, neglecting to say, as the law required, that he had once been convicted of a federal offense.[20]

[18] *Ibid.*; FDA file, Interstate Sample No. 18-317L, FDA Records, Washington; FDA file, Interstate Sample No. 31-968H, *ibid.*; FDA file, Interstate Sample No. 55-529F, *ibid.*; FDA file 14-497L.

[19] *Providence Journal*, Jan. 6, 1953; *Scranton Tribune*, Jan. 6, 1955; *F&D Rev.*, 37 (Sep. 1953), 174; letters to author from two FDA inspectors who observed Hohensee closely, Ralph M. Davidson, Oct. 21, 1960, and Kenneth E. Kimlel, Oct. 27, 1960.

[20] AMA folder; FDA files 55-529F, 31-968H, and 14-497L.

Hohensee's stock in trade, during his early days as lecturer, consisted of a wide variety of nutritional products which he had ordered packaged as the Adolphus Brand, bearing labels of his own design. Included were peppermint, soybean lecithin, B-complex vitamins, wheat germ oil, mineral capsules, calcium tablets, an herb laxative—even a tar shampoo. And Hohensee's own private inquiry into the literature of nutrition had resulted in numerous pamphlets, especially *The Health, Success and Happiness* series, which included such individual titles as *The Normal Ration; High Blood Pressure; Arthritis and Rheumatism; Better Eyes without Glasses;* and *Your Personality Glands.*[21]

Adroitly turning his lecture audiences into customers for both products and pamphlets, Hohensee had scarcely begun his career before he encountered opposition. In November 1943 in Seattle, charged with selling drugs without a license, he pleaded guilty and paid a $50 fine. The next month Hohensee faced the same charge in Tacoma and fought the case before a jury, handling his own defense. He was convicted, and the verdict stood up upon appeal. Wrote a spokesman for the Tacoma Better Business Bureau, "We feel this man, although lacking formal education, is a shrewd, capable adversary, thoroughly unscrupulous and dangerous."[22]

The next spring Hohensee lost two cases in San Francisco, paying a $300 fine for posing as a medical doctor and another $200 for selling drugs without a license. By this time his protracted conflict with the Food and Drug Administration had begun. Just before Christmas in 1943, Hohensee had shipped an enormous quantity of remedies and reading matter from Seattle to Los Angeles. The FDA seized both, charging the former misbranded by the latter under both food and drug provisions of the law. Hohensee did not come by to claim his property, and the court condemned calcium, peppermint, pamphlets, and all to destruction. The next year Hohensee let another large seizure, shipped from Arizona to California, go by default.[23]

[21] Food NJ 7924 and 10893; DDNJ 1357 and 2092.
[22] AMA folder; FDA file 55-529F.
[23] *Ibid.;* Food NJ 7924 and 10893; DDNJ 1357 and 2092.

It was costly to lose his wares in this way, but not a major deterrent. The sales Hohensee made during a series of lectures in a single city, the FDA estimated, might gross 40 to 50 thousand dollars, and a mighty high proportion of the gross was net. At this rate he could well afford to sacrifice a good many seizures. Since the seizures did not keep Hohensee away from his new and profitable mode of life, the FDA began criminal action. "I am going to keep on with this thing," the lecturer had told some Food and Drug officials, "until they get me behind bars."[24]

But Hohensee insisted his procedures did not violate the law. Following the early seizures, he told FDA officials at a hearing while the criminal case was being prepared, he had paid out big money to get all his labels changed. An expert in the field had given his OK. The processors who sold him his products provided the proper guaranty that label claims met the requirements of the law. As to the pamphlets, they were not part of the label "in any way, shape or form."[25]

"These are separate booklets that I have written," Hohensee said, "books that are being sold, not given away. . . . In checking the book nowhere do we refer to Adolphus Brand products. That booklet has nothing to do with the merchandise."

"When you sell these booklets," Hohensee was asked, "do you refer to any of your products?"

"I do not."

"When you sell these products do you refer to any of these booklets?"

"Not that I remember."

For the trial, Food and Drug inspectors found a witness who did remember. Charles Russ had attended every lecture in one of Hohensee's Phoenix series. Hohensee, Russ said, would hold a package of health food in his hand while describing all the wonderful things it would do. Both products and pamphlets were placed on tables at the back of the hall, where they were sold, sometimes in combination offers, a bottle free if a bottle and book were bought together. Russ in fact had purchased everything, he said, acquiring so many Hohensee

[24] FDA files 18-317L and 55-529F.
[25] FDA file 31-968H.

remedies it took three shelves to hold them. He had arranged them in order, so he could take several handfuls of pills in a single session of therapy.[26]

The government used Russ' recollections to good effect, during the trial at Phoenix in February 1948, to demonstrate that Hohensee's pamphlet references to vitamins and minerals, even though they did not mention the Adolphus Brand, were labeling nonetheless. A number of medical experts testified to the absurdity of Hohensee's nutritional doctrines. Despite tribute to Hohensee from several satisfied customers, the jury, whose foreman was a local merchant named Barry Goldwater, found Hohensee guilty of misbranding.[27]

Hohensee's sentence did not put him behind bars: he was fined $1,800. In conformity with his earlier promise, he continued on his lucrative nutritional "crusade." But once more —as in his earlier modifications in his labeling—he changed his tactics. No longer did Hohensee sell his various vitamins and minerals in the halls where he was lecturing. Instead, he arranged for these wares to be stocked in health food stores in the cities where he delivered his speeches. This posed no problem, for the upsurge of nutritional promotion by fringe operators brought with it a great proliferation of health food stores. Selling an incredible assortment of so-called natural foods and vitamin-mineral mixtures, these stores served as rallying points for the growing body of believers in the new nutritional gospel propagated by prophets like Hohensee, a gospel that condemned the normal American food supply and made purchase of special supplements necessary for physical and mental salvation. Those who operated the stores supported the itinerant lecturers, advertising their coming, providing mailing lists for personal invitations to lecture series, and selling their panaceas and books of doctrine.[28]

If Hohensee stopped vending his vitamins in person, he nonetheless kept on collecting money at his lectures. Sale of his booklets brought in a steady flow of cash. The matriculation fees for his paid series of lectures—$25 a person, or $35

[26] *Ibid.*
[27] *Ibid.* Hohensee referred to Goldwater in a 1952 Phoenix lecture and urged the class to oppose his candidacy for the Senate. FDA file 18-317L.
[28] DDNJ 2579; FDA files 14-497L and 18-317L; Deutsch, 215.

[ 345 ]

for man and wife—brought in more. At each free lecture preceding the paid series, Hohensee took up a free will offering to pay rent on his auditorium. He added a series of gadgets for use in preparing food—without which the nutrient qualities were lost: a tenderizer, a blender, a Lucite set of kitchen implements. Prices were high: the tenderizer sold for $195. El Rancho Adolphus, in its owner's glowing words, became a veritable Eden of pristine health. Paying visitors were welcome; lots were for sale. When litigation threatened, Hohensee begged, in his speeches and in the magazine he mailed (for a fee) to the faithful, for contributions to a fund for his defense. Thus life was lucrative for the ex-taxi driver—even aside from his profits on nutritional wares sold by the health food stores.[29]

Master showman that he was, Hohensee's success came in part from the preconditioning of most members of his audiences to his type of nutritional gospel. Already converts to food faddism, they had heard earlier speakers condemn the American food supply and would attend similar speeches by other lecturers after Hohensee had moved on. Women outnumbered men in Hohensee's audiences, many of them single or widowed or married but childless. Elderly couples living on pensions were well represented. Although some young couples came, the age level of the main group of listeners ranged from the late 40's to the early 60's. The general educational background, Food and Drug inspectors judged, was modest, not above the high school level. Those who listened to Hohensee had some money to spend but were not rich. Among the men, some were skilled workers—carpenters, masons, machinists. A good many of Hohensee's hearers came, perhaps, to alleviate boredom. Few appeared to be very sick, although many certainly thought they were, afflicted with the aches and pains and glooms of aging. As they sat waiting for Hohensee to begin his lecture, they complained to each other about their state of health and swapped symptoms.[30]

[29] This paragraph relies on elaborate notes made by an inspector of a Phoenix series of lectures given by Hohensee during February and March 1952, and transcriptions of wire recordings of a Denver series, July-September 1952. FDA files 14-497L and 18-317L.
[30] Davidson and Kimlel letters.

Knowing his listeners' fears and foibles, Hohensee kept them interested—and shelling out money—throughout each evening's two-hour stint of lecturing. His talks were rambling and unstructured, but he was alert to mood and adept at changing his theme or style to keep things lively. His bag of tricks was fully packed. His rapport was excellent. Hohensee called the women "girls" and "sweethearts," got them to asking questions and to testifying to the good they had received from the suggestions he had made on earlier evenings. He often interrupted his monologue to ask questions of his audience, easy questions to which they knew the answers. He mixed humor, most of it corny, with narrative episodes possessing a touch of drama, some of them autobiographical and intended to reflect his own fame. He uttered homilies on human relations and offered a lot of homespun psychology, urging his auditors to perk up, forget their troubles, wax enthusiastic, feel better. Hohensee quoted the Bible frequently, referred often to God's purposes for mankind, which, as to dietary matters, coincided exactly with Hohensee's own. He told suggestive stories (but not too naughty), teased his listeners about their sexual shortcomings, and promised better things—"The sex act itself should last for one hour"—for those who used his wares. He spoke awesomely of his own nutritional experimentation, throwing in jawbreaking scientific words as if he lived with them on very intimate terms. He cited the work of other researchers, picking quotations that suited his purposes from papers by reputable scholars and from government reports. He got what acclaim he could by identifying with other and better known spokesmen for the nutritional fringe, showing his classes, for example, a picture of himself with Bernarr Macfadden.[31]

Hohensee frightened his listeners with frequent references to their proximity to "the Marble Orchard," with vivid descriptions of the horrors of disease, with distorted excursions into anatomy purporting to demonstrate how the normal diet stagnated the blood, corroded the blood vessels, eroded the kidneys, and clogged the intestines with a putrefying mess. Yet

[31] This and the following paragraphs are based on the Phoenix notes and Denver transcriptions, FDA files 14-497L and 18-317L.

he also reassured them: follow his doctrines and use his products and they would live to be 180 and go with him on man's first journey to the moon.

Hohensee paraded himself as a noble man abused by powerful enemies, a gigantic Medical Trust, headed by "the American Murderers Association" and including the drug trade, dominated by the Rockefellers, the Better Business Bureau, and the Food and Drug Administration. The FDA's hatchet men, he said, pursued him and infiltrated his audiences like spies.

In between his diatribes and homilies, Hohensee told his audience simple concrete things to do, explaining precisely why and how these would benefit their health. Hot and cold baths for the hands and feet, for example, would stir up the stagnant blood. Many of Hohensee's fasting regimens, of course, involved Adolphus products for sale at the local health store. Recipes must be cooked in his tenderizer or pulverized in his blender or got together with the aid of his Lucite knife. However dramatic the Hohensee anecdote, however passionate the tirade, a sales pitch of some kind was not far off.

As to the Food and Drug interlopers, Hohensee was right. The $1,800 fine had not deterred him. The agency began to gather evidence for another case. Agents, incognito, began to attend his lectures, even began to take down his words verbatim with wire recorders. In Phoenix once again, during February and March of 1952, an inspector sat through Hohensee's four free and 14 paid lectures, taking copious notes. The first night Hohensee started in an angry mood. The Phoenix papers and a radio station had refused his advertising, for which the Drug Trust and the BBB were certainly to blame. Then Hohensee shifted his attack to the dangers of foods and medicines in widespread use. Packages of some of these products rested on the table beside him. As he named them—Bisquick, Shredded Wheat, Alka-Seltzer, Hadacol—Hohensee picked them up and tossed them behind him to the floor. He paused, surveying the remaining packages carefully, then looked accusingly at the women sitting in the front row. Who, he asked, had taken his bottle of Lydia Pinkham's? He wanted it back so he could throw it away.

Next Hohensee tore open a loaf of bakery bread, pulled out the center and wadded it into a ball, bouncing it on the floor. The bread, he said, had been made from devitamized and demineralized flour. Then he took the intestines from his anatomical manikin named Fanny, held them aloft beside the ball of bread, and asked how a ball like that could ever make it through.

For the benefit of any Food and Drug stooges present, Hohensee declared, he wanted it clearly understood that he was not selling or recommending any product in his lectures. His only goal was to teach a way of preparing and cooking food, to describe a proper diet for eliminating all our aches and pains. Those who resorted to such a diet could rebuild all the organs of the body (except the kidneys), dissolve the incrustations in the brain that prevented adequate thinking, and dissolve incrustations between the laminations of the eyeball which impaired sight and made glasses necessary. God must have known that man would abuse his eyes, Hohensee said, since He placed the ears and nose so conveniently for hanging glasses.

The American diet was sadly deficient in vitamins and minerals, Hohensee told his listeners, and he picked up and read from a government publication to clinch the point. Yet FDA Commissioner Crawford had recently written in a magazine article that Americans were better fed than ever before. Crawford, said Hohensee, was a short and sickly man, constantly puffing on a cigarette. At this point the lecturer sold subscriptions to his magazine, *The Life Span*.

Women at the menopause, said Hohensee, often went to their doctors and got shots. The estrogen in these shots was nothing more or less than horse urine. He had refused to sell urine from El Rancho Adolphus horses to the Drug Trust, which made vaccinations and inoculations from the pus of sick horses. Such injections caused both polio and cancer.

Scrutinizing the faces of his audience at a later lecture, Hohensee told them that 90 per cent of them had worms.

Worms were a major menace. They might be from two to 20 feet long, some with their heads in your stomach and the rest of their bodies in your intestines. His cleansing diet would remove them. This diet was also a preliminary to removing gallstones. Hohensee's gallstone remedy—the resurrection of an old-time patent medicine trick—helped persuade his listeners to willing acceptance of all the rest of his health counsel. He prescribed his laxative and told listeners to follow it up with olive oil. The oil released fluids in the bile duct which formed soapy concretions in the stool. Nobody could miss them. At a later lecture, Hohensee had members of his class testify as to the results. One woman proudly announced that she had counted 120 stones. "Oh, that is wonderful," said Hohensee. "I was very happy to know one of my students will stand up in a class like this and tell them I have eliminated 120 gallstones. Am I right, students?" There was loud applause. "And then you wonder why I come here without fear of the Medical Trust or their rotten bunch of racketeers, the Better Business Bureau?" The applause continued.

Hohensee's basic pattern of fear and hope conformed to, as it helped create, a major nutritional myth. Other lecturers, door-to-door salesmen, writers, TV pitchmen, health food store proprietors, shared in its construction and propagation. Thousands of Americans came to believe in it implicitly, so that they bet their dollars, staked their health, upon its doctrines. They could be roused to fierce antagonism against any scientist, businessman, or government regulator who questioned the myth's basic tenets.

One of the cardinal principles of this myth held that most disease resulted from improper diet. This was, of course, untrue. A few dietary deficiency diseases did exist, but even these had been largely vanquished in America by the nutritional revolution. It was easy, in America, to buy and eat an adequate diet. The nation's citizens, indeed, would have to go out of their way to avoid being properly nourished. Where deficiencies might exist, the proper solution lay not in spending money for expensive food supplements vended by the ill informed, but in eating better. Only a physician could detect deficiencies, in any case, and only he possessed the knowledge to prescribe therapeutic vitamins and other nutrients if needed. Yet the prophets to the faddists, with goods to sell, persevered in blaming all ills on the American food supply.[32]

A subsidiary principle in the faddist's mighty myth blamed soil depletion for the alleged well-nigh universal malnutrition. The land on which food was grown had lost its zip, been drained of the minerals and vitamins which once it held. "Laboratory tests prove," Hohensee wrote in one of his pamphlets, "that the fruits, the vegetables, the grains, the eggs, even the milk and the meats of today are not what they were a few generations ago. . . . No man of today can eat enough fruits and vegetables to supply his system with the mineral salts he requires for perfect health, because his stomach isn't big enough to hold them!"[33] This doctrine too was false. The soil's quality does affect the quantity of the crop grown, but has very little influence on its quality. Unless the necessary elements are present in the soil, crops will not grow. Only with respect to iodine has there been depletion.

A third aspect of the myth held chemical fertilizers responsible for poisoning the land and the crops grown on it. Here the purveyors of specious nutrition counsel employed an ancient stunt, taking a legitimate concern and distorting it to suit their purposes. Pesticide residues, inadequately removed, did pose a hazard to health. New and more powerful pesticides came increasingly into use, and legitimate scientists expressed alarm. Congress took up the problem and in 1947 and 1954 passed laws to help the Department of Agriculture and the Food and Drug Administration exercise more effective control.[34] The faddists, however, did not relax. Their

[32] A number of efforts have been made to present the structure of the myth underlying food faddism. I rely in this and the succeeding paragraphs on Joseph R. Bell, "Let 'em Eat Hay," *Today's Health*, 36 (Sep. 1958), 22-25, 66-68. An excellent recent article is Fredrick J. Stare, "Sense and Nonsense about Nutrition," *Harper's Mag.*, 229 (Oct. 1964), 66-70. Helen S. Mitchell has compiled "Nutrition Books for Lay Readers, A Guide to the Reliable and Unreliable," *Library Jnl.*, 85 (Feb. 15, 1960), 710-14.

[33] *What about the Vegetables and Fruits We Eat Today?*, in FDA file 31-968H.

[34] Wallace F. Janssen, "FDA since 1938: The Major Trends and Developments," *Jnl. of Public Law*, 13 (1964), 208.

prophets, like Hohensee, urged the eating of only "natural" foods raised by "organic" farming, in which only animal fertilizer was used. El Rancho Adolphus apple juice, Hohensee told his classes, came only from non-sprayed apples fertilized by animal manure; all other apple juice, he said, was contaminated with insect poisons which would destroy the kidneys.[35] Artificial fertilizers, according to the myth, besides being poisons, devitalized the soil and thus ruined the nutrients in food, making necessary the purchase of food supplements.

Still another facet of the myth, based in part on very old folk beliefs, put great stress on the special dietary value of various "wonder" foods. Hauser had his own particular list, and Hohensee too employed this doctrine. One of his favorites was garlic. "In addition to being good for a specific condition of high blood pressure," he wrote, garlic "also seems to have a profound cleansing effect upon the intestines and, of course, the blood."[36] Among other things, it inhibited growth of the tuberculosis germ. To prove garlic's potency in the system, Hohensee advised putting a piece up the rectum at night: by morning its taste would be apparent in the mouth. These claims for garlic were utter nonsense. Some of the other so-called wonder foods might have some value as foods, experts were willing to agree, but they possessed no miraculous properties and were not indispensable in diet.

One more aspect of the myth held that cooking utensils made of certain metals poisoned the food prepared in them. Aluminum was the particular bugaboo, a scare doctrine at least half a century old. Hohensee had propagated this theory right from the start. He also denounced the hazards of peeling vegetables with metal knives. Like other fringe operators, he had his own "safe" tenderizer and Lucite knives to sell.[37]

Processed foods, according to the myth, possessed a double danger. The milling of cereals, the canning of foods, even the pasteurizing of milk, according to the specious nutritionists, destroyed the natural nutrients. At the same time, food proces-

[35] FDA file 18-317L.
[36] *The Health, Success and Happiness Lectures: High Blood Pressure*, in FDA file 31-968H.
[37] AMA folder; FDA file 18-317L.

[ 352 ]

sors poured into their products a mounting array of additives, chemicals intended to deter spoilage, improve texture, and perform other like functions, although the real result, the faddists said, was the slow poisoning of the public. Reputable nutritionists assured the nation that most food values survived milling, canning, and freezing, and insisted that the nutritional losses from pasteurizing milk were far outweighed by the gains. The health faddist's penchant for raw fruits and vegetables, the experts said, was certainly extreme. As with pesticides, food additives posed a genuine problem, but one which the nutritional lecturer distorted beyond all reason. Congress acted to ensure that substances added to processed foods be proved safe before being permitted in use, passing a law in 1958 giving the FDA jurisdiction in this field.[38] The public debate leading to the law provided many frightening charges to bolster the scare doctrines of nutritional lecturers. Hohensee constantly condemned "dead"—that is, processed—foods and praised the "live" foods eaten at El Rancho Adolphus.[39] He had had excellent fortune, he told his classes, curing cancer with chlorophyll.

A final major principle in the nutritional myth concerned subclinical deficiencies. This represented a clever borrowing of a recognized medical concept: a given person's diet might not contain an adequate amount of a given nutrient, although the amount lacking was so small or had continued for so short a time that no symptoms of deficiency were yet observable. As translated by the fringe operators, almost everybody might be so threatened, and the imminent dangers to health were catastrophic. Going further, they blamed many of life's day-to-day difficulties, like weariness, tension, a sense of discouragement, on subclinical deficiencies. The hypochondriac especially found conviction in this theory. If a doctor had examined him and discovered nothing wrong, when he himself knew in his bones that there must be, it was reassuring to find out from a food supplement salesman that there was such a thing as vitamin deficiencies which even a physician could not detect. The answer, of course, lay in the insurance of multi-

[38] Janssen, "FDA since 1938," 208-209.
[39] FDA file 18-317L.

vitamin mixtures. "Good cheer and optimism," Hohensee asserted, "are impossible if you are suffering from hidden hunger or an undernourished brain."[40]

It must have been with difficulty that Hohensee maintained his own optimism, since regulatory agencies, disbelieving the nutrition myth that underlay his profitable venture, seemed so intent on curbing him. The Federal Trade Commission issued an order forbidding him to continue certain advertising claims. The Food and Drug Administration again hailed him into court. Such Adolphus Brand products as the peppermint, the wheat germ oil, and the herb laxative, the indictment charged, were misbranded, since their labels failed to state the purposes, conditions, and diseases for which they were intended. Intent should be determined, the FDA argued, from the whole host of fantastic claims which Hohensee uttered, night after night, to his classes in Phoenix and Denver. The case came to trial in Scranton in November 1954, but not until after one false start. Although the government had assembled its witnesses, Hohensee appeared without a lawyer and asked for a delay. It was granted. Hohensee then flew out to Denver to finish another class. In his audience appeared a woman who ran a health food store which earlier had been an outlet for Hohensee's products. The government had called her to be a witness in order to prove that Hohensee's wares had moved in interstate commerce. Spotting her, Hohensee publicly proclaimed her to be a rat who had sold him out to the Drug Trust and their hatchet men. "The time is coming," he proclaimed, "just like it was in Christ's time, when anyone who dares to tell the truth, Satan's forces will always find a double-crosser, a Judas, to sell him, who speaks the truth, to his adversaries. . . . But I'm not complaining. My Saviour was willing to be nailed to the cross to help people. Is that right, class? I'm still going strong." Hohensee's good cheer seemed somewhat frazzled.[41]

The Scranton jury found Hohensee guilty. Sixteen months later the judge fined him and sentenced him to a year and a day in prison. Another year went by, after a futile appeal,

[40] *Lecture Series on Health and Progress: How to Think and Attain Success,* in FDA file 31-968H.
[41] 50 *FTC Decisions* 321, Oct. 1, 1953; DDNJ 5385; FDA file 14-497L.

before he began to serve his sentence. In the meantime Hohensee pursued his craft with desperate earnestness, lecturing in many cities around the country.[42] In Houston occurred an episode that may further have dampened his good cheer. Acting on an anonymous tip, reporters and photographers hurried to a restaurant.[43]

"Hohensee sat at a back table," wrote Marie Dauplaise of the *Houston Press*, "all by himself, polishing off a dinner of forbidden fruits. There was fried red snapper. (He'd told us at the lecture when he bounced the 'death-dealing' skillet on the floor that frying destroys the good qualities of food.) There were thick slices of white French bread. ('It knots in a ball in your stomach, and stays there in a big lump.') He was rinsing this down with huge gulps of beer. (He'd characterized his enemies at his lectures as 'alcohol drinkers,' and bad people were 'barflies.') Apple pie was his final gastronomic delight."[44]

Thus surprised, Hohensee grabbed his beer bottle and hid it under his chair, covering his telltale plate with a piece of newspaper. Rolling up another section of the paper into a weapon, he started after one of the photographers. But it was too late. The picture was already in the camera. " 'Nature Doc' Dines Out," ran the headline atop the picture, "and Knocks a Decade Off His 180-Year Life Span!"[45]

Perhaps one reason Hohensee permitted his hunger to override his professed principles lay in his skipping of breakfast a day or two before. The lecturer had spent the night in jail, charged with violating Houston's ordinance against itinerant vendors. When the morning meal was brought him, he refused to touch it. "I won't even drink water," he said.[46]

[42] *Ibid.*; DDNJ 5385. FDA files contain a transcript of the trial, U.S. v. El Rancho Adolphus Products, Inc., a corporation; Scientific Living Inc., a corporation; and Adolphus Hohensee, an individual, in the United States District Court for the Middle District of Pennsylvania, No. 12529 Criminal. For the appeal: U.S. v. Adolphus Hohensee . . ., 243 Fed. (2d) 367.

[43] *Houston Press*, June 1, 1955; Marie Dauplaise, "What's Up, Doc?," *Front Page Detective*, Oct. 1955, 24-27, 85-87.

[44] *Ibid.*, 86.

[45] *Ibid.*; *Houston Press*, June 1, 1955.

[46] Dauplaise, "What's Up, Doc?," 86.

The arrest had taken place in the evening soon after Hohensee had begun to instruct his class. When he saw what was happening, he shouted to his students: "The lecture's over! These men say I'm under arrest! Come down to the station and bail me out." His loyal partisans crowded around the detectives, screaming insults. Some 75 followed their leader down to the station house, where they milled around the halls, rebuking the police, and murmuring about a Communist plot. Hohensee played up to them. Turning to reporters present, he shouted, "How much did the medical trust pay you for this night's work?"

The fierce dedication of Hohensee's supporters was matched by the adherents of other nutritional prophets. Whenever fringe operators went to trial, fans crowded the courtroom. They bombarded Congress, the Food and Drug Administration, and other agencies with bitter cards and letters, condemning the persecution of their heroes, damning an alleged conspiracy against them on the part of the FDA, the AMA, and respectable sectors of the food and drug industries. The angry elements seemed to be merging. "Major food peddlers of nutritional quackery who have been prosecuted by FDA," said Commissioner George Larrick in 1957, "have formed a sort of 'FDA Alumni Assn.' and banded together to fight FDA and effective law enforcement." The pseudo-nutritionists organized effectively and prompted their followers to campaigns of mass protest.[47]

The active antagonism of food faddists was a reaction to increasingly vigorous efforts by the Food and Drug Administration to combat nutritional nonsense. Another major promoter besides Hohensee, V. Earl Irons, who distributed his Vit-Ra-Tox products out of Boston, had been sentenced to jail. And dozens of seizures were taking misbranded food supplements vended by lecturers and door-to-door salesmen off the market. But the job was too big. As always, FDA resources were limited, and nutritional cases complex and difficult to develop and prosecute. Despite the increased regu-

[47] *Drug Trade News*, 32 (Apr. 22, 1957), 34; John L. Harvey, "Progress and Problems," *FDC Law Jnl.*, 12 (July 1957), 436.

latory attention being given it, nutritional quackery grew larger. It had reached the stage, the AMA estimated, of a half-billion-dollar annual racket. "We believe," said Wallace Janssen, FDA's director of public information, "that at present more 'bunk' is being peddled to the public concerning food than on any other subject."[48]

In 1957 the FDA began a major educational campaign to supplement its increased regulatory efforts. Not that public warnings had not come from many quarters throughout the preceding years. From the 1920's on, the AMA's magazines had carried countless articles pointing out the dangers of pseudo-nutritional doctrines. Morris Fishbein avowed in 1938 that "public interest in vitamins has led to a more extraordinary exploitation than in almost any other field of medicine, except perhaps the glands." Hohensee felt constantly the necessity of castigating Fishbein, whom he termed "the medical dictator." University professors of nutrition and of home economics, the American Dietetic Association, the American Public Health Association, organizations of food technologists, the Nutrition Foundation (an industry-sponsored group), the National Better Business Bureau, writers for newspapers and magazines, and other concerned parties also spoke out against the follies of food faddism and particularly the waste in money and risks in health inherent in relying on the expensive products dispensed by the fringe operators. But all these warnings bulked small in mass compared with the total wordage written and spoken by the false food prophets. Millions of Americans did not or would not hear.[49]

[48] DDNJ 5308; *Department of Health, Education, and Welfare 1957 Annual Report,* 200-201; *FDC Reports,* Apr. 8, 1957, 11; *FDC Law Jnl.,* 13 (Nov. 1958), 677-78; Janssen, "Food Quackery—A Law Enforcement Problem," *Jnl. of the Amer. Dietetic Assoc.,* 36 (Feb. 1960), 110.
[49] Examples of articles are "Exploiting the Health Interest: Modern Magic—Some Freaks and Fallacies of the Food Faddist," *Hygeia,* 3 (Jan. 1925), 16-21, (Feb. 1925), 70-75; "Don't Be Misled by Food Fakers," *ibid.,* 8 (Aug. 1930), 722; Fishbein, "Modern Medical Charlatans," *ibid.,* 16 (Feb. 1938), 113-15, 172, 182-83; Lois M. Miller, "The Vitamin Follies," *ibid.,* 16 (Nov. 1938), 1004-1005, 1045; D. W. McCrary, "Food Fads, Fallacies and Facts," *ibid.,* a six-part series from 19 (Aug. 1941), 646-49, through 20 (Jan. 1942), 48-51; Max Millman, "The Facts about Vitamins," *ibid.,* 35 (July 1957), 34-37; W. J. Stone,

More strenuous educational efforts, FDA officials hoped, might reap a larger measure of success. District offices were instructed to make the debunking of false nutritional claims a deliberate campaign. Speeches on the theme before consumer and service groups were increased. Newspapers and radio stations were provided with information. From Washington a new and hard-hitting pamphlet, *Food Facts v. Food Fallacies*, was distributed by the thousands. Writers were given welcome and provided with statistics and case histories. Arthur S. Flemming, Secretary of Health, Education, and Welfare, issued a special release and held a press conference to publicize the issue.[50]

The AMA, like the FDA, had become alert to the growing menace. Inquiries and complaints about door-to-door nutritional salesmen, noted Oliver Field, director of the Bureau of Investigation, had come to bulk the largest of any category in the bureau's files. So the AMA also launched an intensified campaign of education against nutritional quackery, treating the subject in *Today's Health*, the magazine for lay readers, preparing a large display for exhibit at state and county fairs, issuing new pamphlets, and making a movie on "The Medicine Man" for showing before clubs and school and church groups. The film vividly revealed the techniques of a health lecturer

"Dietary Facts, Fads, and Fancies," *JAMA*, 95 (Sep. 6, 1930), 709-15; W. H. Sebrell, "Nutritional Diseases in the United States," *ibid.*, 115 (Sep. 7, 1940), 851-54; "Indiscriminate Administration of Vitamins to Workers in Industry," *ibid.*, 118 (Feb. 21, 1942), 618-21; "Common Sense vs. Food Faddism," 157 (Feb. 5, 1955), 514; Hohensee in FDA file 31-968H; Secretary of Health, Education, and Welfare statement by Arthur S. Flemming, thanking other groups, FDA Press Release, Nov. 19, 1958; various publications by the organizations mentioned. See, for example, a series of articles in *Jnl. of the Amer. Dietetic Assoc.*, 32 (July 1956), 623-35, and 34 (Sep. 1958), 935-37; the Amer. Dietetic Assoc., *Food Facts Talk Back*; "Quackery in the Field of Nutrition," *Amer. Jnl. of Public Health*, 42 (Aug. 1952), 997-98; *The Role of Nutrition Education in Combatting Food Fads*, papers given in 1959 at a joint meeting of the Nutrition Fdn. and the Institute of Food Technologists, Northern California Section.

[50] *F&D Rev.*, 41 (June 1957), 98; (July 1957), 119, 129; *Department of Health, Education, and Welfare 1957 Annual Report*, 194-95, 200-201; Flemming statement, Nov. 19, 1958, press release.

vending his wares. Those who had witnessed Hohensee in action might, in seeing the movie, experience a sense of *déjà vu.*[51]

"The Medicine Man" received its first showing at an AMA Public Relations Institute in Chicago in August 1958. At this meeting the announcement was made that the leading foes of nutritional quackery had organized a united front. Spokesmen for the AMA, FDA, and NBBB reported joint efforts to expand the educational crusade. "It will take widespread and repeated dissemination of literature and other visual aids," said FDA's Kenneth Milstead, "to make an impression on the public."[52]

So battle was joined at a new level between the promoters and the opponents of nutritional nonsense, with the health of the American public at stake. At the time of the Chicago Institute, Adolphus Hohensee had served his sentence and was four months out of jail. Being behind bars had not seemed to quench his fighting mood. He resumed the rostrum and re-entered the fray.[53]

[51] *JAMA,* 166 (Mar. 8, 1958), 26-27; 167 (Aug. 23, 1958), 2088; *Drug Trade News,* 33 (Aug. 25, 1958), 2, 29; (Sep. 22, 1958), 33.

[52] *JAMA,* 167 (Aug. 2, 1958), 1745; *Department of Health, Education, and Welfare 1958 Annual Report,* 197; George Larrick, "Report from the Food and Drug Administration," *FDC Law Jnl.,* 14 (Apr. 1959), 238; *Drug Trade News,* 33 (Sep. 22, 1958), 33.

[53] AMA folder; DDNJ 6709; *F&D Rev.,* 45 (Sep. 1961), 203. In 1962 a California judge sentenced Hohensee to jail for selling "ambrosia of the gods"—honey—with curative claims. The judge recommended that Hohensee be put in charge of the prison beehives. *Washington Evening Star,* Dec. 22, 1962. On appeal this conviction was reversed, mainly because of the way the evidence had been secured; Hohensee had already served 18 months in prison. *NBBB Service Bull.* 1889 (Sep. 1965).

# 17

## "THE MOST HEARTLESS"

*"Of all the ghouls who feed on the bodies of the dead and the dying, the cancer quacks are most vicious and most heartless."*
—MORRIS FISHBEIN, 1965[1]

"SUPPOSE you suddenly discovered that you have cancer. A horrible, crab-like disease has invaded your body, is gnawing your flesh, has pushed greedy tentacles into your vital organs. A loathsome scavenger slowly and inexorably is consuming you alive, cell by cell."[2]

With these stark words one of the 20th century's most successful cancer-treating irregulars opened his autobiography, catching cleverly the fearsome and repulsive image in which mankind has conceived of cancer through the ages. The word "cancer" does derive from the Greek word for "crab."[3] The crawling spread of cancer, whether external and observable or internal and secretive, is relentless, and during long centuries the diagnosis of cancer has amounted to a sentence of death, following a painful and often protracted decline.

During the 20th century, important headway has been made in combatting this ancient disease. The basic processes involved in cancer's various forms are ever better understood. Diagnostic techniques are constantly improving. Great advances in therapy have come through improvements in surgery and in the use of x-rays, radium, and other radioactive substances. "The cold knife and the hot rays" really produce cures. Nearly a third of all patients with cancer are now being

[1] Fishbein, "History of Cancer Quackery," *Perspectives in Biology and Medicine*, 8 (Winter 1965), 140.

[2] Harry M. Hoxsey, *You Don't Have to Die* (N.Y., 1956), 1.

[3] Michael B. Shimkin, *Science and Cancer* (Public Health Service Publication 1162: Washington, 1964), 3.

saved, as judged by the fact that they are still alive five years after diagnosis, and this proportion could be raised to a half with prompt and full application of the knowledge and skills possessed by our specialists.[4]

But the age-old fear of cancer still persists. Indeed, relatively, the image of cancer has grown more grim. For the gains in fighting it have been less dramatic than medical triumphs in other areas, especially with respect to contagious diseases. Despite massive research, chemotherapy for cancer has so far yielded only modest results. Drugs can postpone death in patients afflicted with certain forms of cancer. A few antibiotics have caused some profound remission, if not cure. One rare type of cancer, treated with a combination of drugs, has yielded a high rate of five-year cures. But no chemotherapeutic agent has been found that can vanquish cancer as penicillin can often cure pneumonia. So, in the scale of killers, cancer has risen, now ranking as the number two cause of death, destined to end the lives of one out of every eight Americans.[5]

The fear of cancer has doubtless been aggravated by the very necessary effort to combat it. For the word itself has appeared so often in the press during the last generation that latent concern has been constantly quickened into conscious dread. Educational campaigns have aimed at leading the public to recognize symptoms and to seek diagnosis early enough for surgery or x-ray treatment to be effective. This effort has brought continued life to many who would have otherwise been doomed. Yet an inevitable side effect of increasing cancer-consciousness has been a rise in cancer quackery. For fear of cancer, fear that some ambiguous symptom may mean cancer, fear of surgery and radiation if one has or might have cancer, fear of the waiting period after orthodox treatment to determine its success or failure, fear that discovery has come too late to warrant treatment, fear, agonizing numbing fear, overwhelming the safeguards of rational prudence, sends desperate men and women to the cancer quack.

Not that the cancer quack is a new breed, of course; he has been around almost as long as the malady itself. He flourished in the 19th century, offering his "secret specific" to the fright-

[4] *Ibid.*, 23, 30, 35.     [5] *Ibid.*, 1.

ened, who, "like a drowning person grasping at straws, seize upon the frail hope that is offered by the hand of ignorant charlatanry." Within the 20th century, all foes of the charlatan have been forced to keep him constantly in mind. The Sherley Amendment was provoked by the Bureau of Chemistry's loss of a cancer labeling case. Post Office fraud fighters have won a succession of victories over mail-order "specialists" in treating cancer. But Dr. Cramp, in successive editions of *Nostrums and Quackery*, noticed no diminution in their sordid ranks. Hardly a week passed without the receipt in his office of a letter announcing the discovery of a "sure cure" for cancer. Nor did pseudo-science wither during the decades that science was making its most notable advances. By the 1950's, some 4,000 quacks were fleecing thousands of victims who had or feared they had cancer out of about $50 million every year.[6]

In 1936, the year in which Dr. Cramp published the last green-bound volume in his *Nostrums and Quackery* series, one of the key characters in Cramp's cancer cast showed up in Dallas, Texas. There, in a small one-story building, Harry M. Hoxsey opened a cancer "clinic."[7] This venture, unlike a number of Hoxsey's previous efforts which Cramp had chronicled, turned out to be a major financial success.

Hoxsey had inherited the cancer business. Early in his career he gave his father credit for the discovery of his remedy, setting the date at 1908. Later on Hoxsey told a more grandiloquent tale, pushing the date back to 1840 and transferring the distinction to his great-grandfather, who, on his Illinois farm, observed how his Percheron stallion cured a cancer of the right hock by standing knee-deep in a clump of shrubs and flowering plants. In both accounts, Hoxsey's father, a self-taught veterinarian, employed the secret anti-cancer remedy first on livestock, then on men. The elder Hoxsey died in 1919, and the cause of death was cancer, a fact his son later went to great pains to deny. Harry's mother died two years later, also

[6] Caleb Ticknor, *A Popular Treatise on Medical Philosophy* (N.Y., 1838), 178; *N&Q*, III, 7; L. Henry Garland, "California Outlaws the Cancer Quack," *Today's Health*, 37 (Aug. 1959), 30; Jonathan Spivak, "Crusade on Quacks," *Wall Street Journal*, June 22, 1960.
[7] Hoxsey, *You Don't Have to Die*, 180.

of cancer. In 1921 Harry was 20, and life did not look promising. The youngest of 12 children, Harry had grown up in the rural Illinois village of Girard, had quit school after the eighth grade—he later claimed receipt of a high school diploma from a correspondence school—and had gone to work in the coal mines at neighboring Taylorville, selling some insurance on the side.[8]

Young Hoxsey was an ambitious fellow, "quick-brained" and "ingenious," as a federal judge later remarked, natty in dress, glib and persuasive of speech. As one of his early admirers put it, "Harry is not a man of few words but one of many," and those words, not elegant in grammatical construction, definitely possessed the common touch. His endeavors were early imbued with the spirit of the motto he later displayed on a desk plaque: "The world is made up of two kinds of people—dem that takes and dem that gets took."[9]

Some of his siblings were shortly to sue Harry, accusing him of taking their father's cancer formula for his own profit, after his mother's death, a legacy that should have belonged to them all. The suit was never pushed to a conclusive decision. Harry's story had it that his father, just before his death, had taught him the formula by having him copy it 250 times until he learned it by heart and had given him a dramatic death-bed injunction to devote his career to healing the sick, no matter what opposition he might encounter from "the High Priests of Medicine." In any case, Harry claimed, he had changed the composition of the formula.[10]

[8] *The Hoxsey Method of Successfully Removing Cancer* (Taylorville, [1928]), in Hoxsey folder, AMA Dept. of Investigation; Hoxsey, *You Don't Have to Die*, 62-76. The AMA Hoxsey folder contains much data on the cause of Hoxsey's father's death, and the FDA discovered that Hoxsey wrote the Illinois State Registrar for a copy of his father's death certificate using an incorrect middle initial, receiving a reply that no certificate could be found. The initial was corrected in the copy of the Registrar's letter he reprinted in *You Don't Have to Die*. Interview with Gilbert Goldhammer, Nov. 17, 1960.

[9] Judge William H. Atwell's oral opinion, Mar. 18, 1949, in Harry M. Hoxsey v. Morris Fishbein et al., in the U.S. District Court for the Northern District of Texas, Dallas Division, copy in FDA file, Injunction 232; *Girard* (Ill.) *Gazette*, July 18, 1929; *Life*, 40 (Apr. 16, 1956), 125.

[10] AMA Hoxsey file; Hoxsey, *You Don't Have to Die*, 71-74, 141-53.

About 1922 Hoxsey began to use the formula. As he later told the tale, a Civil War veteran with cancer of the lip had come to him and begged for treatment. Harry had demurred, saying he had no license to practice medicine.[11]

"Nobody needs a license to save lives," the veteran had argued. "If I was drowning would you stand by and watch me go down because a sign on yonder tree says 'No Swimming Allowed'?"

"There's no adequate answer to that kind of logic," Hoxsey said in retrospect, "and I didn't waste any time trying to find one."

He used the cancer paste on the venerable veteran, who thereafter, throughout his life, was willing to testify in public utterance and in print that he had been cured.

While practicing spasmodically in Taylorville, Hoxsey joined up with two Chicago men to form the National Cancer Research Institute, a common law trust to exploit the use of his father's formula. When his associates backed out of this enterprise to give their support to another cancer venture, Hoxsey expanded his Taylorville operations into the Hoxide Institute. Supported by some of the town's businessmen, Hoxsey took over from the Order of the Moose an old frame house and began to advertise his treatment far and wide. "CANCER," the copy read, "Any person suffering from this malady . . . , is invited to apply for authoritative information as to the cures that have been effected and are now being effected at Taylorville, under strictly ethical medical supervision, painlessly, without operation, and with permanent results." Inquirers were told to write the secretary of the Taylorville Chamber of Commerce.[12]

Patients responded to the advertising, and shortly the local paper began to run stories of deaths that were occurring at the Institute. Local doctors began to be concerned. One of them wrote the "high priests" at the American Medical Association telling of examining a man who had received the Hoxide treatment. The paste had been applied to a tumor on the

11 *Ibid.*, 76-77.
12 AMA Hoxsey file; *JAMA*, 86 (Jan. 2, 1926), 55-57.

cheek. "Two days before . . . [the man] died," the doctor wrote, "I was called to see him and found necrosis of not only the soft tissue of his face, but a complete destruction of the malar bone. This man died of hemorrhage at the hospital."[13]

To keep the secret of his medicine, the doctor said, Hoxsey bought the separate ingredients each at a different drugstore. The key ingredient, analysis at AMA headquarters revealed, was arsenic. Thus Hoxsey's vaunted remedy was an escharotic, a corrosive chemical that ate away the flesh. Through the ages physicians had employed such corrosive agents in treating external cancers, but this mode of procedure had become outmoded. "Pastes went out with the bustle," a cancer authority has noted, "so far as scientific medicine is concerned." Such chemicals could not distinguish between tissues that were cancerous and tissues that were sound. The risk of damage to healthy flesh was tremendous. The escharotic might eat into the blood vessels and cause death through bleeding. Surgery was much safer and more certain.[14]

The goings-on at Taylorville brought Hoxsey into conflict both with the AMA and with the law. Dr. Cramp blasted the Hoxide Institute's methods in the AMA *Journal*. Tragedy awaited "sufferers from carcinoma," he wrote, "who are beguiled by false beacons displayed by the highly respectable citizens of Taylorville" into resorting to Hoxsey's treatment. He detailed instances of tragedy that already had occurred. "The promoters of the scheme" were reaping "a rich harvest from gullibility and suffering."[15]

Hoxsey sued the AMA in response to its criticism, asking a quarter of a million dollars libel judgment. The case dragged on, and finally the AMA insisted that it be brought to trial. The Hoxsey Institute was not prepared, and the judge dismissed the suit. In the meantime, Hoxsey had gone to court as defendant instead of plaintiff. Charged with responsibility

[13] *Ibid.*, Samuel B. Herdman, M.D., to Cramp, Oct. 9, 1924, AMA Hoxsey file.
[14] *JAMA*, 86 (Jan. 2, 1926), 55-57; AMA Hoxsey file; Charles S. Cameron, *The Cancer Quacks* (Public Health Service Publication No. 559: Washington, 1957), 3.
[15] *JAMA*, 86 (Jan. 2, 1926), 55-57.

for the death of one of his victims, he was accused of practicing medicine without a license. He pleaded guilty and paid a $100 fine.[16]

The Hoxide Institute in Taylorville closed its doors in 1928, but Harry Hoxsey did not abandon the corrosive legacy inherited from his father. Twice again in quick succession he sought to duplicate his Taylorville venture in Illinois towns, first in Jacksonville, then in Girard. He launched his return to his home town with a mammoth "Hoxsey Day," under the aegis of the Chamber of Commerce, a day that had all the trappings of a Fourth of July celebration. The Girard band played. Living testimonials from among the citizenry, including the Civil War veteran, bespoke their gratitude to Hoxsey before the large audience assembled in the town square under a boiling sun. An eclectic doctor from Indiana lauded the Hoxsey method. A local minister delivered an oration imbued with religious and patriotic zeal. "I love my country," he told the crowd, "because its heroes are such characters as George Washington, Abraham Lincoln, Woodrow Wilson, who love to serve and not to rule. I love Hoxsey because he does not want to rule the world but serve the world."[17]

Hoxsey himself addressed his former neighbors. "There is a lot of knockers," he said, "who do not know what they are talking about, and especially around a man's home town, and if those knockers are here today and have the mind of a six year old child and don't leave here today, a walking, talking dyed-in-the-wool Hoxsey fan and convinced beyond a reasonable doubt that this treatment is a cure for cancer they are either deaf, dumb or blind, or else they are crazy." Regular doctors were "hard-hearted," interested in getting "their hand greased with plenty of money," wanting to drive their Packards and their Stutzes. AMA officials had been invited to attend the rally, but they had not come. "Why don't they fight in the open? Why don't they take this platform? Why don't they prove the Hoxsey affair is a fake as they say? . . . But no, friends, they haven't got the guts to accept this challenge."

And Hoxsey presented his gallery of patients who said they

[16] *Ibid.*, 93 (Aug. 3, 1929), 400-402.
[17] *Ibid.*; *Girard Gazette*, July 18, 1929.

had been cured, quizzing them publicly on the details of their experience. "Anyone in the hearing of my voice," he challenged, "who will prove that the Hoxsey Method does not cure more than 50 per cent of its patients, or if they will prove or show that there is another method under God's skies as good as the Hoxsey, he can receive the reward which we have offered on our large posters."

Applause was frequent, the local editor observed, and when one speaker asked if the audience wished to endorse Hoxsey in his attempts to save lives, "the response was so nearly unanimous that those who remained sitting for any reason could be counted on the fingers."

If the citizens were impressed, the AMA was not. "Perhaps," Cramp wrote, "Girard will flourish briefly—especially the local undertaker and those individuals who have rooms to rent. . . . If that is what the citizens . . . want, the Hoxide fakery will doubtless give it to them. They will also get the doubtful privilege of the reputation of living in a town that fattens off the sufferings of those unfortunates who are lured there by the false hope that an ignorant faker has discovered a 'cure' for one of the most dreadful scourges afflicting the human race."[18]

Hoxsey's Girard endeavors were indeed brief, and twice more he paid a fine for practicing in Illinois without a license. A cooperative venture across the river in Iowa did not work out much better. Hoxsey teamed up in Muscatine with another uneducated promoter of a cancer cure, Norman Baker, but the two fell out, the state stepped in, and Hoxsey was barred by injunction from treating cancer patients. During the next several years, Hoxsey was much on the move. He set up shop in Detroit, in Wheeling, then in Atlantic City. Wherever he went, the AMA dogged his footsteps. Legal actions were sometimes instituted. Finally, in 1936, Hoxsey went south. Dallas promised to be a safer and more prosperous haven, at least for a time.[19]

As had been true beginning with his Illinois enterprises, Hoxsey strove to concentrate on the business and promotional sides of his Dallas clinic, leaving the diagnosing and treating

[18] *Ibid.*; *JAMA*, 93 (Aug. 3, 1929), 400-402.
[19] AMA Hoxsey file; *JAMA*, 133 (Mar. 14, 1947), 774-75; FDA file, Inj. 232.

mainly to a series of eclectic, homeopathic, and osteopathic physicians whom he employed. But he could not bring himself to abstain completely from therapy. Again convicted of practicing medicine without a license, Hoxsey was fined $25,000 and sentenced to five months in jail. A higher court, however, set aside this verdict. Hoxsey managed to acquire an honorary Doctor of Naturopathy degree and was licensed in Texas as a naturopath.[20]

Hoxsey's early years at Dallas coincided with the early years of the chemotherapeutic revolution. His burgeoning business owed not a little of its success to this fact. For, in addition to treating external cancers with escharotic substances, the clinic offered to treat internal cancers by "chemical" means. Hoxsey was to claim that his internal medicines had been used by his father and inherited from him. But the evidence seems to suggest that, in his Illinois days, only the corrosive paste was employed in therapy, used, to be sure, not only in treating skin cancers, but also for cancer—or purported cancer—of the breast and female organs. Exactly when he began using his "tonics" for hidden cancers within the body is not clear. Perhaps he acquired his formulas from Norman Baker during the tempestuous joint operation in Muscatine. At any rate, in his early Dallas days, Hoxsey boasted he could cure internal cancers with medicines. To a public increasingly fearful of cancer and increasingly hopeful of chemotherapy, such an appeal offered a gleam of hope.[21]

The ingredients in Hoxsey's internal medicines, kept secret until revealed in court actions, varied somewhat from time to time. Two liquid mixtures played the central role, one brownish-black in color, the other pink. The brownish-black liquid contained water, potassium iodide (used mainly in medical practice as an expectorant to loosen tenacious sputum in cases of bronchitis), cascara sagrada (an herbal laxative), sugar syrup, and usually prickly ash, buckthorn, alfalfa, and red clover blossoms. The pink liquid, besides the other ingredients, contained lactate of pepsin, a vehicle used to help the stomach tolerate nauseating medicines; the pink variety was prescribed when patients encountered some of the unpleasant side

[20] *Ibid.*      [21] *Ibid.*; AMA Hoxsey file.

effects occasionally experienced when taking potassium iodide.[22]

Why his colored mixtures cured cancer, Hoxsey and his spokesmen were frank to confess they did not completely know. "We have been too busy treating cancer victims—and fighting court battles to keep our clinic open—," he asserted in his autobiography, "to spare the time, personnel and facilities for objective study." His hypothesis, in its bluntest version, held that a major chemical imbalance in the body caused normal cells to mutate into a cancerous form, and his medicines restored the original chemical environment, checking and killing the cancerous cells. This hypothesis could be elaborated at length—as in an address delivered by Hoxsey's medical director—into a complicated fantasy of irrelevant scientific and pseudo-scientific jargon that sounded very impressive to the layman but caused genuine cancer experts to grieve. What made things worse, as the experts assessed the Hoxsey theories, was that the Hoxsey literature condemned the only treatments yet found valid in cancer therapy. "In my opinion," wrote medical director J. B. Durkee, "x-ray and radium have no place in the treatment of cancer. . . . They further upset basic cell metabolism rather than do anything to correct it." Durkee's lecture, in printed form, played a prominent role in Hoxsey's "scientific" confrontation of his would-be patients.[23]

Equally important in that confrontation were testimonials from earlier patients. Just as on "Hoxsey Day" at Girard, so in Dallas Hoxsey could present "satisfied" users of his method, men and women who credited him with saving their lives. They would respond to letters from inquirers, talk to investigating groups, testify in court, and write their touching expressions of gratitude for Hoxsey to print and distribute far and wide.

Hoxsey's promotional documents did not claim that all can-

[22] FDA file, Inj. 232; *JAMA*, 155 (June 12, 1954), 667-68; *Transcript of Record in the United States Court of Appeals, Fifth District, No. 13645, United States of America, Appellant, versus Hoxsey Cancer Clinic, a Partnership and Harry M. Hoxsey, an Individual, Appellees* (Fort Worth, 1951), 69-84.
[23] Hoxsey, *You Don't Have to Die*, 44-46; Durkee address in *Hoxsey Cancer Clinic, Specializing in Cancer*, in FDA file, Inj. 232.

cers could be cured. Indeed, he specifically denied this was the case. Cures were less certain if x-ray or radiation treatment had been used first. But with Hoxsey's "entirely revolutionary" internal medicine, many cancers could be cured. The cure rate for breast cancer, for example, according to Dr. Durkee's speech, was 50 to 60 per cent. And countering his caveats, in the minds of those who read Hoxsey's literature, were the compelling case histories.[24]

When a fearful patient showed up at the door of Hoxsey's first small Dallas clinic, or later at the larger building which growing business led him to acquire, the patient's case history was transcribed by a clerk. The sufferer's own suspicions were taken down, plus a record of anything he had been told by doctors whom he might have consulted earlier. Documentary records of previous diagnosis or treatment, like the results of a biopsy, were solicited. Then came some laboratory tests: various blood studies, a urinalysis, a test for syphilis. Very rarely a biopsy was secured. Chest and pelvic x-rays were made and a general physical examination given by a member of the staff. The medical director reviewed the records and, if cancer was diagnosed, prescribed the Hoxsey treatment. Patients said to have external cancer were treated with Hoxsey's current version of the escharotic powder. They and patients said to be suffering from internal cancer were put on the internal medication, usually the brownish-black liquid first, three teaspoonfuls a day. "Supportive" treatment of vitamins, laxatives, and antacids was also prescribed. Then the patient saw the business manager and arranged for the payment of the clinic's charges: the basic fee in Dallas was first $300, later increased to $400, plus certain other costs. Hoxsey insisted, as he had asserted throughout his career, that many indigent sufferers were treated free.[25]

As the years went by, thousands of patients from all over the nation made the trip to Dallas, learning of Hoxsey through his printed pamphlets or by word of mouth. Some had diagnosed their own symptoms without consulting doctors and had reached the fearful decision that cancer had attacked

[24] *Ibid.*
[25] *Transcript of Record, passim;* FDA file, Inj. 232.

them. Others, with cancer diagnosed by physicians, sought out Hoxsey instead of submitting themselves to surgery. Still others had already undergone operations and x-ray treatments, but in their despair determined to miss no bets. The Dallas methods were also exported to other states. A few physicians and osteopaths around the country, after spending some time in Dallas, returned to their own cities and sought to treat cancer the Hoxsey way, receiving by mail their supply of the brownish-black and pink tonics.[26]

As his clinic prospered, Hoxsey sought to bolster its prestige. In 1945, accompanied by three Congressmen, he showed up at the National Cancer Institute in Washington. The year after Hoxsey had begun his Dallas operation, Congress had created the National Cancer Institute to confront, with all the resources of modern science, a major health problem in which the public was displaying an increasing concern. Besides conducting its own research, the NCI was eager to discover helpful clues wherever they might be found. Suggestions coming from outside the agency were often turned over for appraisal to the National Advisory Cancer Council, a group of the nation's leading experts in the cancer field. To avoid burdening the Council with trivial and patently futile suggestions, criteria had been established to govern which methods of treating cancer, among those proposed, warranted investigation and possible testing. When Hoxsey, the Congressmen in tow, showed up at the Institute, the NCI's chief, Dr. R. R. Spencer, explained these criteria. The Institute, he said, would be glad to present Hoxsey's case to the advisory council if he would furnish certain information. He must reveal his formula and explain his techniques of treatment in detail. He must also present a record of at least 50 cases treated by his method. Each case must represent an individual in whom the presence of internal cancer had been confirmed by competent biopsy, who had been treated by physicians and given up as hopeless, and who then had been treated by Hoxsey and had survived from three to five years.[27]

[26] *Ibid.*
[27] Memorandum by R. R. Spencer, Chief, NCI, of meeting, Oct. 19, 1945, regarding "Bryan & Peak Cancer Clinic, Administering the Hoxsey Method of Treatment," copy in AMA Hoxsey file.

Such stipulations, of course, were much more stringent than those required for publishing testimonials. Hoxsey impressed Dr. Spencer as reluctant to reveal his formula. Nonetheless, after the interview in Washington, Hoxsey went back to Dallas and sent to the National Cancer Institute data on 60 cases. The information did not come near to meeting the criteria. It was too fragmentary and incomplete to warrant investigation. In Hoxsey's view, the NCI did not make a conscientious study of his results because it was under the thumb of the AMA. "I was," he wrote, "bitterly disappointed, disillusioned and shocked."[28]

From Senator Elmer Thomas of Oklahoma, Hoxsey managed to get a more sympathetic response. One of the Senator's constituents credited Hoxsey with saving his son's life and urged Thomas to pay a visit to the Dallas clinic. Thomas came. In a sort of formal hearing, transcribed by a court reporter, the Senator quizzed a group of satisfied users whom Hoxsey had assembled and was obviously impressed. Hoxsey offered to put his treatment to any kind of test the Senator might arrange, and Thomas promised to return to Washington and try to interest government medical experts in such a trial of strength. No test eventuated, but Hoxsey printed up the verbatim testimony of the "hearing" and distributed it far and wide.[29]

Hoxsey's posture on having his methods tested had been used before by the cancer irregulars and would be tried again. Vigorous public protestations that a test was desired, frequently repeated and broadly circulated, impressed the layman, especially when he was desperately seeking help against a dreaded malady for himself or for his loved ones. Such protestations betokened the promoter's self-confidence, his apparent willingness to abide by the rules of the scientific game. The layman could not so easily grasp that the promoter was either too ignorant to understand the real rules of adequate scientific testing or else insincere in his protestations, either

[28] *Ibid.*; "Hoxsey 'Cure' for Cancer," Committee on Cancer Diagnosis and Therapy, National Research Council, Feb. 1, 1951, copy in AMA Hoxsey file; Hoxsey, *You Don't Have to Die*, 200-206.
[29] *Ibid.*, 210-12; FDA file, Inj. 232.

unwilling or unable to provide the type of sophisticated data from which expert scientists could draw valid conclusions. When scientists rejected proffered tests, on grounds that the data were insufficient, it was easy for the promoter to raise the ancient cry of persecution. Physicians did not dare find out the truth, he could say, for fear that their lucrative methods of treatment might become outmoded. This pitch too brought sympathetic response from many laymen, well aware that regular medical treatment often was expensive. Such an appeal played also on a latent suspicion of complicated science that was present, as well as awe and respect, in the mass mind.

Hoxsey continually proclaimed that he wanted tests. In the year that Senator Thomas visited him, Hoxsey wrote the Texas State Medical Board: "If you will come out here to the clinic and we cannot prove to you that we have cured cancer after radium, x-ray, and surgery had failed, we will give you $10,000, or better still, we will take 25 cases of cancer and let the entire Dallas County Medical Society or any doctor in America take 25 cases, and if we do not cure two to their one in sixteen weeks, we will donate $10,000 to any charitable organization in Dallas County." Two years later Hoxsey expressed his eagerness for testing to two scientists who visited the clinic at the behest of the American Cancer Society. The next year he again submitted case data to the National Cancer Institute, and again, after careful appraisal, the Institute determined that the material did not meet its basic requirements. Hoxsey's 77 case reports were accompanied by only six biopsies; only two of these were from patients treated for internal cancer, neither of which revealed anything that could be identified as cancer cells. Despite this, a committee of the National Advisory Cancer Council perused the Hoxsey records case by case. No single case met the Council's criteria. Clinical tests were naturally refused.[30]

By this time Hoxsey had interested another Senator in his operations. William Langer of North Dakota had already gone

[30] AMA Hoxsey file; reports to the American Cancer Society on a visit to the Hoxsey clinic, Feb. 10, 1949, by L. T. Coggeshall and Andrew C. Ivy, attached to "Hoxsey 'Cure' for Cancer," Committee on Cancer Diagnosis and Therapy; J. R. Heller, Director, NCI, to Sen. William Langer [May 1951], copy in FDA file, Inj. 232.

on record as complimenting another unproved cancer remedy. Now he quizzed the National Cancer Institute rigorously on its approach to Hoxsey's problem. After a visit to Dallas, Langer brought Hoxsey much publicity by introducing a resolution in the Senate under which a subcommittee would have been authorized to make "a full and complete study and investigation" to determine if Hoxsey's methods "in the treatment of cancer have proved a cure for such disease."[31]

If Hoxsey had not had tests, he had certainly undergone trials. The results of these court actions in Dallas doubtless had much to do with the buoyancy with which he fraternized with senators and the boldness with which he spoke his mind. A new effort to convict Hoxsey of practicing without a license had come to naught when the jury could not agree upon a verdict. Nor was Hoxsey found guilty in a damage suit brought by a widower who charged that his wife's death had been due to negligent and improper treatment at the clinic. Hoxsey, moreover, won two judgments in libel suits involving Morris Fishbein. And a federal district judge refused the government an injunction to stop Hoxsey's distribution of his tonics in interstate commerce.[32]

The AMA had not forgotten Hoxsey, and in 1947 Fishbein had written an excoriating editorial in the *Journal* entitled "Hoxsey—Cancer Charlatan." To warn a wider audience, Fishbein had also co-authored an article called "Blood Money" for the Hearst chain's weekly magazine section, carried by the *San Antonio Light*. Fishbein repeated the phrase "cancer charlatan" in reference to Hoxsey and termed his father "a veterinarian and dabbler in faith cures" who had himself succumbed to cancer after claiming to have found a cure for it. Hoxsey promptly sued, asking a million dollars libel damages.[33]

He won the case, receiving, however, not a million dollars but only two, one for himself, one for his father. Elderly Judge William Atwell, who heard the case, concluded from the testi-

[31] *Ibid.*; *JAMA*, 137 (Aug. 7, 1948), 1333; Langer to Surgeon General Leonard A. Scheele, May 25, 1951, copy in FDA file, Inj. 232; Sen. Resolution 142, *Cong. Record* (82 Cong., 1 ses.), 5611.

[32] FDA file, Inj. 232; *Dallas Times Herald*, May 25, 1948; *JAMA*, 145 (Jan. 27, 1951), 252-53.

[33] *Ibid.*; Hoxsey, *You Don't Have to Die*, 223-43; *Chicago Herald-American*, Mar. 20, 1949.

mony that Fishbein, acting from "a mistaken sense of public duty" and bearing Hoxsey "no malice," had indeed been guilty of libel. Yet Hoxsey, whose methods of promotion depended in part on making the public believe that the AMA was hounding him, had suffered no serious damage from the article: hence the nominal award. Hoxsey had no license to practice medicine in Texas, and yet he had applied his yellow arsenic powder to the breast of a woman and this had resulted in her death. But, the judge ruled, Hoxsey did have the right to employ physicians, even though they were "not especially learned men," and patients had the right to go to them for treatment. "Pay your money," Judge Atwell said, "and take your choice." The judge seemed to have been much impressed by the testimony of the satisfied users whom Hoxsey had paraded to the witness stand. They said they had had cancer, and they said they had been cured. "Healing," Atwell was persuaded, had occurred, and the circumstances brought to his mind the healing of Christ.[34]

Judge Atwell was also on the bench when, in 1950, the government sought to enjoin Hoxsey from shipping his medicines for internal cancer across state lines. Not until this date had court decisions broadened the definition of labeling under the 1938 law so as to make it seem applicable to Hoxsey's methods of operation. The Food and Drug Administration first instituted a seizure action against tonics sent from Dallas to a Hoxsey practitioner in Denver, but Hoxsey let this action go by default. Now, in Judge Atwell's courtroom, he fought.[35]

Food and Drug officials had worked prodigiously to develop a persuasive case. Their goal was to demonstrate the ineffectiveness of Hoxsey's tonics in treating internal cancer and to disprove Hoxsey's oft-repeated claims that cases had been cured. Dr. David I. Macht, a distinguished specialist in pharmacological and experimental therapeutics, long a Johns Hopkins professor, was called to the stand.[36]

"Doctor," he was asked by the district attorney, "is there any recognized therapeutic use of any of these items [in the tonics],

[34] Judge Atwell's oral opinion, Hoxsey v. Fishbein.
[35] FDA file, Inj. 232; DDNJ 3288.
[36] FDA file, Inj. 232; *Transcript of Record, passim.*

including potassium iodide, or cascara sagrada, or buckthorn, and other items, any therapy for malignant cells, that you are aware of?"[37]

"Absolutely no basis for it," he replied, "and I am speaking not only as a pharmacologist, but as a member of the American College of Physicians."

Potassium iodide, indeed, another specialist testified on the basis of his own researches, "would speed up the growth of cancer." Hoxsey's tonics, still another noted cancer research scientist said, had not cured cancer in mice. In an experiment which he conducted for the Food and Drug Administration, malignant growths in mice treated with the medicine were uniformly larger at autopsy than at the beginning of the tests.[38]

In preparing for the trial, Food and Drug inspectors had tracked down the case histories of scores of Hoxsey's patients. Men, women, and children who had talked with Senator Thomas, those whose names had been used in Hoxsey's promotions, those whose cases had been submitted to the National Cancer Institute, all were investigated. Patients still living were talked with; members of the families of those who had died were interviewed. Physicians with whom Hoxsey's patients had consulted before or after going to the Dallas clinic were queried, their records checked. Hospital records, the records of pathological clinics, were studied. Hoxsey's former employees were questioned. From all this inquiry a pattern emerged. This pattern the government sought to make clear in court. Selecting 16 cases—nine of them persons whose testimony had been given in Hoxsey's pamphlet considered as labeling—the government called to the stand the patients or their survivors, diagnosticians, pathologists, surgeons, and other scientific experts. Hoxsey's claimed "cures" of internal cancer as represented by these typical cases, the government sought to show, all fell into three classes. Either the patients had never had cancer, although treated for it at the Dallas clinic. Or they had been cured of cancer by proper surgical or radiation treatment before consulting Hoxsey. Or they had had cancer and either still were so afflicted or had died.[39]

[37] *Ibid.*, 93.  [38] *Ibid.*, 101-108, 122-33.  [39] *Ibid.*, 156-544.

One of the most poignant cases presented involved a high school boy of 16 who, after a football injury, developed an extremely malignant cancer in a leg bone. When the boy's physician recommended amputation, the parents could not face this prospect and took their son instead to Hoxsey's clinic. The medical director, the father testified, had guaranteed a cure. For some four months the lad took Hoxsey's tonics. They did no good. Several months later the boy was dead. Had the amputation been performed, the physician who had first treated the boy testified, he would have had a fighting chance.[40]

Hoxsey, who did not take the stand himself, based his defense mainly on another round of testimonials. Indeed, some of his former patients who were government witnesses continued, despite the evidence, to express their loyalty to him. Twenty-two other patients took the stand for the defense to bless the Hoxsey treatment. Half of these cases had been treated for skin cancers with Hoxsey's escharotic powders and pastes. The issue of the external treatment was not on trial, but Judge Atwell let these witnesses testify anyhow. Cancer specialists did not deny Hoxsey might cure some cases of skin cancer with his tissue-eating chemicals. The method, however, was outdated and unnecessarily painful and hazardous. Modern surgical and radiation techniques could cure upwards of 95 per cent of such cases more safely and humanely.[41]

Of Hoxsey's 11 patients testifying that they had been cured of internal cancer, the only evidence that three had ever had the disease was their own affirmation. In four other cases, the government introduced rebuttal testimony to show that the patients had been cured before consulting Hoxsey. In the four remaining cases, the sole evidence that the patients had indeed had cancer was the testimony of Dr. Durkee, Hoxsey's medical director. In cross-examining Durkee, the district attorney brought out the inadequacy of his qualifications to speak with authority in this field. A 1941 graduate of a Chicago osteopathic college, Durkee had interned for less than a year at a small unaccredited osteopathic hospital in Nebraska, where he had seen only four or five cases of cancer. Then he had practiced for several years in a Texas village, encountering perhaps

[40] *Ibid.*, 429-46.    [41] *Ibid.*, 544-1065.

10 to 15 cancer patients. In 1946 he had joined Hoxsey's staff. There he had seen some 35 to 50 patients a day, examining each one for an average of five to ten minutes. He did not "need a biopsy to make a diagnosis of cancer," he testified, and rarely used the technique. Biopsies that Durkee had submitted to pathological laboratories, other evidence showed, were so poorly prepared as to be useless. His knowledge of the pharmacological action of the drugs in the Hoxsey tonics was vague, his explanation of the Hoxsey theory of cancer and its cure as fuzzy from the witness stand as in his public address reproduced in the labeling pamphlet.[42]

Despite Durkee's confusion, despite the government's carefully presented case, Harry Hoxsey won the contest. Judge Atwell would not grant the injunction. He could not agree that Hoxsey's treatment was either injurious or futile. "Some it cures," he ruled, "and some it does not cure, and some it relieves somewhat." Its "percentage of efficient and beneficial treatments," the judge decided, was "reasonably comparable to the efficiency and success of surgery and radium."[43]

Atwell's decision did not surprise FDA officials. His admission into the record of the self-diagnosis of cancer by Hoxsey's lay witnesses, his willingness to hear testimony about external cancer, had been straws in the wind. In any case, the Food and Drug men suspected that Atwell himself had once been a Hoxsey patient.[44]

The government appealed. Persuaded that Atwell had been swayed by incompetent testimony, that he had misapprehended the impact of evidence presented by medical experts, the government asked the circuit court to grant the injunction which Atwell had refused. After a careful scrutiny of the two large volumes of testimony, the three-judge court unanimously acceded to this request. A layman's opinion as to whether he had had cancer and been cured, the judges said, was "entitled to little, if any, weight." Only a biopsy could permit accurate

[42] Ibid., 544-1065; U.S. v. Hoxsey Cancer Clinic, a Partnership, and Harry M. Hoxsey, an Individual, 198 Fed. (2d) 273 (1952).

[43] U.S. v. Hoxsey Cancer Clinic, a Partnership, and Harry M. Hoxsey, an Individual, 94 Fed. Supp. 464 (1950).

[44] Goldhammer interview, Nov. 17, 1960; Washington Report on the Medical Sciences, May 28, 1951.

diagnosis. Only surgery, x-ray, and other radioactive substances could cure: such was the judgment of the "overwhelming weight of disinterested testimony." A judge "should not be so blind and deaf as to fail to see, hear and understand the import and effect of such matters of general public knowledge and acceptance." Hoxsey's entire promotional campaign sought to persuade the cancer sufferer that "he had an excellent chance to be one of those cases in which the medicine would be successful." Yet with respect to Hoxsey's own testifiers in his labeling, the government had demonstrated that the brown-ish-black and pink tonics had not proved efficacious. Atwell had erred, therefore, abusing his discretion. He must grant the injunction which the government had sought.[45]

Before Atwell could ponder this directive, Hoxsey asked the Supreme Court to reverse the circuit court's decision. But the highest tribunal would not grant certiorari. So Atwell yielded to the circuit court's demands. The injunction he is-sued, however, followed a form suggested to him by Hoxsey's attorneys rather than the form presented by the government. The decree did not flatly bar Hoxsey's internal medicines from interstate commerce. It forbade their interstate shipment *un-less*—and here was an effort to appeal to the McAnnulty deci-sion of half a century before—*unless* they were labeled to show that there existed a conflict of medical opinion concerning their curative claims. Such a ruling, Food and Drug officials knew, would shut no doors at all.[46]

Since the circuit court had found as fact that Hoxsey's in-ternal remedies could not cure cancer, no legal room existed for the assertion of differences of medical opinion. So the gov-ernment sought from the circuit court a writ of mandamus that would require Atwell to issue the injunction in the proper form. In the legal maneuvering over the writ, Hoxsey again appealed to the Supreme Court and was denied. The circuit court, using a less rigorous remedy than a writ of mandamus, nonetheless made it clear to Atwell that the disputed clause in his injunction was in "direct conflict" with the court's earlier

[45] Circuit court decision, 198 Fed. (2d) 273.
[46] 346 U.S. 897; In Re: United States of America, Praying for a Writ of Mandamus, 207 Fed. (2d) 567 (1953).

ruling—McAnnulty did not apply—and must be excised. In October 1953, nearly three years after the case had gone to trial, Judge Atwell issued the injunction without the "conflict of medical opinion" clause. But the issue was still not finally settled. Hoxsey went to court once more, appealing for a stay of execution of the injunction on the grounds that his constitutional rights had been violated, an appeal the government termed "frivolous." Another year went by before the Supreme Court, refusing to hear the circuit court's denial of Hoxsey's plea, put an end to the extended litigation. In October 1954 the injunction at long last went into effect.[47]

The government's injunction, won at great cost, did not stop Hoxsey's Dallas operation. Two years later, indeed, one estimate put his annual gross at $1.5 million extracted from some 8,000 patients. Curtailing his interstate shipments and exchanging his labeling for a "prescription" approach, Hoxsey continued to manage his clinic, staffed by osteopaths who dispensed the tonics to cancer sufferers much as before. "There's only one way they'll ever close that Hoxsey Clinic," he told one audience, "and that's to put a militia around it." To attract patients to Dallas, Hoxsey set out on a massive drumbeating campaign. He used favorable passages from the trial testimony as "advertising," planting such extracts and laudatory comments in mass-appeal magazines, sometimes in exchange for a fee. He brought to Dallas a group of doctors from around the country—many of whom the AMA considered less than fully reputable—and published their favorable reactions. He went on extensive lecture tours, speaking to fringe groups who shared his antagonism toward organized medicine. He paid a writer to ghostwrite his autobiography and sent a copy to every Senator and Representative. He made motions as if to run for the governorship of Texas. He leagued together with other foes of the FDA and the AMA in accusing these organizations of conspiring to stifle medical freedom.[48]

[47] *Ibid.*; 212 Fed. (2d) 439; 348 U.S. 835; FDA file, Inj. 232; DDNJ 4654.
[48] *Life*, 40 (Apr. 16, 1956), 125; FDA file, Inj. 232; *Findings of the Doctors Who Investigated the Facilities, Procedure and Treatment at The Hoxsey Cancer Clinic April 10th and 11th, 1954; JAMA*, 155 (June 12, 1954), 667-68; FDA file, Interstate Seizure No. 4-052M; *Dallas News*, Apr. 10, 1956.

One of Hoxsey's new allies in his expanded fight was Gerald B. Winrod, the Kansas evangelist. A militant fundamentalist, Winrod had fought modernism in religion during the 1920's. Later he turned his attention to right-wing politics, providing the inspiration for Sinclair Lewis' portrait of "Buzz" Windrip in *It Can't Happen Here*. A visit to Germany in 1934 confirmed Winrod's pro-Nazi inclinations, although he played this down while nearly winning the Republican Senatorial nomination from Kansas in 1938. During the war he was indicted for sedition for expressing views calculated to injure morale in the armed forces, but the death of the judge halted the trial. After the war, Winrod's personal organ, the *Defender*, brought to a hundred thousand subscribers a mixture of fervent fundamentalism in religion and morals, right-wing political extremism, violent antagonism toward Jews and Negroes, hostility to fluoridation and mental health programs. The *Defender* also accepted flying saucers and championed unorthodox healers.[49]

Winrod helped publicize Glyoxylide, the specious cancer remedy devised by a Detroit physician, William Frederick Koch. A group of ministers in Winrod's circle even set up a religious front, the Christian Medical Research League, to market this purported cure. And Winrod also joined hands with Hoxsey. Over many months the Wichita evangelist praised the Dallas clinic in the pages of the *Defender*, in pamphlets, in a book, in radio speeches. Winrod's motives were not unmixed. Although he asserted that he himself, when young, had been cured by the Hoxsey treatment—a tribute which Senator Langer inserted in the *Congressional Record*—Winrod's publicity, whatever his gratitude, was not freely given. According to evidence later introduced in court, Hoxsey paid Winrod over $80,000. This fact was not apparent to *Defender* readers who learned of Hoxsey's marvelous "cures" along with their fundamentalist Sunday School lessons. After a Hoxsey defeat in court, Winrod wrote a letter to his constituency asking them to offer "daily, persistent, argumentive prayer" for Hoxsey, according to Luke 18:1-7. Winrod asked

[49] "Keep Them Out! The Reverend Gerald B. Winrod," *Nation*, 155 (July 4, 1942), 7-9; Roy Tozier, "Mr. Dies Kills an Investigation," *New Republic*, 102 (Apr. 22, 1940), 532; *N.Y. Times*, Nov. 13, 1957; the *Defender, passim*.

more: funds to carry forward Hoxsey's "anti-cancer crusade" and the names and addresses of at least five cancer victims to whom Hoxsey literature might be sent. Winrod signed this appeal "Yours in Christ's Service."[50]

Hoxsey had other similar allies. The American Rally was an isolationist organization, established in 1952 "For Peace, Abundance and the Constitution." Like Winrod's journal, it opposed fluoridation and polio vaccine and believed in flying saucers. In 1955 the Rally's magazine came out for Senator Langer for president in the 1956 election, lauding him as the "Abraham Lincoln of the 20th Century." Shortly the Rally discovered a vice-presidential candidate fit to run with Langer, Harry Hoxsey. Introducing Hoxsey to a Rally convention in Chicago, its executive head said, "The spirit of Lincoln is here tonight." Hoxsey responded with such Lincolnian phrases as: "The AMA killed my daddy . . . the same bunch of rats I've been kicking ever since."[51]

The American Rally shared with other dissident groups belief in "medical freedom," defined as the right of every individual to seek treatment from Hoxsey's clinic and other clinics and practitioners frowned on by the orthodox medical profession. Two such groups were the American Association for Medico-Physical Research and the American Naturopathic Association. Hoxsey and his associates spoke before their meetings. At a naturopathic convention in Chicago, Hoxsey addressed himself to the theme, "Who Are the Real Cancer Quacks and May God Have Mercy on Their Souls." From the same rostrum during this meeting, an address was also given by Fred J. Hart.[52]

[50] *JAMA*, 140 (Aug. 27, 1949), 1352-53; *F&D Rev.*, 45 (Feb. 1961), 27; *Defender*, 1954-1957, *passim*, May 1956, p. 5, on Winrod's boyhood "cure"; *Cong. Record* (84 Cong., 2 ses.), 6296; "Truth Loses at Pittsburgh," a Nov. 28, 1956, Winrod letter to *Defender* readers, in FDA file, Interstate Seizure No. 4-052M; W. F. Janssen, "Quackery and the News," *Public Health Reports*, 74 (July 1959), 637.

[51] American Rally membership card; printed flyer announcing 1955 convention; *American Rally*, Feb.-Mar. and Oct. 1955; announcement of Apr. 1955 Chicago meeting; memorandum on Hoxsey address at Chicago meeting, Apr. 30, 1955. These documents are in FDA file, Interstate Seizure No. 4-052M.

[52] Program for Aug. 1959 convention in Chicago of the American

Hart was one of Albert Abrams' many heirs. Listing his fields of endeavor as "Agriculture and Research," Hart had been associated with the College of Electronic Medicine, which sought to keep Abrams' doctrines flourishing, as early as 1935 and had become president by 1946 when the name was changed to the Electronic Medical Foundation. In 1954 the government had secured an injunction banning shipment in interstate commerce of numerous therapeutic machines fabricated by the Foundation. Hart was the moving spirit, the next year, in creating a new group to fight for "medical freedom," the National Health Federation. Hart became president, one of Hoxsey's lawyers served as legal representative in Washington, and several of the FDA's most stubborn antagonists sat on the Federation's board. At membership rallies in California, Hart pleaded for funds to help Hoxsey carry on his fight, and Hoxsey asserted that he was giving the royalties from his autobiography to help finance the Federation.[53]

The Food and Drug Administration was not an independent agent, spokesmen for the Federation charged. As Hart once put it, Commissioner "Larrick has to do what the medical trust tells him or he'd lose his job and he wouldn't like to wash dishes for a living." The medical profession, the drug industry, the food manufacturers (who added "poisons" to their cans), according to the Federation's journal, were all allied against the people. "The House of Rockefeller" owned "the drug, food, milk, serum, news and money trusts" and it owned the Eisenhower administration too. As a result, the FDA's administrative actions were marked by "viciousness," and the agency allowed its employees "to blackmail and slander firms and individuals without restraint." The Federation aimed at making the FDA "a servant of the people; rather than leaving it as it now is—a ruthless enemy, as tiranical [*sic*] in its actions as any

---

Association for Medico-Physical Research, in FDA Decimal file 045.A; *Naturopath*, 60 (Oct. 1955), 338-43.

[53] AMA folder on Abrams, Albert (College of Electronic Medicine); DDNJ 4667; FDA file, National Health Federation; FDA file, Inj. 232; Ralph Lee Smith, "Amazing Facts about a 'Crusade' That Can Hurt Your Health," *Today's Health*, 44 (Oct. 1966), 30-35, 76.

Russian bureaucrat." The cover of the Federation's magazine in which this statement appeared again appealed to Lincoln, carrying his picture—and Washington's too—and the caption, "They Too Fought for Liberty Against Great Odds."[54]

Federation representatives lobbied on the federal and state levels, seeking an investigation of FDA policies and procedures, striving for the right of other practitioners besides M.D.'s to have access to federal research funds, seeking to limit fluoridation and cancer quackery control measures, trying to secure a ban on publicity by regulatory agencies about court cases until the final judgment was rendered, and much else. The Federation's literature flowed forth in quantity, seeking to win support from such groups as the Gold Star Mothers and the D.A.R. Petitions to Congress were sponsored, many in behalf of Hoxsey, asking an investigation of the FDA. Nearly 200,000 petitions had already reached the Capitol, Hoxsey told a Federation meeting in California in 1957, and this was "driving" the FDA "nuts." Letter-writing campaigns were also stimulated among the faithful. "Using specialists in mass psychology," Commissioner Larrick stated, "the promoters held numerous meetings under the guise of 'scientific lectures' to organize a protest movement among those prejudiced against recognized medical treatment. They used radio, television, circulars, 'religious' publications and even huge barnside signs, to encourage the public to write to Congressmen and the President, demanding investigations of FDA 'persecution' of their leaders." The faithful disciples of Hoxsey and his allies responded eagerly. "We have had," said Larrick, "a torrent of belligerent letters to answer." One result of this deliberate effort to arouse the hostility of common citizens is revealed in a sentence from one woman's letter: "I do not trust the government anymore."[55]

Hoxsey's cancer treatment metastasized from Texas into other states, particularly Pennsylvania. There its chief cham-

[54] *Ibid.*; *NHF Bulletin*, Nov. 1956, Feb. and July-Aug. 1957.

[55] FDA file, National Health Federation, especially NHF Progress Report on work accomplished during 1958 session of Congress; FDA file, Inj. 232; Larrick, "Report from the Food and Drug Administration," *FDC Law Jnl.*, 13 (Mar. 1958), 153. The protest letter is in FDA file, Interstate Seizure No. 4-052M.

pion and promoter was state senator John Haluska. Having lost his mother and a young son from cancer, Haluska gave Hoxsey credit for saving his sister's life after regular doctors had given her up. (Her physicians later testified she had been cured by x-ray before going to Dallas.) Administrator of a hospital in Spangler, Haluska had been ousted for trying to convert the nurses home into a cancer clinic according to the Hoxsey pattern. Then Haluska remodeled an appliance store and garage in Portage, a coal-mining town in the mountains of western Pennsylvania, employed one of Hoxsey's former medical directors, and offered to treat cancer sufferers. The medication was slightly different, not tonics but pills—first red and black pills, then red, green, and yellow pills, the size of small lima beans. The pills contained, however, most of the ingredients in Hoxsey's tonics. When Hoxsey visited Portage, he was welcomed with a motorcade and a banquet at which Haluska apotheosized him as "the greatest man in the country today—greater than President Roosevelt was, and greater than President Truman and President Eisenhower." Similar praise resounded through the chamber of the Pennsylvania senate, with Hoxsey taking a bow from the balcony, as Haluska in a long oration announced the opening of the Portage clinic and lauded the Hoxsey methods. To his fellow senators, Haluska also introduced Kathy Allison, a young girl from Indiana. "Here, Mr. President," he said, taking Kathy into his arms, "is that little angel who, according to medical science, had to meet the angels soon. Today, she is going to school; was X-rayed last week and found to be cancer-free and is playing like any other normal child." Hoxsey had treated her; God had spared her. "Senator Haluska's Great Speech" was published in Winrod's *Defender*, and thousands of reprints spread across the country.[56]

The Portage clinic opened in 1955 to brisk business. One early customer, a perfectly healthy FDA inspector, received an examination lasting a minute or two and was told he had cancer of the prostate. Quickly Food and Drug officials and a federal marshal visited the clinic and, amid a hostile throng

[56] *Ibid.*; *Pittsburgh Press*, Oct. 31, 1958; "Senator Haluska's Great Speech," reprint from the *Defender*, Mar. 1955.

of townspeople, seized half a million pills. After long delay, the seizure action came to trial. Hoxsey, testifying that he was not financially interested in the Portage venture, although serving as adviser, sat out the six-week jury trial at the defense table. Again, as at Dallas, satisfied users praised the Hoxsey methods. Again the government presented medical experts who condemned the Hoxsey medications as useless in cancer and refuted Hoxsey's alleged cures. Even little Kathy Allison, eight months after her touching appearance in the Pennsylvania Senate, had died of cancer of the chest. The jury condemned the Portage pills and ordered them destroyed.[57]

While waiting out the law's delays, the Food and Drug Administration took an unprecedented step. The 1938 law authorized the dissemination of information regarding drugs in situations involving imminent danger to health or gross deception of the consumer. This provision had not hitherto been used. As the Pennsylvania seizure trial kept being postponed, and as cancer victims continued visiting Dallas and Portage, the FDA weighed the value of a major public warning. Might not such an outburst of publicity for Hoxsey, even though critical, do more harm than good, giving a clue to the desperate, who might sense Hoxsey's promises and disregard FDA's explanation of the dangers? On the other hand, a flood of letters was reaching FDA from cancer victims or their families, frightened people who had been advised to consult Hoxsey and were inquiring for the facts. One such letter came from a college girl in California who, while studying a semester in the nation's capital, had heard a speech on quackery by a man from the FDA. Now her father had cancer and was planning to go to Dallas. She wanted "to discover the truth as far as it is known." The official who had made the speech telegraphed her that Hoxsey's treatment was "totally ineffective," sent fuller information by airmail, and wrote that he had talked about her father's case with the director of the National Cancer Institute, to whom her father's physician should immediately phone. Might there not be many such citi-

[57] FDA file, Interstate Seizure No. 4-052M; DDNJ 5212; *Johnstown Tribune-Democrat*, Apr. 5, 1956; *F&D Rev.*, 40 (Dec. 1956), 205, 223.

zens who could be prevented by a public warning from wasting their money and risking their lives? FDA officials decided to act.[58]

In April 1956 the FDA issued its warning, terming Hoxsey's methods "worthless," and "imminently dangerous to rely on . . . in neglect of competent and rational treatment." The basic facts of the Texas injunction trial were tersely given. Besides relying on the daily press, FDA officials made a special effort to circulate the warning notice among farm, lodge, and church periodicals, asking those tempted to try Hoxsey's treatment to write to the FDA first for fuller facts. For months pathetic inquiring letters reached Washington at the rate of 50 to 100 a day. To spread the warning even further, the FDA prepared a "Public Beware!" poster, printed in red and black, which was displayed in the 46,000 post offices and postal substations throughout the land. These warnings, FDA officials concluded, did much good. While they triggered a new barrage of angry letters from Hoxsey's admirers, mailed to Congress, to the FDA and to the press, they cut down on customers in Dallas and Portage. A conservative FDA estimate held that, in the 30 weeks after the first warning, at least 3,000 people had been dissuaded from trying Hoxsey's futile treatment.[59]

Hoxsey sought to enjoin the government from issuing its warnings. But Hoxsey lost his case, just as his Pennsylvania collaborators had lost their seizure action. While the seizure action was still on appeal, the government sought an injunction to stop the Portage clinic from operating in interstate commerce. After the government had presented its case in court, the Portage opposition collapsed. Haluska and his aides agreed to the injunction, promised to drop their appeal in the seizure case, and offered to withdraw a suit they had launched to stop further FDA investigations of their clinic. In October 1957 the FDA could issue a new release stating that the government had "now been successful in all pending Fed-

[58] Janssen, "Quackery and the News"; FDA file, Inj. 232; FDA release, "Public Warning against Hoxsey Cancer Treatment," Apr. 4, 1956.
[59] Ibid.; Janssen, "Quackery and the News"; FDA release, Jan. 28, 1957; Janssen interview, July 25, 1956; *Drug Trade News*, 32 (May 6, 1957), 26.

[ 387 ]

eral court actions involving the 'cancer remedies' known as the Hoxsey treatment."[60]

The release, despite its announcement of victories, contained a somber note. "The public should know . . .," the text read, "that such actions will not end the menace of this treatment since the Federal Government does not have the power to stop a clinic in any State from treating cancer patients within that State with the nostrums which comprise the Hoxsey treatment. Millions of copies of false promotional literature are still in circulation; much of it reporting cures of persons who are now dead."[61]

But Hoxsey's tide had turned. The Portage clinic closed shortly thereafter. At his home base the pressures mounted inexorably. Texas court actions revoked the licenses of Hoxsey's doctors and granted a permanent injunction to prevent his practicing medicine in Texas. Hoxsey then leased his clinic to another operator. Again the FDA moved in. The agency secured a supplemental consent decree of permanent injunction by which this operator promised to write all persons who had employed the Hoxsey treatment since 1957 that it could no longer be obtained. Since late 1960, therefore, except for a sporadic instance here and there about the country, the Hoxsey method of treating cancer at clinics has disappeared. Testimonials from patients claiming "cures" by the method, however, have continued to appear in the pages of health magazines, along with formulas for the Hoxsey medications and the addresses of herbalists who will supply the raw ingredients from which the medications may be made.[62]

The decade of litigation against Hoxsey had cost the federal government perhaps a quarter of a million dollars.[63] This

[60] Harry M. Hoxsey v. Marion B. Folsom . . . and George P. Larrick, 155 Fed. Supp. 376 (1957); U.S. v. Hoxsey Cancer Clinic, John J. Haluska, et al., Civil Action No. 15807, Western Dist., Pa., Oct. 2, 1957; DDNJ 5202; FDA release, "Report on Legal Actions against the Hoxsey Cancer Treatment," Oct. 24, 1957.

[61] *Ibid.*

[62] FDA file, Inj. 232; FDA release, Sep. 21, 1960; DDNJ 6316 and 6317. In 1962 Utah enjoined a clinic of which a former Hoxsey nurse was a proprietor for using the Hoxsey method. *F&D Rev.*, 47 (Jan. 1963), 6; American Cancer Society, *Unproven Methods of Cancer Treatment* (N.Y., 1966), 53.

[63] Goldhammer interview, Nov. 17, 1960.

expensive victory did not provide a shield against any other wares than the clinic-prescribed brownish-black and pink tonics and the variously colored pills. While Hoxsey had been the largest unorthodox cancer promoter of the 1950's, he had had competitors. During the efforts to close the Portage clinic, a world-noted cancer authority, Dr. David A. Karnofsky, had addressed the American Cancer Society's Pennsylvania division.[64] Besides Hoxsey's treatment, he said, 13 other major promotions were available to Americans who feared they had cancer. In 1966 the American Cancer Society, issuing a catalogue of *Unproven Methods of Cancer Treatment,* came up with a list twice as long as Dr. Karnofsky's.

While the scientific search went on, in public and private laboratories, for chemicals that might better aid in controlling cancer, the unscrupulous and misguided continued to tell Americans that the miraculous discovery had already occurred. Among the fearful and the desperate, these false prophets continued to find victims for their worthless wares.

[64] *Pittsburgh Press,* Nov. 11, 1955.

# 18

# ANTI-QUACKERY, INCORPORATED

*"We hope . . . [this meeting] will be the beginning of a hard-hitting and revitalized crusade by private and governmental agencies against the hucksters of pseudomedicine."*

—C. JOSEPH STETLER, AMERICAN MEDICAL ASSOCIATION, 1961[1]

JUST as, a little later, it was with a sense of shock that an affluent America rediscovered poverty, so was it with shock that, in the mid-1950's, a scientific America rediscovered quackery. Not that either poverty or quackery had been gone or really forgotten. Major emphases, main preoccupations, had just lain in other directions. For both physician and layman, from the late 1930's on, the engrossing theme had been *real* cures through the miracle of chemotherapy. Was it not a fair assumption that, as the sulfas, penicillin, and other potent new drugs expanded their zone of lifesaving power, the territory should shrink in which quacks could profitably operate? Was it not to be anticipated that earnest enforcement of the new laws which Congress had given to the Food and Drug Administration and the Federal Trade Commission in 1938 would reduce the amount of quackery, perhaps virtually eliminate it altogether?

This did not happen. Widely advertised proprietaries sold to the layman for self-dosage did improve, both in therapeutic quality and in the restraint—if not always in the taste—of advertising claims. Many dangerous deceptions and valueless products were banished from the market. But unscrupulous promoters of pseudo-medical wares had always been agile, and once again, as so often in the past, they adjusted to new

[1] *Proceedings, National Congress on Medical Quackery*, Oct. 6-7, 1961 (Chicago, 1962), 1.

demands. Preceding chapters offer ample testimony to their resourcefulness. They enhanced the subtlety of their appeals. They entered grey therapeutic zones where medical knowledge was still ambiguous, regulatory authority still untested. They even profited from the widespread public eagerness to embrace the chemotherapeutic revolution, realizing that John Doe did not possess the judgment to differentiate between a true miracle drug and a false article offered with miraculous claims. Thus pseudo-medicine continued to prosper.

The professional foes of quackery had never been beguiled into thinking quackery dead or even moribund. They met too many cases in their day-by-day routine. Regulators at the FDA, the FTC, the Post Office Department, officials at the AMA, the American Cancer Society, the Arthritis and Rheumatism Foundation, the National Better Business Bureau, all recognized that quackery was very much alive. But even they, in the mid-1950's, began to exhibit some surprise at quackery's immensity and truculence. That the "good old days" of quackery were still, "to a very great extent," extant in 1955 impressed the Food and Drug Commissioner as an "amazing fact." That medical mail frauds had never before been so great in compass struck the Postmaster General in 1957 as a matter of awesome import. That so many arthritics were being deceived by quackery to such a great degree in 1959 seemed to an Arthritis and Rheumatism Foundation researcher "astonishing." When the separate pieces of pseudo-medical deception were put together by one of the first of a new wave of nostrum muckraking journalists, the total cost to the American public came to a billion dollars a year.[2]

It was not size alone that shocked quackery's most knowledgeable enemies into reassessing its significance. The belligerence with which major promoters fought back against regulatory attack was likewise astounding. Nor were these engagements separate and isolated battles. The foe seemed intent on leaguing together. Harry Hoxsey's conduct was the major

[2] George Larrick, "Our Unfinished Business," *FDC Law Jnl.*, 10 (Mar. 1955), 168; Arthur Summerfield, cited in Post Office Dept. release, May 12, 1957; Ruth Walrad, *The Misrepresentation of Arthritis Drugs and Devices in the United States* (N.Y., 1960), 98; *N.Y. Post*, May 20, 1957.

case in point. He persuaded and bought allies where he could, from the naturopaths and chiropractors, from the device promoters and the nutritional proprietors, from the radical fringe of religion and politics, from the Senate of the United States. Hoxsey worked hand in glove with the National Health Federation, formed by leading gadget and food fad promoters also under pressure from regulatory agencies. Waving the banner of "medical freedom," these groups spent thousands for propaganda in an appeal to millions of Americans who were in some way disenchanted with life—the sick, the unhappy, the ignorant, the illogical, the fearful, the bored, the lonely. As the hundreds of angry letters and petitions deluging Washington gave proof, such propaganda found ready converts, men and women willing to believe that the evil conspiracy with respect to American health lay not among the medical irregulars, but among bureaucrats, doctors, and makers of drugs. That such a significant segment of the public could be brought to believe such a colossal reversal of the true facts deeply disturbed all those whose task it was to combat quackery. Somehow, despite their successes, they had failed.[3]

What those closest to quackery came to realize about its tenacity, magnitude, and arrogance, the broader public eventually came to know. The hazards of pseudo-medicine became a theme widely treated in printed and broadcast journalism. This came in part from deliberate efforts by government, medical, and business groups, themselves newly aware of the threat, to sound a broader alarm. The revived anti-quackery crusade was also furthered by journalists who recognized an important and newsworthy theme, some of whom criticized federal agencies for falling short in their efforts to subdue the charlatans.

With respect to the Food and Drug Administration, it was not journalists only who raised the point as to whether the agency's educational efforts against quackery had been sufficient. A Citizens Advisory Committee, appointed by the first Secretary of Health, Education, and Welfare, Oveta Culp Hobby, concluded in 1955 that the FDA had fallen short of its goal. Most Americans, the committee believed, were "very

[3] See ch. 17.

poorly informed" both about hazards in the food and drug
field and about the FDA's protective role. Americans, indeed,
were probably less aware of such crucial matters in 1955 than
they had been in 1906 when the first national law was passed.
The educational campaign should be markedly increased, the
committee counseled. Action must be taken to "inform the
public in specific terms against quackery, especially where
real hazard to health is involved."[4]

To be sure, the FDA's resources for this and all its tasks
were "woefully inadequate." Fewer enforcement personnel
manned the agency in 1955, the committee pointed out, than
in 1941. As the agency's job had grown, its funds had fallen.
Ironically, a major reason for this state of affairs had been the
FDA's enforcement vigor. Although the Citizens Advisory
Committee did not say so, the trade press speculated that, as
had happened before, members of Congress had taken offense
at some of the actions brought by the FDA and had retaliated
by cutting appropriations. Recent low budgets, drug reporters
surmised, were largely the result of displeasure on the part of
key members of the House Appropriations Committee at the
FDA's seizure of some Mountain Valley Mineral Water. The
beverage was widely used by Congressmen, and, as President
Eisenhower told a press conference, he drank it himself. The
FDA had charged that pamphlets promoting the water bore
false therapeutic claims and that the labels did not conform
to regulations governing special dietary uses.[5]

The FDA eventually won the mineral water case, and the
Citizens Advisory Committee report persuaded most members
of Congress that starving the FDA posed grave threats to the
national health. Appropriations started upward, and the FDA
reinvigorated both its educational and its regulatory campaigns against medical quackery. Public awareness of the

[4] *Citizens Advisory Committee . . . Report,* House Document 227 (84
Cong., 1 ses., 1955).

[5] *Ibid.; FDC Reports,* Jan. 23, 1954, white 13; Nov. 6, 1954, pink 3;
June 11, 1956, 9; *Drug Trade News,* 17 (Aug. 26, 1957), 12. During
1954, Congress, in passing a bill to re-codify food and drug law, had
modified the language so as to eliminate FDA's authority to employ its
multiple seizure weapon. At FDA's request, Eisenhower vetoed the
bill. *FDC Reports,* Sep. 4, 1954, white 12; Sep. 11, 1954, white 9.

agency's mission gained, during 1956, from the commemoration of the golden anniversary of the first Pure Food and Drugs Act. A portrait of Harvey Washington Wiley, the redoubtable old warrior who had fathered the law, even appeared on a postage stamp. By mid-1957, the agency could report "more defendants . . . serving jail sentences for false curative claims than at any time in FDA history." A Division of Public Information, organized the next year, increased the outflow of press releases. A new Secretary of Health, Education, and Welfare, Arthur Flemming, made headlines by holding press conferences pointing out the dangers of quackery in the nutrition and weight-reducing fields.[6]

Obesity deception concerned the Blatnik subcommittee also, at its hearings in 1957, and this stimulated more publicity. The hearings provided choice quotations and vivid facts for journalists, who in any case had already been alerted to the quackery theme by such official expressions as the Postmaster General's pronouncement on its magnitude. Exposure of nostrum frauds had not ceased completely during the years that quackery had been "forgotten." Reporters in various cities— Chicago, Cleveland, San Francisco, Memphis, for example— had occasionally called attention to some particularly egregious evil. Radio programs had now and then warned of charlatanism. *Consumer Reports* and *Consumers' Research Bulletin*, organs of the successors of the guinea pig muckrakers, had cautioned readers against continuing hazards associated with self-dosage products. In the mid-1950's, as officialdom expressed ever graver concern that the "good old days" had by no means been banished, so too did journalism.[7]

[6] Food NJ 26597; DDNJ 6023; Larrick, "Report from the Food and Drug Administration," *FDC Law Jnl.*, 13 (Mar. 1958), 151-52; Wallace F. Janssen, "Public Information under the Federal Food, Drug, and Cosmetic Act," *ibid.*, 12 (Jan. 1957), 57-61; (Feb. 1957), 93-98; (Apr. 1957), 229-35; (Sep. 1957), 566-76; Cincinnati District annual report, 1957, FDA Decimal file .053, FDA; *1957 Report of the Food and Drug Administration*, 193, 194; *1958 Report*, 196; HEW press releases, Nov. 18, 1958, Jan. 13 and Sep. 2, 1959.
[7] See ch. 14. *JAMA*, 144 (Oct. 28, 1950), 764, summarizes several recent newspaper attacks on quackery. *F&D Rev.*, 35 (Nov. 1951), 248, and 37 (Sep. 1953), 176, tells of anti-quackery radio programs. *Consumer Reports*: "The Antihistamines," 15 (Jan. 1950), 710; "Chloro-

Typical of the rising tide of nostrum muckraking was a 1957 *New York Post* series, whose chief author was James Cook. It was he who totted up the staggering monetary total of the nation's nostrum bill: "You spent," the first article began, "a billion dollars for 'patent medicines' in the last year." Cook's ire was not aimed solely at the most extreme examples, like Hoxsey and his "witch-doctor brew." Cook raised grave doubts about self-medication drugs much more respectable: "cold 'remedies' which do not cure colds," "old-fashioned bromides and anti-histaminics" masquerading as "the new 'tranquilizer' drugs," vitamin and mineral mixtures peddled with false nutritional claims. "Many laxative manufacturers," Cook asserted, "are blasting the nation's insides with questionable products while blasting the nation's ears with questionable data on the digestive tract." He named names—Citroid, Sleepeze, Sominex, Geritol—in his critique, and wondered if regulatory laws were strong enough, regulatory officials bold enough, to combat the "quackery, hijinks, and razzle-dazzle" that played consumers for suckers.[8]

In *Remedies and Rackets, The Truth about Patent Medicines Today,* Cook revamped and amplified the *Post* series into a hard-hitting book. Bolstered by data from the Blatnik hearings and from the increasing flood of articles written by fellow journalists, he told the nation what he had earlier reported to New Yorkers. By now, Cook said, America contained "170,000,000 Guinea Pigs," and, although regulatory agencies provided some protection, "in the patent medicine jungle" it was "every man for himself." Consumers, he argued, should insist on stronger laws and better enforcement of existing laws, through bigger appropriations to the agencies and "more skill and energy" from the regulators. But basically the health-pursuing public needed to rely on their own protective efforts. They should learn where they could find out the truth about self-

---

phyll: Latest Drug Fad" (Oct. 1950), 458-59; "An FTC Failure" and "An FTC Success," 16 (June 1951), 268-77; "Another Obesity 'Cure,'" 17 (July 1952), 347-48; "Coughs and Cough Remedies," 19 (Jan. 1954), 336-40. *Consumers' Research Bulletin*: comments in "The Consumers' Observation Post," 27 (Apr. 1951), 4; (Sep. 1951), 3; 29 (Apr. 1952), 29; 35 (Feb. 1955), 3.

[8] *N.Y. Post*, May 20–June 2, 1957, *passim*.

medication wares and then apply that knowledge in their own buying. Above all, skepticism and caution were required.[9]

In the reviving anti-quackery crusade, others besides governmental officials and muckraking journalists shared. The National Better Business Bureau, while not displaying the suspicion of virtually all self-medication wares which some critics manifested, took note of the "frightening increase in the number and flamboyancy of fraudulent or misleading advertisements for over-the-counter drug products." Reflecting both the state of the market and the level of public concern, complaints to the Bureau reached an all-time high. In 1958 the NBBB reported five times as many inquiries about drug and cosmetic advertising as three years earlier. "Lamentably," their bulletin stated, complaints were ten times as great. Maye Russ, the dedicated and competent director of the Bureau's food and drug division, set up in 1956, proved a star witness at the Blatnik hearings. Miss Russ saw to the issuance of an increasing stream of bulletins to the Bureau's clientele, reporting on a wide spectrum of health deceptions—obesity drugs and devices, cold remedies, "royal jelly" rejuvenators, bust developers, a book of advice to arthritics, a polio preventive scheme.[10]

Besides urging advertising media to bar disreputable health advertising, the National Better Business Bureau sought to persuade newspapers, magazines, radio, and television to raise standards so that promotion of legitimate drug products might become less offensive. In this campaign, the NBBB received both prodding and backing from the AMA. Some changes occurred in media advertising codes as a result. But the basic problems of excessive implied claims and of questionable taste in such proprietary advertising continued.[11]

[9] James Cook, *Remedies and Rackets* (N.Y., 1958), especially 219-37. Along with the extensive newspaper and magazine exposure, another key book appeared: Ralph Lee Smith, *The Health Hucksters* (N.Y., 1960).

[10] NBBB release, "False Advertising of Over-the-Counter Drugs," Oct. 27, 1958; *False and Misleading Advertising (Weight-Reducing Preparations): Hearings before a Subcommittee of the Committee on Government Operations, House of Representatives* (85 Cong., 1 ses., 1957), 27-53; NBBB *Service Bulletin*, Nos. 1478, 1541, 1550, 1551, 1566, 1573, 1589, 1593, 1613, 1614, 1626, 1630, 1662 (1954-1959).

[11] See ch. 14. Advertising Advisory Committee to the Secretary of

The American Medical Association also took note of and responded to the burgeoning quackery of the mid-1950's. Oliver Field, one of Dr. Cramp's successors at the helm of the Department of Investigation, found, as he opened his mail, cancer, nutritional, and device quackery to be the major areas of pseudo-medicine about which his correspondents were inquiring. A lawyer and former Food and Drug inspector, Field markedly increased the pace of his peregrinations around the country, speaking in his genial way to hundreds of lay and medical audiences, showing them examples of quackdom's most ludicrous but dangerous inventions. The AMA assembled exhibits designed to warn the public about "Mechanical Quackery," to reveal how charlatans went about "Fooling the Fat," to expose the tricks of "Modern Medical Pitchmen." These exhibits were shipped to meetings and conventions and, in time, were translated first into color slide-film presentations, then into movies. Old anti-quackery pamphlets were updated, and new ones written, and were distributed by the thousand. The pages of the AMA's popular health magazine for laymen, *Today's Health,* successor to *Hygeia,* began to reveal much greater emphasis than in many years on anti-quackery themes. In 1960, AMA officialdom called on all physicians to join in a national campaign to alert the public to the wasted money and blighted hopes resulting from reliance on medical quackery and food faddism.[12]

Voluntary health associations also responded with reinvigo-

---

Commerce, *Self-Regulation in Advertising: A Report on the Operations of Private Enterprise in an Important Area of Public Responsibility* (Dept. of Commerce: Washington, 1964); Irving Ladimer [of the NBBB], "Advertising of Drugs to the Public: Ethical and Social Considerations," in Francis X. Quinn, ed., *Ethics, Advertising and Responsibility* (Westminster, Md., 1963), 65-66; Daniel J. Murphy [of the FTC], "Truthful Advertising," in *ibid.*, 137.

[12] "Reports of the Bureau of Investigation" folder [reports, 1950-1959], in Dept. of Investigation, AMA; "New AMA Campaign," *AMA News,* 3 (Oct. 3, 1960), 4. Examples of articles in *Today's Health* are Max Millman, "The Reducing Racket," 32 (Jan. 1954), 18-19; Veronica L. Conley, "Quackery and Baldness," 33 (Jan. 1955), 37; "What Does Quack Mean to You?," (Apr. 1955), 56-57; Conley, "Don't Abuse Your Skin," 34 (Mar. 1956), 49; Jack Kytle, "Don't Help the Quacks" (Nov. 1956), 13; Charles W. Hock, "Laxatives: A \$148-Million Fraud?," 38 (Oct. 1960), 30-31.

rated efforts to expose and oppose quackery's growing menace. Especially significant were continuing campaigns by the American Cancer Society and the Arthritis and Rheumatism Foundation. In 1955 the American Cancer Society created a Committee on Quackery. Desiring to place emphasis on unproved methods rather than on unorthodox persons, and wishing to remain open-minded about the possibility that a valuable agent might come from an unlikely source, the Society soon changed the name to the Committee on New and Unproved Methods of Cancer Treatment. Information was gathered on medically unrecognized drugs and regimens vended for use in cancer therapy which had been on the market for years or were newly appearing. A similar catalogue had been in the process of compilation since 1950 through the investigations of the Committee on Cancer Diagnosis and Therapy of the National Research Council. In 1957 this committee was dissolved, and its data were transferred to the American Cancer Society's growing storehouse of information. On the basis of this evidence, the committee began the issuance of a series of factual, sober reports, to the medical profession and to the public. No unheralded miracle treatments for cancer were discovered. Reports invariably concluded, "After careful study of the literature and other information available to it, the American Cancer Society has found no acceptable evidence that treatment with . . . [this method] results in any objective benefit in the treatment of cancer in human beings."[13]

The committee also prepared background reports on cancer quackery for the press and warning pamphlets for the common citizen. It urged upon state medical societies the creation of cancer committees and the need for more effective state laws. Several states, most notably California, enacted legislation strong enough to ferret out and stop the impositions of quacks. The committee spurred local branches of the Ameri-

[13] Roald N. Grant, et al., "Progress against Cancer Quackery," *JAMA*, 175 (Feb. 4, 1961), 401-402; Grant, "Worthless Cancer Remedies—A Challenge to Society and Medicine," undated mimeographed text of speech; L. Henry Garland, "Investigation of Cancer Remedies," *National Academy of Sciences–National Research Council News Report*, 7 (Sep.-Oct. 1957), 73-77; "Unproven Methods of Cancer Treatment" are published periodically in *Ca—A Cancer Jnl. for Clinicians* and distributed as reprints.

can Cancer Society to intensify the educational campaign, through radio panels, the showing of movies, the distribution of warning literature. Yet after five years of diligent effort, the committee's director, Dr. Roald Grant, concluded that "the steps so far taken" had "only pointed the way in the struggle to control cancer quackery."[14]

Arthritis quackery shared abundantly in the new boom days of pseudo-medicine. In one year a single firm spent as much money to promote its arthritis medicine over network television—the sum was $800,000—as the Arthritis and Rheumatism Foundation dispensed for arthritis research. Like the American Cancer Society, the Foundation sought to intensify its campaign of educating the public against hazards inherent in self-treatment. As part of this campaign, the Foundation sponsored the first systematic study, with respect to a single disease, of the magnitude of the problem. Making national estimates on the basis of a survey of 3,000 arthritic sufferers, Ruth Walrad concluded that "arthritics spend their drug money not wisely but too well." The disease in its various forms provided a well-nigh perfect field for the impostor to exploit. Excruciatingly painful, arthritis drove its victims to almost any expedient in the hope of relief. For the major forms of the disease, professional medicine had found no cure. Frequently the disease waxed and waned in intensity. If a sufferer had used a specious drug or device just prior to a period of remission, he credited the treatment with his relief and often became an enthusiastic proponent for the treatment among other arthritis victims. Since 11 million Americans—one out of every 15—had arthritis, the potential market for misrepresented wares was great. Some forms of arthritis become worse as the victims advance in age, so the growing ranks of America's senior citizens proved especially vulnerable to this form of quackery.[15]

[14] Grant, "Progress against Cancer Quackery"; Garland, "California Outlaws the Cancer Quack," *Today's Health,* 37 (Aug. 1959), 30-31, 68-71; pamphlets entitled "Unproved Cancer Therapy a Continuing Challenge" and "I Have a Secret Cure for Cancer!"; Roald Grant and Irene Bartlett, "Unproven Cancer Remedies—a Primer," *Unproven Methods of Cancer Treatment,* 2-20.

[15] Kenneth N. Anderson, "What You Should Know about Phony Arthritis Remedies," *Today's Health,* 39 (July 1961), 32-33; Walrad, *The Misrepresentation of Arthritis Drugs,* 1-4, 67-71.

A conservative estimate, Miss Walrad concluded, of the annual sum spent by arthritis sufferers for proprietary products (excluding plain aspirin) and for treatment at clinics and spas amounted to $435 million. Over half of this amount, she wrote, some $252 million a year, was wasted, spent on drugs and devices whose value was misrepresented. Five million of the nation's 11 million arthritis victims fell prey to such deceptions.

In the pages of her book, Miss Walrad proceeded to describe many of the exotic drugs, "glorified aspirins," food supplements, devices, treatment centers, books of advice, either harmful and worthless or oversold with exaggerated promises, which contributed to the quarter-of-a-billion annual arthritis cheat. Building on the solid factual basis of Miss Walrad's research, the Arthritis and Rheumatism Foundation enlarged the scope of its publicity. With press releases and speaking tours by its officials, especially by Dr. Ronald W. Lamont-Havers, its medical director, the Foundation sought to apprise the nation about the magnitude of arthritis quackery. Through a steady flow of Medical Department Memos and Product Bulletins to its local chapters, the Foundation strove to increase similar educational efforts on the regional level.[16]

Thus, as the 1950's drew to a close and gave way to the 1960's, the United States witnessed a heavier and more persistent barrage of criticism aimed at medical quackery than ever before. Regulatory agencies also kept scoring direct hits on specious promotions by means of victories in court. The Food and Drug Administration, as the previous chapter indicates, after a decade of litigation had by 1960 stopped Hoxsey's cancer activities in both Texas and Pennsylvania and had brought his method of treating cancer virtually to a halt. The FDA had likewise closed in on several of the National Health Federation's major members. When Fred Hart, the Federation's president, violated a 1954 injunction forbidding shipment of his electronic instruments in interstate commerce, the FDA launched criminal contempt proceedings which Hart did

[16] *Ibid.*, 67-100; Arthritis and Rheumatism Foundation Memos, Sep. 29, 1958–Sep. 15, 1960; Committee on Arthritis Advertising of the Arthritis and Rheumatism Foundation, Product Bulletins, May 11, 1961–June 15, 1962, provided by the Foundation.

not contest. In 1961 Royal Lee, one of the Federation's board
of governors, acquiesced without fighting in a sweeping injunction forbidding him and his assorted corporations from distributing in interstate commerce more than 115 falsely labeled
special dietary products. Another of the Federation's governors, Earl Irons, also a nutritional promoter, served a term in
jail.[17]

But as the foes of pseudo-medicine surveyed the battle-
ground, they questioned seriously whether the tide was running in their favor. While injunctions stopped new interstate
shipments of medical gadgetry, hundreds of quack devices
remained in use by deluded or unscrupulous practitioners, who
seemed to have no trouble finding eager patients. As old promotions of futile remedies for treating cancer, arthritis, and
alleged nutritional deficiencies were brought under control,
new ones took their place. Nutri-Bio became a national mania.
Creating a sales force built like a military hierarchy, the Nutri-
Bio general staff had soon enlisted an army of salesmen that
outnumbered all the employees of the Food and Drug Administration by a ratio of 40 to one. Dan Dale Alexander's *Arthritis and Common Sense,* a book of "worthless advice" in Miss
Walrad's judgment, soared to the best-seller list and was read
by at least a million and a half arthritics, then reached more
through serialization in the press. Krebiozen was rising to the
level of the most publicized unorthodox cancer treatment in
the whole span of American history. Brought to this country
from Argentina by two Yugoslav brothers named Durovic,
Krebiozen, a whitish powder said to have been extracted
from the blood of horses which had been injected with a mi-
cro-organism responsible for "lumpy jaw" in cattle, was presented by its promoters as a cancer cure. It won the dogged
allegiance of one of the nation's outstanding scientists, Dr.
Andrew Ivy, and of Senator Paul Douglas, although the American Cancer Society considered its claims unproved. While
insisting upon governmental tests, the Durovics and Dr. Ivy
resisted meeting the National Cancer Institute's testing criteria, criteria which Dr. Ivy had earlier helped formulate. Can-

[17] DDNJ 4667 and 7303 (Hart); DDNJ 7077 (Lee); DDNJ 5308
(Irons).

cer victims who thought they had been helped by Krebiozen developed into a vocal pressure group at least as powerful as that which had petitioned and picketed for Hoxsey.[18]

Faced with this disturbing state of affairs, quackery's foes drew together more solidly. All along regulatory agencies had exchanged information, and among them and voluntary organizations a mutually helpful interchange of data concerning quackery had existed. Fraud fighters at the FDA, the FTC, and the Post Office Department often received tips on new and suspicious promotions from the NBBB, the AMA, and other health associations. Frequently, when investigating a case, federal agencies inquired what information the NBBB and the AMA's Department of Investigation might already have available in their files. In turn, many releases and publications issued by the private associations were devoted to disseminating word of actions launched or completed by men in the agencies of government. To some members of the anti-quackery forces it came to seem desirable, even mandatory, to work toward even closer collaboration, to present to the American public in some dramatic way a show of unity. Such a grand gesture might help to awaken the public to quackery's size and style and ever-threatening danger more effectively than the separate warning campaigns had so far done.[19]

Prime movers in this venture were the AMA's Oliver Field and the FDA's Director of Public Information, Wallace Janssen. Convincing their superiors of the value of such an enter-

[18] George P. Larrick to author, Apr. 21, 1964; "A Background Paper on Krebiozen from the American Cancer Society," June 19, 1959; "Unproven Methods of Cancer Treatment: Report on the Current Status of Krebiozen," *Ca—A Cancer Jnl. for Clinicians*, 13 (1963), 76-78; Warren R. Young, "What Ever Happened to Dr. Ivy," *Life*, 57 (Oct. 9, 1964), 110ff.; interview with Morris Fishbein, May 15, 1961; NBBB *Report*, Oct. 25 and Nov. 9, 1961; FDA news releases, Nov. 27 and Dec. 7, 1961; *Newsweek*, 58 (July 31, 1961), 60; James L. Trawick (FDA), "Modern Faces of Quackery," typed copy of Apr. 15, 1966, speech; Walrad, *The Misrepresentation of Arthritis Drugs*, 79; Ernest Havemann, "No More a Headache, Book Business Booms," *Life*, 50 (May 12, 1961), 117; *Unproven Methods of Cancer Treatment*, 62-64.

[19] Reference to information provided federal agencies by the NBBB and AMA appears in the Blatnik subcommittee hearings, p. 28, and in the AMA "Reports of the Bureau of Investigation" folder. Files of all the voluntary agencies' reports to their membership summarize actions taken by FDA, FTC, and the Post Office Department.

prise, Field and Janssen began the planning of a National Congress on Medical Quackery, under the joint sponsorship of the AMA and the FDA, to be held in Washington. The goal was to secure widespread coverage of this Congress in news media by reason of the prominence of the speakers who would address it, and to achieve a longer lasting effect by inviting to listen to the speakers opinion leaders from all over the nation concerned with public health and with the integrity of American business.[20]

To the National Congress on Medical Quackery during October 1961 came some 700 men and women, from state medical societies and licensing boards, Better Business Bureaus and trade associations, federal and state agencies, medical and pharmacy and nursing schools, health insurance companies, research institutes, women's clubs, societies concerned with arthritis, cancer, diabetes, nutrition. Even a few quacks slipped in under assumed names, pretending to be members of the press.[21]

Delegates studied exhibits demonstrating the quack promoter's ingenuity. They saw a "horse collar" that was supposed to cure disease by magnetizing the blood's iron. They pushed a doorbell and heard the actual recorded pitch of a salesman touting a vitamin and alfalfa mix as a sure-fire panacea. They looked at a wooden hut—resembling an old-fashioned privy—in which the patient sat to let "orgone energy" accumulate for banishing his ills. They saw countless pills and potions labeled with shrewd but futile therapeutic claims.[22]

The delegates listened intently to a day and a half of speechmaking by veteran fighters against pseudo-medicine. Government officials, while not neglecting their successes, made clear their plight. The record of FDA court victories, Commissioner George Larrick noted, was "very small" compared with the total extent of food quackery. In the device field, even after the FDA had secured numerous injunctions against shippers of falsely labeled gadgets, some 3,000 to 5,000 practition-

[20] Interviews with Field and Janssen, Oct. 6, 1961.
[21] *Ibid.* as to quacks attending. "Those in Attendance," *Proceedings, National Congress on Medical Quackery,* 94-113.
[22] Notes made at the Congress.

ers, especially chiropractors, continued using bogus electrical machines. And whatever kind the case, Larrick said, FDA's burden in court was getting ever more difficult, as proprietors drafted labeling and advertising ever more subtly.[23]

This last point was elaborated by William Goodrich, General Counsel for food and drug matters in the Department of Health, Education, and Welfare. In the field of medicine, he reminded his audience, claims for the efficacy of a drug were presumed false until established as true by sufficient pharmacological and clinical evidence. In law, however, a medical claim was presumed to be true until the government proved its falsity by a preponderance of the evidence beyond a reasonable doubt. This put a staggering burden upon the FDA—proof that the remedy or gadget in question would *never* work for the purposes claimed. And this had to be done "in terms that a jury of laymen can grasp." If one juror remained unconvinced, a strange anomaly resulted: the drug or device, although believed by all reputable scientists to be devoid of value, continued in the eyes of the law as useful for health. Physicians were too often reluctant to waste time testing therapeutic wares which they viewed as transparent hoaxes. Yet if hard quackery cases were to be won in court, doctors had to be willing to help regulatory agencies by making such tests and then by testifying. Too "many doctors fear the witness chair almost as much as lawyers fear the operating table."[24]

Other speakers before the Congress raised more serious questions regarding the relations of the medical profession and quackery. Commissioner Larrick condemned the occasional doctor who engaged in " 'rigged research'—the study that was set up and written to support a claim, rather than to seek for scientific proof." Such a study need not be conclusive. Indeed, in its very inconclusiveness lay its value. "Only enough work is done to point in the proper direction and to get the report published in a medical journal; only enough to raise a doubt, or to put the Government to the task of proof by a preponderance of evidence." Maye Russ of the NBBB cited specific ex-

[23] *Proceedings, National Congress on Medical Quackery*, 12-18.
[24] *Ibid.*, 19-23.

amples of such specious research and made clear that some doctors were still directly engaged in quackery. One recent boom had seen sea water promoted as a virtual cure-all. "The incorporators of one of these firms included four physicians, and its President was an officer of the local medical society."[25]

Physicians came in for other criticism. Dr. Henry Garland condemned "the incompetent or conscienceless fringe" who used orthodox methods of treating cancer but used them incompetently, such as the surgeon who removed only part of an excisable tumor. Dr. Lamont-Havers spoke sadly of physicians who, by their "disinterest and frustration" in treating arthritics, drove dissatisfied patients plagued by pain into the arms of quacks.[26]

Criticism was pointed in other directions as well. Too many newspapers and magazines printed flamboyant stories about medical advances that turned out to be specious promotions. "Unquestionably," Dr. Morris Fishbein said, "editors seeking for sensational discoveries will accept articles from science writers who have not been capable of evaluating scientific evidence or who have been led by too persuasive publicity hounds into lending their space to unwarranted exploitation." Book publishers, too, Dr. Lamont-Havers observed, too often published dangerous tomes, their "desire to profit from the gullibility of the arthritic . . . overrid[ing] any feeling of compassion."[27]

Federal agencies were also accused of falling short. In view of the vast quantity of false nutritional claims soaring forth over the nation's airwaves from radio and television stations, Dr. Fredrick Stare of Harvard concluded, the licensing policies of the Federal Communications Commission were much too lenient. Considering that nutritional quackery bulked largest of all forms in money terms, it was regrettable that the FDA, during the previous year, had been able "to devote the services of only eight people to the investigation of lecturers, spielers, and canvassers" in this crucial field of deception.[28]

Whatever failings physicians, or regulatory agencies, or self-regulators had been guilty of, the basic evil lay with the greedy

[25] *Ibid.*, 17, 54-59.  [26] *Ibid.*, 46, 52.
[27] *Ibid.*, 53, 90.  [28] *Ibid.*, 66-71.

quacks themselves. In the continuing confrontation with this enemy, more vigorous law enforcement, supported by more ample funds, was a prime essential. On this the Congress speakers agreed. Self-regulation by media with respect to advertising needed tightening too. Equally fundamental was "an all-out campaign . . . of public education."[29]

Why earlier warnings, issued in such vast quantities by so many agencies, had not so far achieved a greater measure of success was a question not confronted so explicitly by the Congress speakers as it might have been. Some conclusions could have been inferred, perhaps, from references to the deep and complicated phenomenon of which the proneness to quackery consisted. Many speakers alluded to facets of this theme, and an articulate Texan, Dr. William H. Gordon, elucidated with vivid, imaginative case histories various deep forces in human nature to which the quack appealed. Dr. Gordon began his address by citing from Dr. Cramp's favorite book. "One can't believe impossible things," Alice had said. But the White Queen had answered: "I daresay you haven't had much practice. . . . When I was your age . . . I believed as many as six impossible things before breakfast."[30]

So many people believed so many impossible things about their health, and they seemed ever anxious, for the most compelling reasons, to believe so many more—the countless glittering but impossible promises urged upon them by quackdom's host of clever schemers. The separate educational campaigns by public and private agencies had doubtless done much good, but not enough. Could an intensified educational crusade, spurred by the National Congress on Medical Quackery, using the same techniques of the smaller, isolated campaigns, be expected to succeed much better? Some spoke of quackery as, in some measure, an unyielding accompaniment of human existence. But most speakers took a more optimistic tone, seeming to consider quackery's "final eradication" at least a possibility.[31] The Congress might well have devoted

[29] *Ibid., passim,* quotation from p. 59.
[30] *Ibid.,* 49-55. Dr. Gordon's address, "The Keys to Quackery," is reprinted, 33-41.
[31] All speakers at the Congress believed it possible to reduce quackery

more attention, in view of the complex motivations that prompted people to fall prey to quackery's appeals, to considering ways of fashioning the ongoing educational crusade more subtly.

The nation's news media did give the Congress much publicity. The 700 delegates went home much better informed than they had come, doubtless to use this knowledge in fighting charlatans on the local scene. The desire for unity among quackery's foes persisted. Two years later, again in Washington, a Second National Congress on Medical Quackery convened. This time delegates listened to a more probing analysis of the deep currents of human nature so fundamental to quackery's continuing appeal.[32]

---

substantially. Some talked as if quackery might in time be completely eradicated: *ibid.*, Abraham Ribicoff, 4; Dr. Leonard W. Larson, 7; Herbert J. Miller, Jr., 11; Goodrich, 19. Other speakers suggested that a complete victory could never be won: Paul Rand Dixon, 54; Russ, 59; Field, 64; Dr. Harold E. Jervey, Jr., 84.

[32] See, for example, articles in *Atlanta Journal-Constitution*, Oct. 1, 1961; *N.Y. Times*, Oct. 7 and 8, 1961; *Wash. Post*, Oct. 7 and 8, 1961; *This Week Magazine*, Oct. 8, 1961; *Medical Tribune*, Oct. 23, 1961. *Proceedings, Second National Congress on Medical Quackery*, Oct. 25-26, 1963 (Chicago, 1964). See ch. 20.

# 19

# TURMOIL ON THE DRUG SCENE

*"A . . . unique characteristic [of prescription drugs] is the difference between buyer and orderer; in the words of Chairman Kefauver, 'He who orders does not buy; and he who buys does not order.' . . . Hence in ethical drugs the ability of the ordinary consumer to protect himself against the monopoly element inherent in trademarks is nonexistent. The consumer is 'captive' to a degree not present in any other industry."*

—REPORT OF THE KEFAUVER SUBCOMMITTEE, 1961[1]

*"Americans are now paying the greatest price they have ever paid for worthless nostrums, ineffectual and potentially dangerous devices, treatments given by unqualified practitioners, food fads and unneeded diet supplements, and other alluring products or services that make misleading promises of cure or end to pain.*

*"It is incredible that a wealthy nation, priding itself on its enlightenment and its thirst for progress, should pay such a heavy penalty for ignorance or lack of adequate enforcement."*

—REPORT OF THE WILLIAMS SUBCOMMITTEE, 1965[2]

TO COMBAT the menace of quackery, Secretary of Health, Education, and Welfare Abraham A. Ribicoff told the delegates to the 1961 Congress on Medical Quackery, his Department and the American Medical Association could cooperate wholeheartedly. "It is a well-known fact," he also said, "that we do not always agree on every subject—the AMA and myself."[3]

[1] *Administered Prices: Drugs*, 87 Cong., 1 ses., *Senate Rep.* 448 (1961), 3.

[2] *Frauds and Deceptions Affecting the Elderly*, 89 Cong., 1 ses., Committee print of a report of the Subcommittee on Frauds and Misrepresentations Affecting the Elderly to the Special Committee on Aging, United States Senate (1965), 1.

[3] *Proceedings, National Congress on Medical Quackery*, 3.

This remark brought a chuckle from Ribicoff's audience, well aware that the power struggle over Medicare, quiescent during the Eisenhower years, was, with John F. Kennedy's accession to the presidency, beginning to heat up. The President would shortly present to the Congress a wide-ranging plan of legislative and executive action to protect more adequately the consumer's interests, a plan in which the tighter control of drugs held high priority. A new period of reform was dawning in America, and central to the design of the New Frontier was improvement of the nation's health. The thrust of the Kennedy years would continue in Lyndon B. Johnson's striving toward the Great Society. "The Department of Health, Education, and Welfare," stated John W. Gardner, one of Ribicoff's successors, in 1966, "is a partner in a historic effort in health, an effort that will mean a more rewarding life for each individual in our society and for society as a whole. But the partnership will work only if all of the elements with which the Federal Government has allied itself enjoy continuing strength and vitality—and that includes state and local agencies, public and private hospitals, professional associations and private practitioners. All of them must play a creative and independent role."[4]

Ways in which a partnership to curtail the hazards of pseudomedicine might enhance the public health had formed the agenda of the 1961 Congress on Quackery. But as the overall drug problem was coming to be viewed, quackery was only one of many serious issues which required attention. As to prescription medication, critics were charging, the chemotherapeutic revolution had produced a "therapeutic nightmare."[5]

[4] *N.Y. Times,* Mar. 16, 1962; Gardner, "The Creative Partnership for Health," *Medical Tribune,* June 22, 1966, 1, 11.

[5] Morton Mintz used *The Therapeutic Nightmare* as the title for his book critically surveying the period (Boston, 1965). The discussion below is derived mainly from two sets of Senate committee hearings, presided over by Senators Estes Kefauver and Hubert Humphrey respectively; the printed hearings contain not only the testimony of witnesses but also a rich assortment of documents taken from the files of pharmaceutical manufacturers and of the FDA, as well as a reprinting of articles from the press and many journals: *Administered Prices: Hearings before the Subcommittee on Antitrust and Monopoly of the Com-*

Academic physicians initiated the criticism, and their somber judgments were picked up by lay journalists and Congressional committees. No one denied the tremendous benefits that a generation of new drugs had brought in saving lives, easing pain, reducing the population of mental hospitals. But the valuable new therapeutic agents had proved to be so powerful that, when improperly used, grave consequences, sometimes long delayed, ensued. Some patients, because of personal idiosyncrasies, could not take drugs others could use with safety and displayed dangerous, sometimes fatal, reactions. Some drugs had cumulative toxic effects. Other drugs, once effective, lost their value as germs mutated into new and resistant strains. Drug-induced ailments of various kinds became an increasingly urgent problem as the statistics of "therapeutic misadventure" mounted.

Some risk was inevitable in drug therapy, the critics said, a chance necessarily taken when striving to achieve a cure. But various developments had ballooned the risk beyond all need. Many practicing physicians must share in the blame. They sometimes prescribed drugs when none was needed. They used too potent and hazardous drugs for conditions which might be served by medicines less potent and hazardous. They tried out new therapeutic agents without adequately informing themselves about the potential dangers in their use. To be sure, the task of keeping up to date was well-nigh impossible for the average doctor. New drugs were marketed in such a bewildering array and in such numbers—some 400 a year—that had a doctor sought to read all the pertinent scientific literature, much of which, in any case, was published after the drugs became available for use, he would have had no time to see his patients. What bothered the academic critics most was

---

mittee on the Judiciary, *United States Senate* (86 Cong., 1 and 2 ses.), Parts 14 through 26 (1960-1961), cited below as Kefauver hearings; *Interagency Coordination in Drug Research and Regulation: Hearings before the Subcommittee on Reorganization and International Organizations of the Committee on Government Operations, United States Senate* (87 Cong., 2 ses., and 88 Cong., 1 ses.), Parts 1 through 4 (1963-1964), cited below as Humphrey hearings. See also the essays in Talalay, ed., *Drugs in Our Society,* and Louis Lasagna, *The Doctors' Dilemmas* (N.Y., 1962).

that too many physicians did not resort to the most authentic sources to keep themselves informed. They relied too heavily on the promotional literature with which they were deluged by pharmaceutical manufacturers and on the counsel of these companies' traveling salesmen, called detailmen.

Drug manufacturers received sharper criticism than did doctors. To be sure, they were engaged in a highly competitive business with wares that rapidly became obsolete. Much of their expensive research seeking to find new agents of value went for nought, since most prospective medicines turned out to be ineffective or too toxic to market. Thus, when they found a drug that showed commercial promise, they wanted to cash in on it before another drug from another pharmaceutical house replaced it. Critics charged, indeed, that too little of the research budget of such companies went for basic research to seek genuinely needed new drugs and too much of the budget went for seeking minor modifications, which might be patentable, of competitors' drugs that had achieved outstanding commercial success. Critics also held that, in the rush to get drugs to the market, some pharmaceutical manufacturers did not engage in adequate testing programs, either in animals or in man, to establish as securely as was desirable the safety and efficacy of their new wares. Some of the clinical testing that took place, critics believed, smacked more of promotion than of science, being an effort to acquaint doctors with the product prior to its release for sale by the FDA.

New prescription drugs had as part of the labeling enclosed with each package a brochure, which the FDA had to approve, describing the therapeutic indications for the drug's use, informing about the proper dosage patterns, and also providing warnings and contraindications. But, since the drug went from the manufacturer to the pharmacist, many doctors did not see this brochure as a matter of course. A few companies mailed copies to physicians, but many did not. They did send, however, lavishly printed literature stressing the drug's merits but playing down, or omitting altogether, commentary on the risks. Nor did drug advertising in most medical periodicals provide a balanced picture of the good and bad. Some detailmen, it was discovered, had been instructed, even after a new

and more vigorous warning had been required in a drug brochure by the FDA, to minimize the warning in their conversations with physicians. Pharmaceutical companies were also
guilty, the critics said, of placing research papers in medical
journals that fell far short of meeting sound scientific canons.
And the companies sometimes went to elaborate lengths to
plant stories of some soon-to-be-released drug in the popular
press or in a family magazine, presumably with the hope that
patients would bring pressure on their doctors to prescribe it.

Pharmaceutical companies, moreover, the more severe critics
held, charged too high a price for drugs. Drug industry
profits ranked highest among all American industries, and promotional costs were certainly near the top, needlessly high.
Trade-name pharmaceuticals which were patented held the
same price level for years, despite economies of production,
and sometimes this occurred when there were several trade-
name pharmaceuticals made by different companies useful for
essentially the same therapeutic purposes—they all remained
for a long span of time stable in price, a price virtually identical from brand to brand. Institutional buyers, such as governmental agencies, sometimes found that bids for contracts from
several competing companies were identical; at other times, it
seemed, bids revealed that companies could make profits from
drug prices incredibly lower than those the individual consumer was required to pay.

Whatever the degree of validity in these various charges—
and they launched a great debate as the groups criticized
sought to defend themselves—it was apparent that much was
amiss. Instances of greed, deception, and inexcusable careless-
ness were definitely established. But basically the revelations
during these years showed that old ways were not sufficient for
a new day. All along the line, from the discovery and testing
of new drugs to their promotion, prescribing, and use, a caution, a scientific sophistication, was demanded much beyond
the level required in the era before the wonder drugs had appeared. The speed with which the chemotherapeutic revolution had remolded therapy, the complexity of the chemical
and physiological problems involved, the optimism warranted
by the new drugs' lifesaving potency which tended to becloud

the sober later awareness of the risks had created the need for agonizing reappraisal. This reappraisal took place in full public view, for news of the dangers inherent in drug use came to concern the nation's people as earlier news of drug miracles had cheered them. What came to seem like guilt, from the perspective of the new criticism, had been in some measure an unawareness of the high level of scientific rigor required in the production and use of the new therapeutic agents.

While there had been some popular writing on this crucial theme earlier, and the Blatnik subcommittee had concerned itself with tranquilizing drugs, the hearings presided over by Senator Estes Kefauver, between December 1959 and September 1960, made headlines that turned prescription drug practices into a national issue. The Tennessee Senator introduced a strong remedial bill, but, despite the public concern his hearings had aroused, the bill, weakened by amendment, languished in the Senate Judiciary Committee. As prior to 1906 and 1938, it was to take a stupendous threat to the public health—this time, happily, a "might-have-been"—to ensure legislative action.[6]

The Food and Drug Administration did not escape unscathed during the agonizing reappraisal. The Citizens Advisory Committee of 1955 had urged a marked improvement in the FDA's scientific competency, through increasing the stature and prestige of the professional staff, inaugurating greater cooperation with other federal health agencies, and engaging in more research on the side effects of dangerous drugs. Other CAC suggestions aimed at helping industry by expediting the processing of new drug applications. Later critics wondered if the FDA had not helped business much too much at the expense of the drug-consuming public. In conformity with the general governmental climate during the Eisenhower years, relations between the regulators and the regulated had been generally cordial. In retrospect, from a

[6] *False and Misleading Advertising (Prescription Tranquilizing Drugs)*: *Hearings before a Subcommittee of the Committee on Government Operations, House of Representatives* (85 Cong., 2 ses., 1958). An illuminating account of the Kefauver hearings and of the legislative history of the Kefauver bill, written from a position of sympathy with the Tennessee Senator's objectives, is Richard Harris, *The Real Voice* (N.Y., 1964).

more reformist perspective, this seemed a fault. Some FDA doctors, processing new drug applications, believed that industry representatives had exerted too great and constant pressure on them to rush the applications through, and thought also that their own administrative superiors had not shielded them adequately from such pressure. The entire agency, in its posture toward business, was brought under a cloud as a result of a revelation made by the Kefauver subcommittee. Following up a clue presented by John Lear in the *Saturday Review,* the subcommittee discovered that FDA's director of the Division of Antibiotics, Dr. Henry Welch, had engaged in an enterprise that certainly aroused the suspicion of conflict of interest. Dr. Welch had secured permission from his superiors to edit two journals in his field in exchange for an "honorarium." No one had raised the question as to what size this presumably modest sum might be. As it turned out, Dr. Welch had received, during a seven-year span, an amount exceeding $280,-000. This income came mainly from a percentage on drug advertising carried in the journals and a percentage on reprints of journal articles bought by drug manufacturers for use in their promotion. Although scrutiny by a blue-ribbon committee selected by the National Academy of Sciences revealed no evidence that Welch's "honorarium" had influenced his official decisions in evaluating antibiotics, the Welch case obviously injured the FDA's prestige and made it easier to interpret the agency's relationships with business in a critical light.[7]

The lack of sufficient scientific competence within the FDA received increasing criticism. A new Citizens Advisory Committee in 1962 rebuked the agency for having failed to follow up adequately suggestions for strengthening its scientific resources made by the earlier committee in 1955. Nor did scientists within the agency, medical and Congressional critics charged, carry the weight they should have in making key decisions. "The Food and Drug Administration," Senator Hu-

[7] Pertinent excerpts from the 1955 Citizens Advisory Committee report and from a series of internal and external critiques of FDA during the years that followed are brought together in the Humphrey hearings, Part 2. Kefauver hearings, Parts 22 and 23, are concerned with the Welch case. John Lear, "The Certification of Antibiotics," *Sat. Rev.,* 42 (Feb. 7, 1959), 43-48.

bert H. Humphrey asserted, "has been looked upon as a 'police' department, rather than as an agency of scientists and other professionals with a broad variety of health-related skills." Drugs had been approved which the FDA admitted should not have been, because proof of their safety had not been adequately demonstrated. Drugs had been kept on the market long after accumulating evidence had shown their hazards. Perhaps if scientists had played a more decisive role in the decision-making, such contingencies would not have occurred. "The New Frontier," said Humphrey, had "yet to make its mark on . . . [the] 54-year-old effort" to regulate food and drugs. "The Food and Drug Administration should be upgraded. There should be some 'new blood,' some new endeavor, some new action, some new spirit."[8]

Humphrey's Congressional inquiry, which revealed some of the FDA's shortcomings in evaluating new drugs, had arisen, ironically enough, from one of the agency's great triumphs. The shrewdness and firmness of an FDA woman physician had kept the United States from sharing in a terrible medical disaster.

A drug with the generic name thalidomide had been marketed in West Germany in 1957. By 1960 its sales had skyrocketed and, through leasing arrangements between the manufacturer and foreign drug companies, thalidomide had become purchasable in Britain, Canada, Portugal, and other countries. Used as a sleeping tablet, sedative, and anti-emetic in pregnancy, thalidomide became renowned for a certain sort of safety: unlike most other sedatives, it did not, when taken intentionally or accidentally in large doses, cause death. In September 1960, after nearly two years of animal and clinical testing, an American drug company submitted to the FDA a new drug application to market thalidomide under the trade name Kevadon. So confident of quick approval was the company that it gathered key detailmen together the next month to send them forth on a major pre-clearance campaign of lining up hospital doctors for a final round of clinical trials.

[8] Citizens Advisory Committee, *Report to the Secretary of Health, Education, and Welfare on the Food & Drug Administration* (Washington, 1962); excerpts in Humphrey hearings, Part 2, 428-47. Humphrey cited, *ibid.*, 583, 588.

The purpose, in a minor way, was "confirmation" of thalidomide's already established usefulness, the salesmen were informed. "But the main purpose is to establish local studies whose results may be spread among hospital staff members. You can assure your doctors that they need not report results if they don't want to. . . ." In all, more than 1,200 investigators were given free samples, nearly 20,000 patients treated.[9] .

But in the FDA's Division of New Drugs, Dr. Frances O. Kelsey, who was given the application to process, did not believe that the evidence submitted by the company demonstrated beyond question the drug's safety. Despite a succession of letters, phone calls, and personal visits from company officials, she would not grant acceptance and asked for more data. Her precautionary hunch ·was confirmed by a doctor's letter to the editor in the *British Medical Journal*, wondering if thalidomide might not be responsible for four cases he had observed of peripheral neuritis, a deterioration of the nerves in the hands and feet. A similar discovery in West Germany led to the changing of thalidomide's status from over-the-counter to prescription sale. Dr. Kelsey wondered, if thalidomide produced such an ailment, might it not be hazardous to the unborn child?

About the time the American drug company was briefing its detailmen, two cases of phocomelia were presented by a German doctor to a pediatric convention. As an American physician later reported the episode, "Photographs and X-ray pictures showed that the long bones of the infants' arms had almost completely failed to grow; their arms were so short that their hands extended almost directly from their shoulders. Their legs were less affected but showed signs of a similar distortion of growth. Both infants were also marked by a large hemangioma (strawberry mark) extending from the forehead down the nose and across the upper lip; one of them was also found to have a duodenal stenosis, that is, a constriction of the beginning of the small intestine."[10] Phocomelia, a name

[9] Humphrey hearings, Parts 1 and 2, are concerned with the thalidomide case, and contain not only testimony but a vast assortment of documents, including reprinting of comment from magazines and the press. The William S. Merrell Co. document appears in Part 1, 259-70.
[10] Helen B. Taussig, "The Thalidomide Syndrome," *Scientific Ameri-*

derived from two Greek words meaning "seal" and "limb," had been so rare an affliction that most doctors had never encountered it during a lifetime of practice. But babies by the hundreds began to be born in Germany thus terribly malformed. By November 1961, a German physician suspected the culpable agent to be thalidomide taken during the first three months of pregnancy. Hearing a rumor of this widespread affliction, Dr. Helen B. Taussig, of the Johns Hopkins University pediatrics department, went to Germany immediately for an investigation on the spot and came home to spread the word through letter, public address, and print of thalidomide's horrifying potentiality. Dr. Kelsey went to Baltimore to learn first-hand from Dr. Taussig her disquieting intelligence. On March 8, 1962, the American drug company asked Dr. Kelsey that its new drug application be withdrawn.

Had Dr. Kelsey been less adamant and had Kevadon been released, some 10,000 deformed babies would have been born in the United States before the danger was known. That a smaller-scale disaster did not take place was remarkable, considering the widespread distribution of Kevadon by the American company to clinical "investigators." Much of the record-keeping by these doctors was non-existent or shoddy, and the FDA had a difficult task making sure that all supplies of the drug had been recalled or destroyed. As it was, only a few cases of phocomelia occurred in America, mostly from thalidomide secured abroad.

The story of Dr. Kelsey's determined opposition to the marketing of thalidomide was first publicly reported by Morton Mintz in the *Washington Post* in mid-July.[11] This news story precipitated a tidal wave of national publicity and numerous editorials of gratitude for Dr. Kelsey's perceptive contribution to the American people. President Kennedy presented her with the Gold Medal Award for Distinguished Civilian Service. The thalidomide episode focused scientific attention on the problem of teratogenicity: could other drugs taken during pregnancy also make monsters of babies who would be born?

---

*can*, 207 (Aug. 1962), 29-35, reprinted in the Humphrey hearings, Part 1, 108-14.

[11] July 15, 1962.

The episode also called into question anew, as during Senator Humphrey's hearings, the practices of drug companies in testing their drugs prior to marketing and the procedures by which the Food and Drug Administration evaluated drugs which they released for sale. The FDA issued new regulations seeking to control clinical testing sponsored by manufacturers prior to their submission of new drug applications. If the FDA had had such authority under the 1938 law, Senator Humphrey questioned, why, in view of the way thalidomide had been distributed for testing to so many doctors who could by no means be classified as "experts," had not the agency promulgated such regulations much earlier?

The thalidomide near-disaster, like the meat-packing scandals of 1906 and the sulfanilamide tragedy of 1937, forced the Congress to enact a major new protective law. The languishing bill was revived, its weakened clauses restrengthened, and on October 10, 1962, the Kefauver-Harris Drug Amendments passed both Houses of Congress unanimously. Although provisions dear to Senator Kefauver's heart aimed at reducing drug prices did not find their way into the law, the measure markedly improved the FDA's control over the marketing and promotion of prescription drugs. Henceforth the FDA must approve all plans for clinical testing, must be assured that clinical investigators were scientifically qualified to conduct the tests. An investigator was required to inform his patient that he was taking part in an experiment involving an investigational drug unless, in the doctor's judgment, this was not feasible or would not be in the patient's best interest. The new law also required that no new drug could be released to the market unless the manufacturer had submitted to the FDA substantial evidence that the drug was not only safe—the 1938 law had required this—but also efficacious for treating the ailments for which it was designed as therapy. Both during clinical trials and after marketing, drug companies were required to notify the FDA immediately—as they had not always done before—should they receive reports of any adverse effects caused by a drug. All drug manufacturers were required by the new law to operate according to good manufacturing procedures, and the scope of the FDA's factory inspection was enlarged in plants making prescription drugs. An effort failed to put into the law the same inspection rigor for plants making proprietary products. Pre-marketing certification by the FDA was expanded from five antibiotics to all of them. And prescription drug advertising, hitherto the Federal Trade Commission's prerogative, was brought within the jurisdiction of the FDA. Each advertisement was required henceforth to present truthfully a brief summary of known side effects and contraindications, as well as information about the drug's effectiveness.[12]

As Food and Drug Administration officials sought to implement the new law, they did so in a goldfish bowl. Seven years before the public may have been largely unaware of the agency and its mission, but the Kefauver hearings, the thalidomide headlines, and the new law greatly enhanced the newsworthiness of the agency. In the years that followed, reporters and Congressional committees kept the FDA under constant and critical scrutiny.[13]

Such was the broader drug scene within which the continuing contest with medical quackery took place. Amid all the testifying about prescription drug difficulties that preceded the 1962 law, Congressional committees occasionally heard the shortcomings of over-the-counter medication mentioned. Arthritis and Rheumatism Foundation spokesmen, for example, described for the Kefauver subcommittee the broad range of deceptive remedies offered for direct sale to arthritis sufferers. And the editorial director of Consumers Union, Mrs. Mildred Brady, expressed her sympathy with the doctor's dilemma. "We who listen hours a day," she said, "to the conflicting claims made by various brands of deodorants, cold remedies, toothpastes, hair dyes, headache remedies and laxatives—claims made frequently by the same companies who also promote and sell brand name prescription drugs to doctors—we television viewers and radio listeners cannot help but feel a sympa-

[12] 76 Stat. 780; Harris, *The Real Voice, passim*; George P. Larrick, "Appraising Drug Safety and Efficacy," *Emory University Qtly.*, 21 (Summer 1965), 88-96.
[13] For an example of hearings, see *Drug Safety: Hearings before a Subcommittee of the Committee on Government Operations, House of Representatives* (88 Cong., 2 ses.), Parts 1 and 2 (1964).

thetic uneasiness for our physicians, subject as they are to equally intensive and extravagant hard sell directed at them."[14]

The main thrust of the hearings, however, as of the law, aimed at abuses associated with prescription drugs. The new law, nonetheless, provided important weapons against quackery. The new proof-of-efficacy pre-marketing standard applied to all drugs, not just prescription products. No promoter could henceforth seek to sell direct to the lay public any new drug that had not met this rigorous provision without quickly facing a Food and Drug action he could not hope to win. Nor would it any longer be possible for a specious promotion to masquerade for years under the guise of pre-marketing clinical trials, distributing "medicine" in exchange for a "contribution" to help cover the firm's expenses, a contribution that might really include a large margin of profit. Now the promoter would have to present to the FDA his plan for clinical trials and must persuade the agency that his experts were properly qualified, or else stop distributing his wares in interstate commerce. On this rock were wrecked the hopes of Krebiozen, proved by FDA scientists to be nothing more than mineral oil and creatine, a common laboratory chemical. A committee of 24 cancer experts, chosen by the National Cancer Institute, reported in 1963, after surveying the records of 504 patients treated with Krebiozen, that the drug was ineffective in treating cancer. The committee strongly recommended that no clinical trial was warranted. Dr. Durovic filed with the FDA a plan for the investigational use of Krebiozen, required by the Kefauver-Harris law. But a month later Durovic withdrew his plan. Thus he failed to meet the new law's standard and could no longer distribute Krebiozen as an investigational drug across state lines. This ban held, even though the government failed to convict Krebiozen's promoters in a criminal case decided by a Chicago jury in 1966.[15]

[14] Kefauver hearings, Part 14, 7975-94; Part 21, 11536.

[15] George P. Larrick, "Changes in the Status of Proprietary Drugs under Federal Law," mimeographed text of May 11, 1964, address; *Ca—A Cancer Jnl. for Clinicians*, 13 (1963), 76-78; Dept. of HEW release, Oct. 16, 1963; *Medical World News*, Aug. 2, 1963, 41, and June 3, 1966, 25; *Newsweek*, 67 (Feb. 14, 1966), 65-66; American Cancer Society, *Unproven Methods of Cancer Treatment*, 62-64. An

In a pioneering case under the Kefauver-Harris law, the Food and Drug Administration took successful action against another unproved cancer remedy, Mucorhicin. This substance, extracted from a mold grown on a mixture of wheat, salt, yeast, and water fermented in a pan, had neither been proved effective nor been produced under good manufacturing practices. So it too was barred from interstate commerce.[16]

The 1938 law formed the legal basis for precedent-setting victories in the device and nutritional fields: the Micro-Dynameter and Vitasafe cases broadened the scope of the FDA's control over these critical areas. It began to appear as if the Food and Drug Administration, through the new law and accumulating judicial precedents, had gained enough legal authority to prevent the promotion of an unquestionably ineffective drug aimed at the consumer market from growing to gigantic proportions, as had so often happened in the past.[17]

A myriad of small and border-line deceptions, however, continued and were born anew: a Cincinnati promoter, for example, advertised that he could counteract the hazardous effect of thalidomide. Legal procedures still could drag. FDA resources, while expanding, hardly kept up with its growing obligations. Quackery practiced solely within the borders of the individual states remained immune to federal restraint. "In my experience," stated John W. Miner of California, the only prosecutor in the nation specializing in medicolegal crimes, "less than 10% of quackery cases could be filed in federal courts or reached by federal agencies." Speaking before the Third National Congress on Medical Quackery held in Chicago in 1966, Miner termed earlier estimates of quackery's financial toll too low. "An overall annual quackery take of two or more billion," he asserted, "would be a reasonable guess."

---

expert summary of the Krebiozen events, entitled "The Krebiozen Story: Is Cancer Quackery Dead?," was presented on Oct. 7, 1966, to the Third National Congress on Medical Quackery by Dr. James F. Holland of the Roswell Park Memorial Institute of Buffalo, *Papers, Third National Congress on Medical Quackery* (Chicago, 1967), 48-59.

[16] *Ca*, 11 (1961), 17-18; FDA release, Mar. 7, 1964.

[17] Micro-Dynameter: see ch. 11; Vitasafe: 226 Fed. Supp. 266 (1964); 235 Fed. Supp. 84 (1964); 345 Fed. (2d) 864 (1965); 382 U.S. 918 (1965).

Quackery "channels an amount equal or more to 2% of our national budget into the pockets of criminals."[18]

Other experts, seeking to balance regulatory gains and losses, agreed that quackery had not diminished in size. Henry B. Montague, Chief Postal Inspector, thought fraudulent schemes still on the increase. The Arthritis Foundation, in 1966, raised its estimate of the annual sum spent by arthritics on misrepresented wares to a new high of $310 million. AMA headquarters, judging by letters of complaint received, considered cancer quackery the number one medical fraud, and the American Cancer Society issued its updated survey of the wide range of unproved remedies from whose appeals victims—or frightened self-diagnosers—of cancer might choose.[19]

Thus, despite very real regulatory gains, quackery remained a major social problem, "a criminal activity as harmful as any in society," in John Miner's words, "but against which the law has done the least." And despite mounting campaigns to warn the public against the hazards of pseudo-medicine, many citizens of this "wealthy nation, priding itself on its enlightenment and its thirst for progress," continued to hunt health in unenlightened ways. What was there about John Doe that made him such a perennial victim?[20]

[18] *F&D Rev.*, 47 (July 1963), 191; Miner, "The Costs of Quackery," mimeographed text of Oct. 8, 1966, address.

[19] *Health Frauds and Quackery: Hearings before the Subcommittee on Frauds and Misrepresentations Affecting the Elderly of the Special Committee on Aging, United States Senate* (88 Cong., 2 ses., 1964), Part 3, 286; *Medical Tribune,* July 23-24, 1966, 15; American Cancer Society, *Unproven Methods of Cancer Treatment.*

[20] Miner, "The Costs of Quackery"; *Frauds and Deceptions Affecting the Elderly,* 89 Cong., 1 ses. (1965), 1.

# 𝟚𝟘

## THE PERENNIAL PRONENESS

---

*"There is a class of minds much more ready to believe that which is at first sight incredible, and because it is incredible, than what is generally thought reasonable."*

—OLIVER WENDELL HOLMES, 1842[1]

---

"QUACKERY . . . is the legitimate offspring of ignorance." So asserted an orator at the opening of a new medical school in Nashville in 1851. Certainly ignorance has ever been and remains one of medical quackery's major props. "Many people . . .," asserted a recent Food and Drug Commissioner, "know little more about the human body than if they had lived a hundred years ago." Much of what is "known" is what *was* known a century ago, traditional lore, handed down from generation to generation by precept and example, some of it going back centuries, even millennia, or at least resembling medical lore cherished in those remote days. One scholar has done an intriguing job of tracing back the supposed aphrodisiac properties of the mandrake root, which was a popular article long before Machiavelli wrote his play centered on this theme. The same might be done with other aspects of medical and nutritional folk belief. False beliefs about health and therapy derive in part from outmoded theories of orthodox physicians. Such antiquated theories, for example, provide the base for a great deal of today's arthritis quackery. "The rag-bag of folk-medicine," wrote the historian Edward Eggleston, "is filled with the cast-off clothes of science."[2]

[1] Holmes, *Medical Essays*, 33.
[2] *Addresses Delivered by Professors* [Charles K.] *Winston* and [Paul F.] *Eve at the Opening of the Medical Department of the University of Nashville* (Nashville, 1851), 9-10; George P. Larrick, "Quackery as a

Part of the untrue knowledge concerning health that handicaps laymen is the incorrect relationship among facts. Man's reasoning seems to flounder particularly, commented a 19th-century observer, when the issues relate to matters medical, the "most difficult, obscure, and complicated" of all branches of human learning.[3] It remains true that, in this vast morass, he who seeks to guide himself by the same commonsense cause-and-effect logic he applies to certain other aspects of life may well get stuck.

"Ailment plus medicine equals cure" is an equation widely cherished as true. But the algebra is not so simple. Countless times, of course, the true equation is "Ailment plus Nature equals cure," and if any drug is added its value is zero. Why, a physician once asked, was quackery more prevalent in medicine than in other areas of science? "Because," he answered himself, "the medical quack attributes to himself what is due to Nature. Nature can not build a railway, but she can very often cure disease."[4] Quacks have harvested countless testimonials from customers whose gratitude was thus misplaced.

Another version is this: "symptoms equal disease," hence, add medicine to produce cure. A vastly confusing aspect of medical science, to physician as well as to layman, is the way so many ailments, major and minor, are heralded by the same symptoms. An Atlanta chest specialist, checking medical textbooks, found 56 different causes for spitting blood, 76 different causes for pain in the chest, 137 different causes for coughing.[5] The quack has taken advantage of such confusion, claiming that his bottled remedy has cured a dread disease at the

---

Public Health Problem," mimeographed text of Oct. 23, 1957, address; C.J.S. Thompson, *The Mystic Mandrake* (London, 1934); F. William Saul, *Pink Pills for Pale People* (Philadelphia, 1949), 100-104; Ronald W. Lamont-Havers, "Quackery in Arthritis," *Proceedings, National Congress on Medical Quackery* (1961), 51; Edward Eggleston, *The Transit of Civilization from England to America in the Seventeenth Century* (N.Y., 1900), 60.

[3] Paul F. Eve, *The Present Position of the Medical Profession in Society* (Augusta, Ga., 1849), 22.

[4] Francis J. Shepherd, "Medical Quacks and Quackeries," *Popular Science Monthly*, 23 (June 1883), 162.

[5] Andrew Sparks, "How Good Are Physical Checkups?," *Atlanta Journal and Constitution Magazine*, Apr. 15, 1956, 26.

serious end of the cough spectrum—say, tuberculosis—when in fact a change in the weather has dried up postnasal drip. To the quack and his most susceptible victims, all coughs are consumption, all lumps cancer, all backache kidney disease.

Since "symptoms equal disease" in the mathematics of credulity, the quack can go a step further in tampering with the equation. He can, through his promotion, substitute false symptoms for real symptoms. He can convert normal physiological conditions, like low spirits, tiredness, mild insomnia, spots before the eyes, into dire harbingers of syphilis and insanity. Therefore, in the patent medicine algebra, "non-symptoms equal disease," *ergo,* add Helmbold's Extract of Buchu to produce cure.

It is not fair, to be sure, to characterize this artificially stimulated malaise as non-disease. For it is every bit as traumatic, although of emotional origin, as if caused by germ or virus and may indeed display marked physiological effects, like stiffness, pain, and rash. Half of current sickness, according to the widespread generalization, has a psychogenic component. Certainly the placebo effect has been a subject of recent earnest inquiry in reputable medicine. Henry K. Beecher, the Harvard anesthesiologist, has written that placebos appear to cause improvement in some 35 per cent of all cases, no matter what the affliction.[6] Obviously countless ailments throughout history have been relieved by nostrums or by the ministrations of quacks because the sufferers have had faith in the process. The assurances in printed advertising, or the comforting attentions of self-promoting healers, are sufficient to reverse, at least temporarily, the emotional tides.

In this province of ill health, then, a series of suggestions and counter-suggestions may, in the very susceptible, actually create an ailment where none existed and then remove the ailment, all for a price. Such was the mechanism of the New York "clinic" which frightened healthy young men into thinking they had syphilis or grievous ailments resulting from masturbation, then relieved their fear by electric therapy so vigor-

[6] *Atlanta Journal,* Feb. 22, 1962; *Medical Tribune,* Feb. 15, 1963; *Drug Trade News,* 30 (June 20, 1955), 50; Henry K. Beecher, "Quantitative Effects of Drugs on the Mind," in Talalay, ed., *Drugs in Our Society,* 84.

ous as to persuade its chastened victims they certainly must
have received a cure.[7]

The Nashville orator of 1851, after calling quackery "the
legitimate offspring of ignorance," went on to say that quackery could "only be abridged by elevating the standard of medicine and disseminating a correct public sentiment." In "an intelligent community," he added, reflecting an optimism often
echoed since, quackery could not flourish. Medicine has certainly been elevated since this orator spoke, and education
vastly augmented. Since, in view of this, quackery has not been
vanquished, commentators have raised the question as to
whether ignorance alone is a sufficient explanation for quackery's persistence, or at least whether ignorance must not be
defined so as to include something more than mere lack of
adequate facts plus fuzzy logic. The respectable medical historian, Fielding H. Garrison, referred to a "fetichistic instinct,"
a "primitive craving for the supernatural which is ever latent
in man." This craving he saw as a common aspect underlying
primitive medicine and modern quackery. It is sometimes
tempting to believe in an emotional vaulting toward the occult,
something positive in itself and not merely an act of bad judgment made on the basis of wrong premises and incorrect information. Rabbits' feet afford a steady market in America, at
prices ranging from a dime to five dollars. Charms, voodoo
bags, and love potions have been said to bring in a million
dollars a year from residents of Alabama, Mississippi, and
Louisiana alone. And a Missouri root doctor found customers
for three magical remedies, a cathartic, an emetic, and—as he
called the third—a "rank pizen," all made from the very same
root. *Hibobalorum* was prepared by peeling the bark down-
ward, *Lobobahirum* by peeling it upward, and *Hi-lo-bustem*
by peeling it around.[8]

[7] See ch. 11.
[8] *Addresses Delivered . . . at the Opening of the Medical Department of the University of Nashville*, 9-10; Garrison, "On Quackery as a
Reversion to Primitive Medicine," *Bull., N.Y. Academy of Medicine*, 2s,
9 (Nov. 1933), 601-12; *Atlanta Journal*, Feb. 1, 1948; Willis F. King,
*Quacks and Quackery in Missouri* (St. Louis, 1882), 23-24. See also Paul
G. Brewster, " 'Witchdoctor Advertising': Folklore in the Modern Advertisement," *N.Y. Folklore Quarterly*, 14 (1958), 140-44.

If not so deeply implanted as an instinct, the proneness to quackery may often be related to personality structure. Among the victims of medical charlatanry are many who make their decisions on grounds almost belligerently anti-intellectual. Before elaborating this point, it needs to be stressed that "intellectuals" are not immune to quackery. "I do not know," Erasmus wrote centuries ago, "whether out of the whole world of mortals it is possible to find one who is wise at all times of the day." The quack can erect a beautifully logical structure on the basis of one false but plausible premise. Countless intelligent and educated men have missed the premise, admired the logic, and been trapped. Indeed, it has been argued that the highly literate man, familiar with words and self-assured about their use, may be even more susceptible than his less literate fellow when approached outside his field of expertise with a well-structured and persuasive piece of prose. In his "fantasy life," a Temple University professor has written, the American business executive possesses the same craving for magical cures as does "the Zanzibar pygmy." And Dr. Walter Alvarez insists that "university towns are hot-beds of quackery."[9]

Suffering, of course, may also sweep aside the intellectual defenses of the very bright. Jerry J. Walsh, executive director of the Illinois chapter of the Arthritis and Rheumatism Foundation, himself an arthritis victim, explained for some Senators how this might be.[10]

"But I can guarantee any of you gentlemen . . . ," he said, "that if you are in this bed of pain with arthritis, you will try anything to stop the pain, at any cost. You say, 'What have you got to lose?'

"I know that I went from copper bracelets to buckeyes trying to find a cure. I've tried vibrating machines and diets, and had a chiropractor break one of my legs with his special treatment. Yet, continually, I went back, maybe to the tune of

[9] Erasmus, *The Praise of Folly*, in *Introduction to Contemporary Civilization in the West*, i (N.Y., 1946), 424; "Ex-osteopath," *Quacks and Grafters* (Cincinnati, 1908), 38-40; Alvarez, "The Appeal of Quackery to the Nervous Invalid," *Minnesota Medicine*, 16 (Feb. 1933), 87.

[10] *Frauds and Quackery Affecting the Older Citizen, Hearings before the Special Committee on Aging, United States Senate* (88 Cong., 1 ses., 1963), Part 1, 9-10.

$2,000 or $3,000 more. You don't keep track of the dollars, and in fact you like to forget them. You are always looking for relief. . . .

"If someone would approach me today offering me, with a glib tongue and all, the opportunity of getting better, even better than I am right now, I am sure that I would think it over maybe for a couple of days. If I could do it in the back room unbeknown to you gentlemen, and I wouldn't have much to lose in time or money—and I don't know where I would draw the line on time or money, $200 or $300—I am sure that I would sneak a treatment."

It is sad enough that men of high intelligence and great capability should, through such suffering or through a distortion in their perception, become merely the customers of pseudo-medicine. It is even sadder that the gifted but misguided have now and again used their great influence to champion the quack or even, like the engineer who devised the Micro-Dynameter, to enter upon dubious careers. As has been suggested, dedicated members of Congress, because of a sort of blindness in one sector of their awareness, have given specious drugs strong support and have thus created much belief in the popular mind. Nor has this troublesome astigmatism been absent from the judicial bench.[11]

No one, therefore, can afford complacency, thinking himself forever immune from the quack's ingenious appeals. Yet there are not enough errant intellectuals among us to keep quackery flourishing. The poorly educated do after all pay most of the bills. Among them is a group motivated, it would seem, by something more than sheer lack of knowledge. Some sort of alienation, some sort of perversity, drives these people to follow the most extreme pathways. Often they share with others not so far out as themselves a deep resentment against orthodox authority. Physicians have always been highly vulnerable to attack. They have an impossible job to do: keeping mankind out of the grave and well. Yet they often make pronouncements with an ex cathedra air, and by no means always in the field of their own expertness. They earn more and live better than most of their patients, engendering envy. The high

[11] See ch. 11; William W. Goodrich, "Searching for Medical Truths in the Courtroom," FDC Law Journal, 11 (Sep. 1956), 481-85, 492.

pressure under which they live often leads to a manner resembling brusque busyness, so that intruding upon their time is done uneasily. The therapy they prescribe may be unpleasant and protracted. Some patients are easily frustrated and cannot muster "the patience, discouragement, and degree of cooperation" necessary "in the course of receiving scientific medical care." Much medication, any doctor knows, is prescribed but never taken. Through the centuries physicians have had a hard time with their public image, and motivational research reveals the same today. Through the centuries the quack has played on this widespread latent suspicion of the regular doctor.[12]

Besides criticizing reputable medicine, the quack also lauds his own alleged miraculous cures. Here too he finds an eager hearing with a segment of the people. "There is a class of minds," wrote Dr. Oliver Wendell Holmes over a century ago, "much more ready to believe that which is at first sight incredible, and because it is incredible, than what is generally thought reasonable. *Credo quia impossibile est.*"[13] That class of minds is still extant. Although, through the years, Holmes and other commentators have reflected fruitfully on this phenomenon, not until recently have the insights learned through the modern study of personality been turned toward understanding the quackery-prone mind.

Delegates attending the Second National Congress on Medical Quackery, held in Washington two years after the first Congress, and likewise sponsored by FDA and AMA, listened to one such significant effort at explanation. Dr. Viola Bernard, professor of psychiatry at the Columbia University College of Physicians and Surgeons, recognized that "economic, ethical, socio-cultural and educational factors," all intertwined and reinforcing each other, are deeply involved in the quack victim's motivation. She sought to probe, however, in her address, "the psychological component of this broad issue."[14]

Some emotionally immature people, Dr. Bernard suggested,

---

[12] Viola W. Bernard, "Why People Become the Victims of Medical Quackery," *Proceedings, Second National Congress on Medical Quackery* (1963), 53-56; Ernest Dichter, "The Doctor's Human Relationships," *Medical Annals of the District of Columbia*, 27 (Sep. 1958), 493-94.

[13] Holmes, *Medical Essays*, 33.

[14] Bernard, "Why People Become the Victims of Medical Quackery."

carry over into adulthood the magical thinking common in childhood, "along with an excessive inner sense of their own vulnerability and a corresponding exaggeration of the power of others to harm or protect them." When trouble comes— sickness or stress of some other kind—their fear of death or bodily harm may be exaggerated to an excruciating degree. So too may their trust be exaggerated in him who offers a "get well quick" solution. Reliance on a quack seems to provide a hopeful alternate course to the "effort, frustration and risks of failure which are essential to realistic success in overcoming or improving the stressful situation." The "Medicine Man" is endowed in the believer's mind with the childhood image of "parental omnipotence" over life and death.

The sense of hopelessness making some people prone to quackery, Dr. Bernard asserted, may rest in various emotional problems, much of the mechanism unconscious. Some persons are frustrated because their fantasies of achievement far transcend their capabilities to perform. Their goals, indeed, may be impossibly idealistic, involving "cravings for 'perfect beauty' or other forms of inordinate excelling." Other people "have come to feel it futile to compete in ordinary ways for the rewards of a hostile rejecting society." Among the various categories of the hopeless, with nothing to lose and everything to gain, are to be found the most committed of quackery's converts. People of this personality type can seldom be weaned away from their loyalty by rational appeals; a challenge to their delusion only strengthens its hold. Such converts—as we have seen with Hoxsey's army of dedicated disciples—often treasure a wide assortment of irrational health biases. "There is a close resemblance—and often actual identity—between those who are fervently *for* some medically unauthorized health 'causes' and those who are as fervently *against* certain health programs under medical auspices."

Discussing the same problem in its broader dimensions, the historian Richard Hofstadter has commented that the "most malign forms" of anti-intellectualism are found in a small but "vociferous" segment of the American people, possessing what

---

See also: "Why Do People Detour to Quacks?," *Psychiatric Bull.*, 4 (Summer 1954), 66-69.

he calls "the one-hundred percent mentality—a mind totally committed to the full range of dominant popular fatuities." For this group, imbued "with obscure and ill-directed grievances and frustrations," hatred becomes a kind of creed. A whole host of enemies threaten and evoke their ire. Their leaders, sharing these fears and hates, play on them, provoking letter-writing campaigns and worse. Case histories have been well told in Ralph Lord Roy's *Apostles of Discord* and the techniques of such agitation lucidly analyzed in Leo Lowenthal and Norbert Guterman's *Prophets of Deceit*. Their gospel is perversely irrational. As Hofstadter says, using a Latin phrase very like that cited a century earlier by Oliver Wendell Holmes, *"Credo quia absurdum est."*[15]

The modes of thought, feeling, and action of those committed to the most extreme pathways are often reflected not only in the pursuit of health but also across the whole range of life's concerns. The implications are significant not merely for those who would seek to counter quackery by education, but also for those dedicated to preserving a healthy democracy.

While Dr. Bernard was addressing the delegates attending the Second National Congress on Medical Quackery, down the avenue at another Washington hotel speakers of contrary view were talking before a competing Congress on Health Monopoly, sponsored by the National Health Federation. "Freedom of choice is the American heritage," a former Federal Trade Commissioner was saying, and that freedom should extend to use of Krebiozen. "Personally," the ex-commissioner remarked, "if I like to take two yeast tablets I want no damned bureaucrat breathing his fluoridated breath down my neck."[16]

Dr. Bernard, in seeking to provide insight into why people fall prey to quackery, employed psychoanalytical theory. The use of modern behavioral science research techniques might also furnish enlightening facets of an answer to this disturbing question. In the summer of 1966 such a research project got under way. Instigator of the project was Senator Harrison A.

[15] Hofstadter, *Anti-Intellectualism in American Life* (N.Y., 1963), 20, 37, 42, 118-19, 136; Roy, *Apostles of Discord* (Boston, 1953); Lowenthal and Guterman, *Prophets of Deceit* (N.Y., 1949).

[16] *Wash. Evening Star*, Oct. 25, 1963; *Wash. Post* and *Baltimore Sun*, Oct. 26, 1963.

Williams, Jr. As a member of the Senate's Special Committee on Aging, he had listened to expert witnesses describe how the elderly were being victimized by medical fraud. As chairman of a Subcommittee on Frauds and Misrepresentations Affecting the Elderly, he had explored the matter further. Senator Williams' subcommittee report, issued in January 1965, recommended "a broad research study on consumer attitudes" as fundamental to the proposition that "educational efforts should receive at least as much attention at the Federal level as enforcement efforts." The next month Senator Williams requested the National Institute of Mental Health to help launch such a survey of consumer attitudes relating to medical quackery. During the following year seven federal agencies pooled their planning talents and their funds, the Food and Drug Administration serving as coordinator. In June 1966 a contract was signed with a private research agency to conduct the study. A broad-scale survey of 3,000 citizens selected at random so as to represent a cross-section of the population, the study ambitiously sought to probe many aspects of "Susceptibility to Health Fallacies and Misrepresentations." What role did family and educational background, previous health experiences, age, and psychological orientation have to play in determining susceptibility? How did a person develop the particular pattern of beliefs he had come to hold about sickness and the actions he should take, the practitioners he should consult, to overcome it? It was the hope of the agencies sponsoring the project that profiles of proneness might emerge from the research, a more sophisticated understanding that might permit the fashioning of educational antidotes for quackery more perceptively—and hence successfully—than had yet been possible.[17]

[17] *Frauds and Deceptions Affecting the Elderly*, 89 Cong., 1 ses. (1965), 17; Memorandum of Meeting, Health Fads and Fallacies Survey, Dec. 7, 1965; Dept. of HEW release, May 10, 1966; *FDC Reports*, July 11, 1966, T&G 2. Besides FDA, other agencies supporting the survey were the Administration on Aging, National Institute of Child Health and Human Development, National Institute of Mental Health, Vocational Rehabilitation Administration—all within the Department of Health, Education, and Welfare—the Agricultural Research Service of the Department of Agriculture, and the Veterans Administration.

The letting of the contract for this study happened to coincide with the 60th anniversary of the enactment of the first Pure Food and Drugs Act. To commemorate this pioneering statute, Food and Drug Administration officials hung in the lobby of their new building a portrait of their first chief under this first law, Dr. Harvey Washington Wiley. The man who in 1966 occupied the post of authority which Wiley first had held was another physician, Dr. James L. Goddard, the first physician in more than four decades to head the FDA. Like Dr. Wiley, Dr. Goddard spoke out forthrightly, creating national headlines, and took brisk regulatory action. Prescription medication continued to be the most pressing area of the agency's drug concern, but not the only one. Long dormant, proposed regulations with respect to special dietary products sold direct to consumers were updated and announced: their enforcement, even in the modified form that might result after hearings and court action, would no doubt put a heavy brake on nutritional nonsense. Dr. Goddard raised doubts about therapeutic claims suggested or implied in some proprietary advertising, and he and FTC chairman Paul Rand Dixon got their heads together about how better to cooperate in confronting this problem. Increasingly rigorous enforcement of the laws could be anticipated.[18]

The millennium, of course, will never come. Knaves there will always be, and fools—whatever the justification for their folly—and, therefore, pseudo-medical deception. Yet there is room for guarded optimism that the high tide of medical quackery at the middle of the 20th century might be at least pushed back. Ever stronger federal regulation, more rigorous state laws better enforced, education more appropriately aimed than in the past, an increasing adequacy of sound medical care for a larger portion of the population, these forces might be expected eventually to reduce in some measure quackery's enormous toll in wasted dollars and frustrated hopes for health.

[18] N.Y. Times Magazine, May 15, 1966, 23, 80-102; Advertising Age, 37 (May 30, 1966), 1, 64; (June 20, 1966), 50; FDC Reports, May 2, 1966, 22; June 20, 1966, 3-9; July 4, 1966, T&G 6.

# AFTERWORD

ON a Saturday afternoon in June 1990, on a Chicago El train rumbling from Wrigley Field back to the Loop, a friendly, well-dressed woman handed another passenger a single sheet of paper crowded with suggested uses for aloe vera, plus three telephone numbers from which that botanical in its various processed forms might be ordered. As juice, gel, lotion, facial, shampoo, and activator, aloe vera, according to this simple document, could come to grips with over a hundred health problems, external and internal, from scalp sores to athlete's foot, from migraine headaches to intestinal flu.

From the earliest times, aloe has played a multiple role in medication, favored by Dioscorides and Galen.[1] The aloe vera variety was introduced at least as early as the sixteenth century to the Dutch West Indies, where it was grown on the island of Curaçao. Official from the first edition of the *United States Pharmacopeia*, aloe was prescribed by physicians and was included in such popular patent medicines as Brandreth's Vegetable Universal Pills and Kickapoo Indian Sagwa.[2] Aloe may still be found in the 1990 edition of the *United States Pharmacopeia Drug Information* volume on *Advice to the Patient*, as one of two botanical laxative ingredients in an over-the-counter medicine called Nature's Remedy.[3]

The vast variety of therapeutic values once ascribed to aloe in regular medicine, and still retained to a considerable extent in folk belief, has, under scientific scrutiny, shrunk to a bare minimum.[4] Internally, the dried latex (juice) of aloe has cathartic power. Externally, the fresh gel or mucilage (often confusingly called juice) may be of use in treating minor burns and bruises.

[1] John Uri Loyd, *Origin and History of All the Pharmacopeial Vegetable Drugs, Chemicals and Preparations* (Cincinnati, 1921), vol. 1, 4-14.

[2] Charles W. Oleson, compiler, *Secret Nostrums and Systems of Medicine* (5th ed., Chicago, 1894), 18-19, 22.

[3] United States Pharmacopeial Convention, *USP DI*, vol. 2, *Advice for the Patient* (Rockville, 1990), 801.

[4] Varro E. Tyler, *The Honest Herbal: A Sensible Guide to the Use of Herbs and Related Remedies* (Philadelphia, 1982), 23-24; Varro E. Tyler to author, July 2, 1990.

[ 435 ]

Commercial fabrications, however, have not necessarily shown such dermatological benefits and, indeed, have been toxic to cultured cells on which tests have been made.

Scientific medicine would certainly give no credence to the implied claims on the Chicago handout that aloe vera would prove useful in treating arthritis, asthma, baldness, cancer of the skin, coronary thrombosis, diabetes, female problems, gallstones, glaucoma, psoriasis, and stomach ulcers. Passengers suffering from such severe ailments who yield to the El train softsell promotion and purchase aloe vera for their ills contribute to the nation's multibillion-dollar annual quackery toll.

Just how many billions quackery's bill amounts to can only be estimated. A quarter-century ago, despite the most intensive regulatory and educational campaign against health fraud in the nation's history, the figure approximated, according to an informed public official, "two or more billion" a year, and it was growing.[5] Hardly anyone, however, anticipated the rapidity of its expansion.

By 1984 a subcommittee of the Select Committee on Aging of the House of Representatives, chaired by Claude Pepper of Florida, concluded after a four-year staff study that quackery afflicting the elderly alone added up to "A $10 Billion Scandal."[6] For the population as a whole, testified Victor Herbert at a hearing held by the subcommittee, the annual sum was two-and-a-half times as great.[7] Early in 1990, other expert observers put the figure at $28 billion.[8]

Dr. Herbert, a professor of medicine at the State University of New York Downstate Medical Center, a lawyer, and one of the nation's most dogged foes of quackery, had in his testimony broken down his $25 to $26 billion yearly health fraud total into

[5] See above, 421-22.

[6] *Quackery: A $10 Billion Scandal, A Report by the Chairman of the Subcommittee on Health and Long-Term Care of the Select Committee on Aging,* House of Representatives (98th Cong., 2d sess., May 31, 1984). Hereafter, *Quackery: A $10 Billion Scandal* (Report).

[7] *Quackery: A $10 Billion Scandal, Hearing before the Subcommittee on Health and Long-Term Care of the Select Committee on Aging,* House of Representatives (98th Cong., 2d sess., 1984), 88-91. Hereafter, *Quackery: A $10 Billion Scandal* (Hearing).

[8] James A. Lowell and Alison E. Lowell for the American Council on Science and Health, *Quackery and the Elderly* (New York, 1990), 1.

its component parts.[9] Six billion dollars, he told the House sub-committee, went for "food supplement, pill, powder and potion quackery." About $3 billion each were expended for arthritis, cancer, and heart disease quackery. Several complex categories each accounted for $2 billion: (1) "quack diagnostic tests, such as specious computer questionnaires, hair analyses, cytotoxicity testing, kinesiology, iridology"; (2) "naturopathic, herbalist, oc-cult healing and other cult quackery"; and (3) "clinical ecology, hypoglycemia, nontoxic, metabolic, and natural quackery." In the $1 billion range fell three more quack genres: (1) false treat-ment for Alzheimer's disease and mental illnesses; (2) "quackery-promoting literature"; and (3) diploma mills providing false cre-dentials to those offering dubious regimens of treatment. Thus the terrain of quackery had become broader and more costly than ever and, Dr. Herbert charged, more adept at its ability to "maim and kill."

How to explain the two-decade boom in pseudomedicine? Why did the guarded optimism among fighters opposed to health fraud in the late 1960s dissipate, to be replaced by gloom in the mid-eighties? In part, currents in the broad environment were responsible. On a narrower front, the cohesion and vigor of antiquackery efforts diminished, while the energy, ingenuity, and collaborative efforts of those promoting unproven therapies expanded considerably.

As the century wore on, philosophical currents presented and the impact of events revealed human nature in a less optimistic way than when the century had begun.[10] Error was more firmly rooted than it once had seemed to be, less easily eradicated by that universal panacea, education. Progress, once deemed well-nigh inevitable, had slowed, if not reversed itself. Lookers to-ward the future "shifted their gaze from utopias to dystopias."[11] Many of the disillusioned, especially among the young, came to distrust reason and to flirt with wild varieties of unreason. As-trology soared, not as a pastime but for real: publishing houses

[9] *Quackery: A $10 Billion Scandal* (Hearing), 88-91.

[10] In what follows I rely somewhat on two of my articles, "The Persistence of Medical Quackery in America," *American Scientist* 10 (1972), 318-26, and "The Foolmaster Who Fooled Them," *Yale Journal of Biology and Medicine* 53 (1980), 555-56.

[11] Harry Levin, "The Great Good Place," *New York Review of Books*, March 6, 1980, 47-49.

minted millions from it; almost every campus had a peripheral
course in reading the stars; in time its influence invaded the
whitest houses in the land. Tarot cards, numerology, and palm-
istry flourished. Paperbacks on these themes were among the
hottest-selling items in university bookstores from Cambridge to
Berkeley.[12] A popular magazine announced: "Witches are surfac-
ing everywhere."[13]

Vietnam and Watergate left a legacy of disillusionment with
big government, including its regulatory function. Environmental alarms, especially with regard to nuclear energy, increased
skepticism of big science, including government's scientific
role.[14] An ironic expression of this perspective came in a 1979
commencement address by Kurt Vonnegut. "We would be a lot
safer," the novelist told the graduates, "if the Government would
take its money out of science and put it into astrology and reading palms."[15]

The distrust harbored by citizens went beyond government.
"There is virtually no one," columnist Erma Bombeck asserted,
also in 1979, "who is beyond question or suspicion."[16] Scientists,
Carl Sagan observed, had acquired a negative image in the public mind.[17] Physicians became more vulnerable to sometimes
querulous suspicion. Following a television program in 1978 presenting the perspectives of the medical profession, hundreds of
viewers wrote letters voicing a wide variety of complaints.[18] The
year before, patient visits to orthodox physicians had declined by
eleven percent.[19]

Consumer literacy regarding medicine and science generally,

[12] Bennett Kremen and Peter Collier, "Unrequired Reading: East and West," *New York Times Book Review*, February 15, 1970, Part II, 5, 24, 26.

[13] Brian Vachon, "Witches Are Rising," *Look* 35 (August 24, 1971), 40-44.

[14] Allan Mazur, "Public Confidence in Science," *Social Studies of Science* 7 (1977), 123.

[15] Cited in James Wolcott, "Mod Apostle," *New York Review of Books*, November 22, 1979, 11-12.

[16] Erma Bombeck, "Will America Regain Its Trust?" *Newsweek*, November 14, 1979, 138.

[17] Sagan on MacNeil/Lehrer News Hour, PBS, February 9, 1983.

[18] James T. Patterson, *The Dread Disease: Cancer and Modern American Culture* (Cambridge, Mass., 1987), 262-63.

[19] "The Rise of Alternatives to Drug Therapies and the Implications for Pharmaceutical Research and Development," Foresight Seminars on Pharmaceutical Research and Development, Institute for Alternative Futures, Antioch College, Washington, D.C., undated, 6.

critics charged, had seriously declined. Sagan considered the level of science education in the schools abysmal.[20] John Allen Paulos blamed widespread mathematical illiteracy for muddled judgments in many areas, not least in health.[21] "Today," complained a psychology professor, "we can go from kindergarten through graduate school without having to take a single course in the sort of logic, scientific methods and self-understanding which would help protect us from quackery."[22] John C. Burnham, tracking the theme of popular science and health through American history, compressed his sobering conclusion into his title, *How Superstition Won and Science Lost.*[23]

Whatever their capacity for being confused, Americans had entered upon a period of great preoccupation with keeping fit. Taking control of one's own health, in a variety of ways, amounted to a public passion. "Running," Lewis Thomas wrote in one of his perceptive essays, "a good thing for its own sake, has acquired the medicinal value formerly attributed to rare herbs from Indonesia."[24] But beyond exaggerated expectations lay false advice and fraudulent products. A healthy attitude could be twisted into unhealthy buying. Taking charge of one's health could get distorted into handing that health into the custody of an unscrupulous marketer and paying dearly for the deception. Promoters of specious wares plugged into self-help psychology. A firm vending a fake vitamin, brought to court by the Food and Drug Administration, chose to simplify the confrontation in a publicity release by terming it "Self-help v. 'Doctor knows best,' " thus sneaking its specious product, condemned by scientific medicine, under a rubric invested with popular enthusiasm.[25]

While the cultural climate became more hospitable to irrational ventures, both the criticism and the regulation of health quackery declined from the high plateau of intensity reached in

[20] Sagan on MacNeil/Lehrer News Hour.

[21] John Allen Paulos, *Innumeracy: Mathematical Illiteracy and Its Consequences* (New York, 1988).

[22] Ray Hyman, "Occult Healing," in Stephen Barrett, ed., *The Health Robbers* (2d ed., Philadelphia, 1980), 34.

[23] John C. Burnham, *How Superstition Won and Science Lost: Popularizing Science and Health in the United States* (New Brunswick, 1987).

[24] Lewis Thomas, *Medusa and the Snail* (New York, 1979), 21.

[25] FoodScience Laboratories news release, November 30, 1979.

the 1960s. The American Medical Association, dominant in the realm of nostrum fighting since early in the century, while not abandoning the role completely, in 1975 abolished its quackery committee and closed down its Department of Investigation.[26] The major joint educational campaign against quackery, sponsored by regulatory and voluntary health associations during the sixties, had no counterpart in the seventies. The interpretation of unorthodoxy in the popular media, print and electronic, shifted away from skepticism, often toward drum-beating support. One rare critic wondered if a great many of the self-help health books universally available were not a "$R_x$ for Disaster."[27] David Leff described the science in the checkout-counter tabloid press as a "neo-medieval fantasy world of magic, mystery and miracle."[28] Even mainstream newspapers and magazines have been known to curb their critiques of quackery in order to avoid the threats of economic and legal reprisals.[29] Television and radio talk shows have often given promoters of unscientific health ideas and products a welcome warm enough to constitute endorsement.[30] Some television programs, indeed, have masqueraded as entertainment, even hiring out-of-work actors to serve as studio audience. In fact, however, these programs are nothing but half-hour or hour-long commercial pitches for obesity, baldness, and impotency "cures."[31]

Regulatory control of quackery also receded in the seventies. To make this point starkly was one of Claude Pepper's main goals in his 1984 subcommittee report and hearing.[32] The Postal Ser-

[26] Robert C. Derbyshire, "The Make-Believe Doctors," in Stephen Barrett and Gilda Knight, eds., *The Health Robbers: How to Protect Your Money and Your Life* (Philadelphia, 1976), 88.

[27] "Self-help Health books: $R_x$ for Disaster?" *American Council on Science and Health News & Views* 1 (1979), 1.

[28] David Leff, "Four Wondrous Weeks of Science and Medicine in the Amazing, Incredible Supermarket Press," *National Association of Science Writers Newsletter* 2 (1980), 3.

[29] Max Gunther, "Quackery and the Media," in Barrett and Knight, *The Health Robbers*, 283-300.

[30] Victor Herbert and Stephen Barrett, *Vitamins and "Health" Foods: The Great American Hustle* (Philadelphia, 1981), 141-42; *National Council Against Health Fraud Newsletter* 9 (May/June 1986), 3. Hereafter, *NCAHF Newsletter*.

[31] Ibid., 13 (May/June 1990), 4; Richard Cleland in *1988 National Health Fraud Conference Proceedings*, 30.

[32] *Quackery: A $10 Billion Scandal* (Report), 3-4, 161-79, 190-91; *Quackery: A $10 Billion Scandal* (Hearing), 1-8, 13-16, 134-88.

vice, aided by a 1983 law increasing penalties on repeat offenders, had continued to perform with skill and diligence, although its enforcement officials could handle only a fraction of fraudulent promotions introduced into the mails. Otherwise, federal antiquackery efforts had become "minimal." The Food and Drug Administration spent only .001 percent of its budget combating health fraud. Although possessing an earlier proud record, the FDA's current efforts, in the subcommittee's judgment, "resemble indifference and neglect." The Federal Trade Commission's role in seeking to restrain false advertising related to health also had shrunk to the extent that it had become "almost non-existent, . . . imperceptible." The Commission seemed "strangely paralyzed." Were the federal agencies doing a satisfactory job? "In a word, no." Nor were state and local antiquackery endeavors any more vigorous.

Government inaction, testified a former committee aide, had given a green light to quackery and the perception that "the law of the jungle" was legitimate; it was "open season to rip off the elderly."[33] Congressman Pepper agreed: the recent boom in quackery resulted from its "immense profitability and apparent absence of risk."[34]

The regulatory agencies could make a plausible case that their resources had not been adequate for the broad scope of the responsibilities assigned them by the Congress, and that quackery cases were complex, difficult, and expensive to investigate and litigate.[35] Food and Drug Commissioner Arthur Hull Hayes, Jr., for example, confessed in 1983 that the agency was "simply overmatched. . . . There are too many quacks, too skilled at the quick change of address and product name, for the cumbersome procedures of the FDA." The 1962 Kefauver-Harris Amendments had vastly increased the FDA's obligations for controlling prescription drugs and had prompted a retrospective review—begun in the early seventies and still under way—of over-the-counter medicines, to assure their safety, their efficacy, and the truthfulness of their label claims.[36] The results of this review

[33] Val J. Halamandaris testimony, ibid., 14.
[34] Ibid., 2.
[35] *Quackery: A $10 Billion Scandal* (Report), 169.
[36] James Harvey Young, *American Self-Dosage Medicines: An Historical Perspective* (Lawrence, Kans., 1974), 51-52.

would help curb quackery in the long run, but in the meantime it absorbed much agency time. So too did implementing the Medical Device Amendments that became law in 1976.[37]

As a result of its accumulating duties, the Food and Drug Administration had accorded quackery a lower priority.[38] Moreover, a modification of the way in which the FDA conducted its business made its control of quackery arguably less effective. Partly as a result of advice given the agency by two Citizens Advisory Committees, the FDA began to regulate more by education and less by litigation, becoming, as it were, more of a counseling agency helping legitimate industry untangle its complex problems, and less of a police force. Crises arose from industry's excessive zeal or unwitting accidents, and usually got settled without going to court. Recalls boomed; prosecutions plummeted.

For most of the FDA's mission, involving legitimate drugs, devices, and food additives, the highly scientific, collaborative, rarely litigious approach may well have been the most efficient and effective way. However, to protect the public from old-fashioned, bare-bones, hard-core quackery, as well as from new-fashioned, ingenious, ruthless, hard-core quackery, some critics both within and without the FDA came to believe, required the return to a greater reliance on criminal prosecutions. Victories in court, especially those imposing heavy fines and imprisonment, would cause other promoters with similar operations to stop or to modify their procedures. Court victories would also provide greater credibility to the FDA and others in carrying on expanded antiquackery educational campaigns. Such legal decisions would further help shield critics of quackery from nuisance libel suits.

With the ambient cultural climate favorable and regulators greatly preoccupied with other tasks, proprietors of questionable and specious health products increased the vigor and blatancy of their promotions. They met their would-be customers at all the

[37] Peter Barton Hutt, "A History of Government Regulation of Adulteration and Misbranding of Medical Devices," *Food Drug Cosmetic Law Journal* 44 (1989), 99-117.

[38] James Harvey Young, "The Regulation of Health Quackery," *Pharmacy in History* 26 (1984), 3-12; notes taken at FDA Policy Board Quackery Go-Away, March 25, 1983.

old places. Health food stores boomed, and survey after survey around the country revealed the distorted, often dangerous, counsel offered by the clerks. After AIDS had been identified, for example, Dr. John H. Renner sent students to health food stores in Kansas City to ask if they had products that would help ward off that dread disease, and fifteen of sixteen managers said they did.[39] Many of the herbs for sale in such stores, even herbs with ancient reputations in folk tradition, posed grave hazards to health.[40]

Pyramidal schemes for the vending of nutritional supplements to friends and neighbors, who would then be recruited as salespersons, resurfaced in an inflated way.[41] A newer form for face-to-face selling expanded: the alternative therapy convention, at which a wide variety of wares was displayed at booths, and occasional lectures were delivered to those in attendance. Typical was a cancer-nutrition convention held in Detroit in 1978, boosting such unorthodox modalities as reflexology, iridology, ionization, kinesiology, chelation, and transcutaneous nerve stimulation, plus a broad gamut of vitamin and mineral supplements.[42] Clinics, as will be seen below, also proliferated, both within the nation and outside its borders, a way of reducing or escaping regulatory attack.

Advertising ran rife in specialty catalogs, the magazines of unorthodoxy, and the scantily self-policed press, as well as over the airwaves. Cautious about claims, advertisers relied on getting their curative messages across in First Amendment–protected feature articles, often in the same journals in which the ads appeared.[43] Sometimes such stories were deliberately planted. In 1986 an officer and a former officer of General Nutrition, Inc., the largest chain of health food stores in the United States and Canada, pleaded guilty to misbranding a proprietary form of eve-

[39] John H. Renner in *1988 National Health Fraud Conference Proceedings*, 51. See also *NCAHF Newsletter* 12 (March/April 1989), 2, and James J. Kenney, "Have You Seen Your Vitamitrician Lately?" *Nutrition Forum* 7 (March/April 1990), 13.

[40] Varro E. Tyler, "Hazards of Herbal Medicine," in Douglas Stalker and Clark Glymour, eds., *Examining Holistic Medicine* (Buffalo, 1985), 323-39.

[41] *Nutrition Forum* 4 (February 1987), 15.

[42] Young, "The Foolmaster Who Fooled Them," 560-64. Most of these modalities are given critical analysis in Stalker and Glymour, *Examining Holistic Medicine*.

[43] Young, "The Foolmaster Who Fooled Them," 564.

ning primrose oil by arranging newspaper and magazine stories and radio coverage that falsely praised the oil's value in preventing such serious diseases as arthritis, hypertension, and multiple sclerosis. This campaign was planned to coincide with company advertising.[44]

Advertising became increasingly sophisticated, often composed by M.D.s and Ph.D.s and crafted with cleverness and skill, making pseudoscience sound like science.[45] The slickness of his advertising, suggested Wilbur J. Blechman, Jr., a longtime observer of arthritis quackery, was perhaps the quack's solitary scientific achievement.[46]

Some advertising sent the reader to a health food store. Other advertising persuaded him or her to mail in money. Since use of the mails for ordering and delivering health wares that might transgress fraud statutes posed some degree of risk for promoters, they sought increasingly to dilute this hazard by resorting to such new inventions as the 800 long-distance number and commercial delivery systems. Other modern devices came into play: computers, banks of WATS-line telephones, customized lists for reaching special groups of likely customers, credit cards. "This is the new electronic midway," the attorney general of Maine wrote for Congressman Pepper's subcommittee. "Two-headed cows are easily ignored compared to the late night phone call to your home by an out-of-state caller who uncannily knows that you are an elderly person suffering from a medical ailment and who can convince you to invest large amounts of money for relief and magic lures."[47]

The new techniques were used to preach and expand old gospels. The nutrition myth, so effective in the 1960s, retained its persuasive power.[48] Indeed, when *A Study of Health Practices*

[44] FDA Talk Paper, November 7, 1986; *NCAHF Newsletter* 10 (January/February 1987), 2.

[45] James C. Arsenau and J. Tate Thigpen, "The New Quack—Pseudoscience, Public Relations and Politics," *Journal of the Mississippi State Medical Association* 22 (1981), 202-7; Sorell L. Schwartz testimony, *Quackery: A $10 Billion Scandal* (Hearing), 107.

[46] Wilbur J. Blechman, Jr., testimony, *Frauds Against the Elderly: Health Frauds, Hearing before the Committee on Aging*, House of Representatives, 96th Cong., 2d sess., October 1, 1980, 54.

[47] James Tierney testimony, *Quackery: A $10 Billion Scandal* (Hearing), 178; Richard Cleland in *1988 National Health Fraud Conference Proceedings*, 88.

[48] See above, 350-54, 432.

*and Opinions*, sponsored by seven federal agencies, appeared in 1972, it revealed that a large proportion of American adults engaged in self-treatment that could be characterized as "rampant empiricism," guided by no coherent body of theory, true or false—except in one signal respect.[49] When it came to self-treatment with vitamins and food supplements, consumers did adhere to a set of doctrines, and these bore a remarkable resemblance to the fake tenets of the nutrition myth. Three out of every four Americans believed that, no matter how nutritionally adequate their diet, using extra vitamins would imbue them with added pep.

Nutritional solutions to health problems developed into the dominant feature of unorthodoxy in the years that followed.[50] Modifications of diet and other lifestyle changes aimed at preventing and ameliorating serious degenerative diseases became an increasing concern of scientific medicine as the major infectious diseases came increasingly under control. As so often before, unorthodox medicine mirrored a theme of mainstream science, distorting it to suit its own promotional purposes. The preoccupations of many consumers made them unusually receptive to such carefully crafted promotions. For those seeking to keep fit by their own efforts, diet was a major mode of self-help. Especially for those desiring to keep thin for the sake of health and beauty, a compelling urge since early in the century and now at a new peak of intensity, promoters vended an incredible

[49] *A Study of Health Practices and Opinions* was conducted by National Analysts, Inc. and published by the National Technical Information Service of Springfield, Virginia. Its conclusions were summarized in J. W. Buchan, "America's Health: Fallacies, Beliefs, Practices," *FDA Consumer* 6 (October 1972), 4-10.

[50] Among the many works relevant to this paragraph are Stephen Barrett, "Diet Facts and Fads," and Victor Herbert, "The Health Hustlers," in Barrett, *The Health Robbers*, 49-68, 173-83; Theodore Berland, *Rating the Diets* (New York, 1980); Editors of Consumer Books, *Health Quackery* (Mount Vernon, N.Y., 1980); Victor Herbert, *Nutrition Cultism: Facts and Fictions* (Philadelphia, 1980); Herbert and Barrett, *Vitamins & "Health" Foods*; Gilda Knight, "The Confused Crusaders," and Jean Mayer, "Weight Control and 'Diets': Facts and Fads," in Barrett and Knight, *The Health Robbers*, 47-59, 175-87; Hillel Schwartz, *Never Satisfied: A Cultural History of Diets, Fantasies, and Fat* (New York, 1986); Daniel Tatkon, *The Great Vitamin Hoax* (New York, 1968); Elizabeth M. Whelan and Fredrick J. Stare, *Panic in the Pantry: Food Facts, Fads, and Fallacies* (New York, 1975); and the newsletter *Nutrition Forum*, Stephen Barrett, ed. *Newsweek*, April 30, 1990, and *U.S. News and World Report*, May 14, 1990, had cover stories on reducing.

range of food supplements, drugs, devices, dietary regimens, and books of advice, promising an easier solution than cutting down on calories through self-restraint. The vitamin and mineral market kept booming, with predictions rosy for continuing growth.[51] In time, quackery related to the most dire of diseases, cancer and AIDS, came to encompass a nutritional component.

Critics continued to expose the fallacies and caution of the hazards in pseudonutrition: that consumers on a rounded diet did not need vitamin supplementation, that megadosing could not ward off dread diseases and might itself injure the body, that certain so-called vitamins were not vitamins at all, that some products sold for weight loss were worthless and others could kill. The warning words of scientific nutritionists, dietitians, consumerists, and regulators, however, were outweighed a thousand or more to one by the printed and oral verbiage of pitchmen. Consequently, as a witness asserted at the Pepper subcommittee hearing, "the biggest area of quackery right now is phony diet pills, phony diet cures," a number of which were on display in the hearing room.[52]

The Food and Drug Administration had been concerned with the disordered state of the nutritional marketplace for a long time. In 1962 the agency had announced its intention to update the regulations for food supplements first put in place after the Food, Drug, and Cosmetic Act had been passed in 1938.[53] This proposal led to marathon hearings that accumulated a record of 32,000 pages. In 1973 the FDA issued revised proposals that it hoped might ultimately rationalize the promotion of vitamins and supplements.

Charging to the attack came the health food industry, led by the National Health Federation, many of whose members would be forced to change drastically their promotional practices should the regulations go into effect.[54] Flying furiously the flag

[51] *FDC Reports*, April 16, 1984, T&G 7.

[52] Val J. Halamandaris testimony, *Quackery: A $10 Billion Scandal* (Hearing), 12.

[53] In the discussion of the background to the vitamin law of 1976 I follow my treatment in *American Self-Dosage Medicines*, 46-50, and in "The Agile Role of Food: Some Historical Reflections," in John N. Hathcock and Julius Coon, eds., *Nutrition and Drug Interrelations* (New York, 1978), 13-16.

[54] For the origin of the National Health Federation, see above, 383-84, 392, 400-401, 431.

of "medical freedom," NHF leaders stirred up their customers into a frightened and frenzied lobbying force of considerable numbers. This development was just what had worried Food and Drug Commissioner Alexander Schmidt the most.

"The opposition with which we are most concerned," Schmidt announced,

> stems from the honest fears of many citizens. Some fear that FDA is going to make certain vitamin pills unavailable or, if available, then only by prescription and at higher cost. Others fear that FDA may infringe on their right to decide what they will eat. None of this is true. The single most important purpose and effect of the regulation is to require full and honest labeling and fair promotion of vitamin and mineral products as the basis for a more informed consumer choice.[55]

The misguided customers of nutritional pseudoscience chose to believe their marketers rather than the regulators. Prodded by the NHF, thousands of common citizens expressed to members of the Congress their anger about the FDA's proposals and their support of a bill that had been introduced by Congressman Craig Hosmer, cosponsored by 150 other members of the House.[56] The bill, if it became law, would not only negate the FDA's attempt to tighten controls, but would cut back the agency's authority to regulate vitamins and food supplements to a pre-1938 level.

In the three-year contest that followed, some two million NHF-generated letters flooded Congress. Some members said that the vitamin-control issue spurred more mail than Watergate.[57] Besides responding to such pressure from constituents, some congressmen were also no doubt voting their own convictions, beguiled by the constant reiteration of the nutrition myth. In 1974 a variant version of the first bill passed the Senate by a margin of 81 to 10.[58]

In the 94th Congress, during the nation's centennial year, a revised Senate version of the vitamin bill became attached as a rider to a "must" bill, the Health Research and Health Services

[55] FDA news release, August 1, 1973.
[56] H.R. 643, S. 2801, *Congressional Record*, 93rd Cong., 1st sess., 53, 40936.
[57] Herbert and Barrett, *Vitamins & "Health" Foods*, 131-32.
[58] *Cong. Record*, 93rd Cong., 2d sess., 7455-56, 32376.

AFTERWORD

Act. The House version passed without the rider, but the conference committee accepted it. Both houses then concurred, and President Gerald Ford quickly signed the bill into law.[59]

Congress cannot be said to have given the issue serious consideration, as indicated by the devious parliamentary strategy. Moreover, the 94th Congress did not hold hearings on the bill, despite strong opposition to it by a wide spectrum of groups, including the American Society of Clinical Nutrition, the Committee on Nutrition of the American Academy of Pediatrics, the American Association of Retired Persons, Consumers Union, and Ralph Nader's associates.[60] A trade newsletter termed the course of events "one of the 'legislative miracles' in a lifetime."[61]

The 1976 amendment to the 1938 act represented the first retrogressive step in federal legislation respecting self-treatment wares since the initial Food and Drugs Act became law in 1906. The amendment, as the Food and Drug Administration viewed it, would bar the agency from "limiting the potency of vitamins and minerals in dietary supplements to nutritionally useful levels; classifying a vitamin or mineral preparation as a 'drug' because it exceeds a nutritionally rational and useful potency; requiring the presence in dietary supplements of nutritionally essential vitamins and minerals; [and] prohibiting the inclusion in dietary supplements of useless ingredients with no nutritional value."[62]

Toward the close of this legislative adventure, Commissioner Schmidt spoke of the then pending bill as "a charlatan's dream."[63] The law did indeed embolden the purveyors of food supplements and accelerated the trend toward moving unortho-

[59] *Cong. Record*, 94th Cong., 1st sess., 1785, 9262, 10023, 10839, 11086; 90 U.S. Stat., 410-13.

[60] *Vitamin, Mineral, and Diet Supplements*, Public Health and Environment Subcommittee of the Committee on Interstate and Foreign Commerce, House of Representatives, 93rd Cong., 1st sess., Committee print No. 11, 1973; *Food Supplement Legislation, 1974, Hearings on S.2801 and S.3867*, Health Subcommittee of the Committee on Labor and Public Welfare, U.S. Senate, 93rd Cong., 2d sess., 1974; C. E. Butterworth, Letter from American Society for Clinical Nutrition to members of Congress, July 8, 1975; M. A. Holliday, Letter from Committee on Nutrition, American Academy of Pediatrics, to members of Congress, June 19, 1975.

[61] *FDC Reports*, September 1, 1975, 5.

[62] Harold Hopkins, "Regulating Vitamins and Minerals," *FDA Consumer* 10 (July/August 1976), 10-11; FDA Talk Paper, 1976.

[63] Ibid.

[ 448 ]

dox pills and potions from risky "drug" status into the presumably safer "food" category.

The National Health Federation lobbied strenuously for more forthright legislation to give consumers access to products regulators could otherwise deny them. Senator Steven D. Symms introduced such a bill into the 94th Congress. It would have repealed the requirement of proving to the FDA's satisfaction the efficacy of a drug for its indicated uses before a promoter could market it in interstate commerce.[64] This stipulation had been added to food and drug law by the Kefauver-Harris amendments of 1962. The bill did not pass, but others followed it, introduced by Senator Jesse Helms and by Congressman Lawrence McDonald, a physician and adviser to an NHF publication.[65] The NHF also pushed a "Foods are not Drugs" bill that would bar the FDA from taking actions against manufacturers or distributors of foods who made claims that their products would "prevent, cure, or mitigate disease."[66]

Sometimes the NHF sought to keep legislation from passing, or even from being considered. In connection with his hearing in 1984, Congressman Pepper introduced three bills to strengthen in various ways government's authority to control health fraud.[67] The NHF termed the proposals "lysenkoism," and, when they did not pass in that session, worked hard to persuade Pepper not to introduce them in the next.[68] "NHF President Maureen Salaman," reported William T. Jarvis in the *National Council Against Health Fraud Newsletter*, "went so far as to buy a plane ticket on a flight with Mr. Pepper and arranging to have her seat assignment next to him and bent his ear all the way to his destination."[69] Probably sensing the futility of the effort, Pepper did not reintroduce his bills.

---

[64] H.R. 12573, 94th Cong., 2d sess., 6564; Herbert and Barrett, *Vitamins & "Health" Foods*, 132. NHF legislative representative Clinton Miller presented his defense of such a bill at the Pepper subcommittee hearing. *Quackery: A $10 Billion Scandal* (Hearing), 112-13.

[65] S. 1683, *Cong. Record*, 95th Cong., 1st sess., 18628; Barrett, *The Health Robbers*, 254.

[66] *NCAHF Newsletter Bulletin Board* 8 (June 1985).

[67] H.R. 6049, 6050, 6051, 98th Cong., 2d sess., 21714; *Food Chemical News*, August 6, 1984, 49-50.

[68] NHF publication cited in *NCAHF Newsletter Bulletin Board* 8 (June 1985).

[69] *NCAHF Newsletter* 9 (March/April 1986), 3; *NCAHF Newsletter Bulletin Board* 8 (June and August 1985).

The National Health Federation promoted a number of crusades.[70] It fought the extension of fluoridation tooth and nail. It campaigned against state laws to license scientific nutritionists and to bar the untrained from using the designation. It took a stand against such established health measures as milk pasteurization and vaccination for smallpox and polio. It supported an expansive gamut of unorthodox health doctrines and practices in its publications, special mailings, and convention programs. It helped fund litigation involving persons whose causes it favored. For most of its members, Stephen Barrett concluded, "Nutrition is a religion, not a science." The NHF also sought to blame the nation's health ills on organized medicine and its conspiratorial allies. "The biggest and the most costly and the most dangerous quackery rampant in the United States today," NHF's legislative representative, Clinton Miller, charged at the Pepper subcommittee hearing, "is the medical quackery inside organized medicine as represented by the American Medical Association."[71]

The NHF and its allies in the nutritional products industry also counterattacked those who criticized their policies. William Jarvis, recipient of the NHF's initial "Health Bigot of the Year Award," told of a conversation with Clinton Miller in which the latter said, "There is nothing personal in all of this, but when you are the enemy, we have to clobber you."[72] Such blows included comparing Jarvis, Stephen Barrett, and Victor Herbert to Hitler, Goering, and Goebbels. Herbert told the Pepper subcommittee of an interview, appearing in an NHF publication, with Robert Atkins, formulator of a diet disparaged by scientific nutritionists.[73] Atkins had stated that Herbert "house[d] an evil spirit that needs to be exorcised." Soon thereafter Herbert had received death threats by mail and phone.

The NHF placed on its board of governors David T. Ajay, president of the National Nutritional Foods Association, a trade

[70] Stephen Barrett has discussed the NHF program in chapters entitled "The Unhealthy Alliance" in Barrett and Knight, *The Health Robbers*, 189-201; Barrett, *The Health Robbers*, 244-56; Herbert and Barrett, *Vitamins & "Health" Foods*, 116-38 (quotation at 138); and in his *The Unhealthy Alliance: Crusaders for "Health" Freedom* (New York, 1988).

[71] *Quackery: A $10 Billion Scandal* (Hearing), 111.

[72] *NCAHF Newsletter Bulletin Board* 9 (January/February 1986).

[73] *Quackery: A $10 Billion Scandal* (Hearing), 91.

association of health food producers, distributors, and retailers.[74] In 1978 Ajay proclaimed "Operation Counterattack," a series of lawsuits against critics of the industry. The next year Ajay and two other distributors launched a libel suit for themselves and the NNFA against Elizabeth M. Whelan, executive director of the American Council of Science and Health, and Fredrick J. Stare, Emeritus Professor of Nutrition of the Harvard School of Public Health, both sharp critics of nutritional quackery.[75] None of the plaintiffs was mentioned in the publications at issue, and a judge eventually threw the case out of court. For the defendants it was a welcome, if time-consuming and costly, victory.

In the 1970s, the National Health Federation, with its aggressive leadership, more than a hundred local chapters, and 25,000 members, increased its influence by allying with the expanding ranks of the supporters of Laetrile, an unproven cancer remedy.[76] In the early days of the NHF, its founder, Fred J. Hart, had collaborated with Harry Hoxsey, then the most prominent figure in cancer unorthodoxy, who was locked in a struggle with the Food and Drug Administration he was to lose in 1960.[77] Hart, during this period, testified against a bill being considered by the California legislature aimed at curbing cancer quackery.[78] Another hostile witness was Ernst Krebs, Jr., codeveloper, with his father, of Laetrile. When the FDA forced Hoxsey to abandon his Dallas clinic, his successor began treating cancer patients with Laetrile.[79] The FDA made its first seizure of Laetrile at the clinic in 1960. A nurse who had long been on Hoxsey's staff carried his medications across the border to Mexico, where they are still prescribed for cancer.[80] That is true also of Laetrile, but be-

---

[74] Barrett, *The Unhealthy Alliance*, 7.

[75] James Harvey Young and Robert S. Stitt, "Nutrition Quackery: Upholding the Right to Criticize," *Food Technology* 35 (December 1981), 42-46, 64.

[76] Gerald E. Markle and James C. Petersen, "Resolution of the Laetrile Controversy: Past Attempts and Future Prospects," in H. Tristram Englehardt and Arthur L. Caplan, eds., *Scientific Controversies: Case Studies in the Resolution and Closure of Disputes in Science and Technology* (Cambridge, 1987), 326.

[77] See above, 383-88.

[78] San Francisco District Report, December 9, 1957, San Francisco District File, CF 10 183, John Beard Memorial Foundation, vol. 4, Food and Drug Administration Records (San Francisco).

[79] FDA Drug and Device Notice of Judgment 6543 (1960).

[80] Ken Ausebel, "The Troubling Case of Harry Hoxsey," *New Age Journal*, July/August 1988, 43-49, 78-79, 86; James A. Lowell, "Hoxsey Treatment Still Available," *Nutrition Forum* 4 (December 1987), 89-91.

AFTERWORD

fore its almost complete exile Laetrile provoked "one of the most politicized medical disputes in American history."[81]

The Laetrile of commerce was amygdalin, a chemical first isolated from bitter almonds in 1830 by two French chemists, although the product Ernst Krebs, Jr., trademarked as Laetrile had a slightly different structure.[82] The significant ingredient was cyanide, some six percent by weight,[83] and by centering on this poison Krebs fashioned his first explanation as to how Laetrile combated cancer.[84] When the Laetrile molecule reaches the cancer site, Krebs argued, an enzyme especially abundant in cancerous areas splits the molecule, releasing hydrogen cyanide to kill the cancer. Another enzyme protects normal cells, detoxifying any cyanide that strays into them. Thus Laetrile purportedly fulfills a prime objective of cancer chemotherapy: specificity of action. An impressed business manager for a group of doctors opined that Krebs had made a major step toward receiving a Nobel Prize. Soon, however, cancer specialists were to deny Krebs's premise. The normal cells turn out to contain more of the molecule-cleaving enzyme than do neoplastic tissues. Indeed, Laetrile administered by injection undergoes scarcely any metabolic breakdown and is excreted virtually intact in the urine. Laetrile taken orally, however, can be split by ingredients in food, releasing its poison and placing the person at grave risk. Indeed, both Laetrile and apricot kernels from which it was made killed a number of people.[85]

Under the management of the two Krebs, father and son, Laetrile developed modest sales but encountered increasing criticism from cancer scientists and the beginning of legal restraints from both California and federal regulators. Indeed, in time, the would-be Nobelist spent several months in jail.[86]

[81] James C. Petersen and Gerald E. Markle, "Expansion of Conflict in Cancer Controversies," in Louis Kriesberg, ed., *Research in Social Movements, Conflict and Change* (Greenwich, Conn., 1981), IV, 164.

[82] Food and Drug Administration, *Laetrile: The Commissioner's Decision* (Rockville, 1977), 4-10. Hereafter, FDA, *Laetrile*. This document is reprinted from the *Federal Register*, August 5, 1977.

[83] Herbert, *Nutrition Cultism*, 15-32.

[84] The narrative account of Laetrile is drawn principally from my chapter "Laetrile in Historical Perspective" in Gerald E. Markle and James C. Petersen, eds., *Politics, Science, and Cancer: The Laetrile Phenomenon* (Boulder, 1980), 11-60.

[85] Herbert, *Nutrition Cultism*, 23-32.

[86] *San Francisco Chronicle*, May 13, 1983.

## AFTERWORD

A series of happenstances lofted Laetrile into the national limelight. As the Krebs pair faltered, a Canadian adventurer, Andrew R. L. McNaughton, took control of Laetrile's destinies. He trumpeted his discontent when he failed to secure an Investigational New Drug exemption from the Food and Drug Administration, even though he had not submitted adequate evidence. He expanded his drum-beating, placing in the Hearst *American Weekly* articles penned by G. D. Kittler, the man who thought Krebs, Jr., should win a Nobel Prize. This admirer then published a paperback, promising that Laetrile would "be to cancer what insulin was to diabetes."[87] McNaughton gained a recruit from within the cancer research establishment, Dean Burk, who gave Laetrile a semblance of scientific legitimacy. McNaughton sought to escape rising regulatory pressures by establishing manufacturing and treatment facilities in Tijuana, to which American patients began to go and from which Laetrile was smuggled into the United States and distributed clandestinely.

To McNaughton's assistance came a growing network of institutional support. The first patient treated in Tijuana established the International Association of Cancer Victims and Friends to publicize Laetrile, help cancer victims get to Mexico, and fly the flag of medical freedom. This organization and another that seceded from it, the Cancer Control Society, had unusual success in bringing Laetrile's message to members of the middle class, including some with considerable education.[88] More important still for Laetrile's expansion of social and political influence was the arrest in 1972 of a California physician, John A. Richardson, for prescribing Laetrile in violation of the state's antiquackery law. Two trials ended with hung juries. The California Board of Medical Quality Assurance then stepped in and revoked Richardson's license on grounds of incompetence and gross negligence.

These events upset some of Richardson's fellow members of the John Birch Society. Such dedicated disciples of freedom-

---

[87] G. D. Kittler, *Control for Cancer* (New York, 1963).

[88] Gerald E. Markle, James C. Petersen, and Morton O. Wagenfeld, "Notes from the Cancer Underground: Participation in the Laetrile Movement," *Social Science and Medicine* 12 (1978), 31-37; Morton O. Wagenfeld, Yvonne M. Lissing, Gerald E. Markle, et al., "Notes from the Cancer Underground: Health Attitudes and Practices of Participants in the Laetrile Movement," *Social Science and Medicine* 13 (1979), 483-85.

from-government doctrine saw in this physician's case a prime example of bureaucratic oppression. Led by Robert W. Bradford, a nuclear technician at Stanford University, Richardson's friends formed the Committee for Freedom of Choice in Cancer Therapy. By 1977 Bradford claimed five hundred chapters with some 35,000 members throughout the nation. Experienced in Birch battles against fluoridation and sex education, Committee members used a wide variety of tactics to condemn the community of cancer scientists, to castigate its allegedly futile therapeutic methods of cutting, burning, and poisoning, and to make any governmental interference with a cancer patient's right to use Laetrile or any other unorthodox treatment seem a violation of the Constitution and the fundamental rights of man.

Laetrile at this time, although still the same substance, had changed guises again. Ernst Krebs, Jr., while retaining much of his original theory as to Laetrile's mode of action, had converted cancer to a deficiency disease and transformed Laetrile from a chemotherapeutic drug to a vitamin, designated B-17. In addition to controlling cancer, B-17 could now prevent it. Nutritional scientists denied that Laetrile fulfilled any of the criteria for a true vitamin. "In short," summed up veteran vitamin researcher Thomas H. Jukes, "nothing could be less like a vitamin than laetrile."[89] Such criticism did not deter Laetrile enthusiasts. Krebs, Jr., testifying before Senator Edward Kennedy's Subcommittee on Health in 1977, termed Laetrile "a scientific revolution as profound as the germ theory of disease . . . and the Copernican theory." What Vitamin C is to scurvy, niacin to pellagra, and Vitamin D to rickets, he asserted, Vitamin B-17 is to cancer.[90] If every American took Laetrile regularly, Dr. Richardson told the subcommittee, "in 20 years cancer would be relegated to the dusty pages of history."

[89] Thomas H. Jukes testimony, vol. 0-1, FDA Administrative Record, Laetrile, Docket No. 77N-0048; National Nutrition Consortium, Inc., Statement on Laetrile–Vitamin B-17, December 21, 1976; Jukes, "Laetrile, the Bogus 'Vitamin B-17,' " in A. Neuberger and T. H. Jukes, *Human Nutrition: Current Issues and Controversies* (Lancashire, 1982), 233-41.

[90] Testimony of John A. Richardson, Robert W. Bradford, Ernst T. Krebs, Jr., and Bruce Halstead, *Banning of the Drug Laetrile from Interstate Commerce by FDA,* Hearing before the Subcommittee on Health and Scientific Research of the Committee on Human Resources, U.S. Senate, 95th Cong., 1st sess., 272-74. Hereafter, Hearing before Kennedy Subcommittee.

Besides fighting a propaganda battle in the arena of public opinion, Laetrile's champions sought victories in legislatures and courts. The main legislative effort came in the states. Alaska passed the first law giving Laetrile special distribution status, and by the early 1980s half the states had enacted statutes, the terms varying from place to place.[91] Members of the Committee for Freedom of Choice played a major lobbying role in the state campaigns.

The most significant judicial encounter began with patients who had returned from Laetrile clinics in Mexico and wanted to prevent the Food and Drug Administration from interfering with their imports of the amygdalin product for continuing treatment. The principal plaintiff who emerged was Glen L. Rutherford, a manufacturer's representative from Conway Springs, Kansas.[92] At the Tijuana clinic, he had been treated with Laetrile and enzymes, and an intestinal polyp had been cauterized. Cancer specialists believed that the excision of a polyp solved the problem in a high proportion of cases, but Rutherford wanted the reassurance of Laetrile. In 1975 he won this right from a federal judge in Oklahoma. Judge Luther Bohanon ruled that Rutherford and all other cancer patients as a class who secured physicians' affidavits designating them as terminally ill could import a limited amount of Laetrile in both injectable and oral forms for their personal use.

Considering the deliberate pace of the law during the process of appeals, that privilege stretched through a dozen years.[93] The Circuit Court, taking into account amygdalin's hazard when ingested by mouth, barred oral dosage forms. The Supreme Court ruled unanimously that the safety and efficacy standards of the law did indeed apply to terminal patients. Despite the Court's failure to address all other issues explicitly, "the tone of the opinion," commentators observed, "left no doubt as to the Supreme

[91] *New York Times*, May 2, August 16 and 25, 1977, June 7, 1978; Status Report of State Legislative Actions Regarding Laetrile, Public Health Service memorandum, January 22, 1988.

[92] Rutherford vs. U.S., 399 F. Supp. 1208 (W.D. Oklahoma, 1975); *Medical World News*, June 28, 1976, 17-20.

[93] 542 F. 2d 1137 (10th Circuit Court, 1976); 424 Supp. 105 (W.D. Oklahoma, 1977); 429 Supp. 506 (W.D. Oklahoma, 1977); 442 U.S. 544 (1979); 616 F. 2d 455 (10th Circuit, 1980); 499 U.S. 937 (1980); FDA, "Laetrile Chronology"; Order No. CIV-75-0218-B, W.D. Oklahoma, March 21, 1987.

Court's determination to uphold the FDA ban on laetrile."[94] The Circuit Court so interpreted the decision and ordered Judge Bohanon so to rule. He finally did so in 1987. The FDA then issued an Import Alert, stating that, as an unapproved drug, Laetrile under its various designations could not be brought into the country.[95]

Along this extended judicial trail, the Food and Drug Administration was ordered to conduct administrative proceedings, and Commissioner Donald Kennedy and his staff turned this task into as thorough and insightful a review of a highly promoted unorthodox drug as could be found in the American literature.[96] The report countered the various claims made for Laetrile's effectiveness in cancer, disputing the shifting theories, remarking upon the inadequate anecdotal character of pro-Laetrile reporting, and citing the lack of promise in numerous well-controlled animal studies made at the National Cancer Institute and private cancer research centers. The report criticized as unpersuasive the few animal tests interpreted as favorable to Laetrile by Dean Burk and others. The commissioner found that Laetrile's appeal lay in the psychology of patients and their families caught in the crushing cancer crisis. The "disparagement of conventional therapy" by Laetrile advocates was "morally reprehensible," leading sufferers away from proven treatment.

Commissioner Kennedy further met the "freedom of choice" argument head-on. Congress had decided, he noted, "that the absolute freedom to choose an ineffective drug was properly surrendered in exchange for the freedom from the danger to each person's health and well-being from the sale and use of worthless drugs." In any case, the choice to use Laetrile, made in an atmosphere of double stress, compounded from the fear of disease and the zeal of Laetrile advocates, with seldom any "rational laying out of competing arguments," could not accurately be described as free.

The litigation and the legislative battles in the states made Laetrile an issue of national concern. News magazines carried cover

---

[94] Jonathan Brant and John Graceffa, "*Rutherford, Privitera*, and *Chad Green:* Laetrile's Setbacks in the Courts," *American Journal of Law and Medicine* 6 (Spring 1980), 151-71.
[95] FDA Import Alert, 62-01 Revision, December 7, 1987.
[96] FDA, *Laetrile*.

stories, and high-ranked television programs looked at Laetrile.[97] Conservative columnists, most notably James J. Kilpatrick, attracted to the freedom of choice theme, gave Laetrile favorable attention.[98] The promoters intensified their own publicity with a series of paperback books.[99] The National Health Federation put leading Laetrile figures—including Andrew McNaughton and Glen Rutherford—on its board of governors and gave the Laetrile cause continuing support with publicity, financing, and legal aid.[100] A majority of Americans came to believe decriminalization of Laetrile would be a good idea.[101] Some Laetrile leaders sounded smug about their prospects.[102]

"Rest assured, gentlemen," Bradford told Senator Kennedy's subcommittee, "that the people demand Laetrile. . . . And they are going to get it whether Big Brother wants it or not. . . . We cannot expect that thousands of American cancer sufferers are going to wait for more long years, while the Federal Government fiddle-faddles through animal tests and more redtape. . . . Do we really want another American civil war?"

Laetrile advocates hoped that they might yet achieve the repeal of the effectiveness provision in the drug law.[103] During the 1980 presidential campaign, Ronald Reagan was quoted in an interview in the National Health Federation journal as favoring such action.[104] Richard Crout, director of the FDA's Bureau of Drugs, feared that this might happen and hoped that, if "the political heat" engendered by Laetrile pressure groups got too much for Congress, the members might choose a less extreme course, exempting Laetrile alone from the effectiveness require-

[97] *Newsweek*, June 27, 1977; *60 Minutes*, CBS, March 31, 1974.

[98] *Atlanta Constitution*, August 21, 1975; February 10, April 1, May 13, 1976; April 19, December 8, 1977; February 9, 1978.

[99] G. Edward Griffin, *World Without Cancer* (Westlake Village, Calif., 1974); Mike Culbert, *Freedom from Cancer* (Seal Beach, Calif., 1976); John Richardson, *Laetrile Case Histories* (New York, 1977); Robert Bradford, *Now That You Have Cancer* (Los Altos, Calif., 1977).

[100] Barrett, *The Unhealthy Alliance*, 9, 11-12.

[101] *Washington Post*, June 27, 1977.

[102] Robert Bradford testimony, Hearing before Kennedy Subcommittee, 272, 310.

[103] H.R. 53, *Cong. Record*, 95th Cong., 1st sess., 127.

[104] *Public Scrutiny*, 3 (August 1980), 1; J. Richard Crout, "The Drug Regulatory System: Reflections and Predictions," *Food Drug Cosmetic Law Journal* 36 (1981), 106-19.

ment. That Dr. Crout should venture to discuss such a worst case possibility suggested its potential for happening.

As public sentiment favoring Laetrile mounted, and as tens of thousands of cancer patients forsook orthodox therapy to rely on Laetrile instead, a debate began within the scientific community. Should the established rules for testing new drugs be firmly adhered to, or, in Laetrile's case, should the rules be breached, with the government itself assuming the testing burden, or even, as the distinguished editor of the *New England Journal of Medicine*, F. J. Ingelfinger, suggested, should Laetrile be made freely available in the marketplace, with detailed records kept of its use?[105] After great deliberation, the middle course was followed. The National Cancer Institute solicited case histories from physicians who had used Laetrile and, in the mass of unchecked data, found the minimal suggestive evidence to warrant proceeding with clinical trials.[106] The FDA doubted that the evidence was sufficient but recognized societal reasons for pushing forward to resolve the issue scientifically.[107]

After consulting with Laetrile physicians, NCI scientists devised protocols that defined Laetrile as amygdalin and included a special diet and numerous vitamins in the regimen, according to then current Laetrile treatment practice.[108] The FDA gave the NCI an Investigational New Drug exemption, thus bringing the experiment under the law. Charles Moertel of the Mayo Clinic led the team of investigators at four cancer research hospitals. With the trials having months to run, Dr. Moertel surprised the scientific community and the nation when, on April 30, 1981, he made an initial report to the American Society of Clinical Oncology.[109] "Laetrile has been tested," he declared. "It is not effective." It did not relieve symptoms of cancer patients or extend

[105] F. J. Ingelfinger, "Laetrilomania," *New England Journal of Medicine* 296 (1978), 1167-68.

[106] Neil M. Ellison, et al., "Special Report on Laetrile: The NCI Laetrile Review," ibid., 299 (1978), 549-52.

[107] *Food and Drug Administration and the 95th Congress* (Rockville, 1978), 116-17.

[108] Charles G. Moertel, et al., "A Pharmacologic and Toxicological Study of Amygdalin," *JAMA* 245 (1981), 591-94; Moertel, et al., "A Clinical Trial of Amygdalin (Laetrile) in the Treatment of Human Cancer," *New England Journal of Medicine* 306 (1982), 201-6.

[109] *Science News*, May 9, 1981, 293-94.

AFTERWORD

their life span. In only one case was there a reduction of tumor size, but it proved temporary.

The fuller published report of the investigative team confirmed and amplified Dr. Moertel's announcement.[110] Laetrile had produced "no substantive benefit . . . in terms of cure, improvement, or stabilization of cancer, improvement of symptoms related to cancer, or extension of life span." Indeed, "patients died rapidly." Oral dosages of amygdalin produced some evidence of cyanide toxicity. In sum, Laetrile failed to meet the FDA's safety and efficacy standards.

Laetrile leaders sought to deny the trial's validity. "The whole thing," charged Robert Bradford, "is a put-up deal to discredit Laetrile. It was a phony test."[111] Despite such disparagement, the failure of Laetrile in the National Cancer Institute clinical trials had considerable impact on public perception of the drug's efficacy. By this time, in any case, Laetrile's image had already gone into decline.[112] The Supreme Court had expressed its skepticism. The campaign for state laws had faltered, and some states had repealed laws earlier enacted.[113] Little Chad Green and actor Steve McQueen, headlined for awhile as successful Laetrile users, had died.[114] Interest in Laetrile did not vanish within the realm of cancer unorthodoxy, but it did diminish. In 1982, shortly after the final National Cancer Institute evaluation of Laetrile was published, Barrie Cassileth of the University of Pennsylvania Cancer Center wrote a short article in the *New England Journal of Medicine* entitled "After Laetrile, What?"[115]

Replacing Laetrile, she explained, was an "unusual" mode, differing from past unorthodoxies and constituting "more of a challenge than did Laetrile or its predecessors." The regimens were multiple and varied, featuring "antimedicines" in the sense that diet patterns, detoxification, and mind control were central

[110] Moertel, et al., "A Clinical Trial of Amygdalin."
[111] *Atlanta Journal*, May 1, 1981.
[112] Irving J. Lerner, "Laetrile: A Lesson in Cancer Quackery," *CA* 31 (1981), 91-95.
[113] Status Report of State Legislative Actions Regarding Laetrile, 1988 PHS memorandum.
[114] Corey H. Marco, "Why Chad Green Died in Mexico," *Legal Aspects of Medical Practice* 7 (December 1979), 35-38; *Quackery: A $10 Billion Scandal* (Report), 152-53.
[115] Barrie R. Cassileth, "After Laetrile, What?" *New England Journal of Medicine* 306 (1982), 1482-84.

to therapy. What brought a certain unity out of complexity, Dr. Cassileth suggested, was theory. The new mode owed much to New Age philosophies and religions from the Far East, as well as to earlier unorthodox traditions that once had great vogue in an earlier America: homeopathic and naturopathic concepts, and the belief that intestinal putrefaction lay at the root of disease. Old cancer quackeries had been medications; the new mode stressed lifestyle changes, adjustments purportedly to restore life to more "natural" patterns. Patients could play an active role in their own healing. The wide scope of ideas fostered an expansive range of disease coverage. Not cancer alone, but other ills fell prey. Since lifestyle was chiefly involved, the new wave was largely beyond the control of licensing and regulatory agencies. Clinics were the customary treatment sites. One of unorthodoxy's zealous journalists had already paraded a series of cancer clinics in the pages of *Penthouse*.[116]

Laetrile's promoters had already recognized advantages in the developing pattern of "total metabolic therapy" and had adopted it. In Robert Bradford's book, *Now That You Have Cancer*, he likened the new therapeutic approach to a crown containing nine jewels, with Vitamin B-17 "the crown jewel within that diadem." The other parts included diet, exercise, vitamins A, C, and E, and another false vitamin, B-15 or pangamic acid, that the Krebses had promoted vigorously. Such a total approach, Bradford insisted, provided "the best chance to *control* cancer." The complexity, it may be presumed, would seem to possess the merit of making Laetrile a less conspicuous regulatory target. To approximate this new expanded regimen surrounding Laetrile, the NCI research team had included the vitamins and enzymes in their protocols.

The 1984 report and hearing of Congressman Pepper's subcommittee unquestionably spurred increased attention to quackery on the part of regulatory agencies, the press, and the public. The tide and temper of concern, however, had already begun to turn. The reporting of events that blackened Laetrile's image played a part in this. So too did the appearance of several books surveying the field of quackery from a severely critical perspec-

---

[116] Gary Null, "Alternative Cancer Therapies," *Penthouse*, November 1979, 107-12, 212.

tive. *The Health Robbers*, engineered by physician Stephen Barrett, had been published in 1976, followed by a revised edition four years later. Also issued in 1980 were Victor Herbert's *Nutrition Cultism* and a collection of hard-hitting articles from *Consumer Reports* entitled *Health Quackery*. Newspaper journalists also displayed a revived interest in investigating quackery's deceptions and hazards. An excellent example was a series by James DeBrosse, researched with the FDA's help and published, despite the threat of multiple lawsuits, by the *St. Petersburg Times*.[117]

Speaking to the Pharmaceutical Advertising Council in 1982, FDA Commissioner Arthur Hull Hayes, Jr., cited Consumer Union's *Health Quackery* and admitted that his agency was doing "not much" about the problem.[118] Dr. Hayes—and later Congressman Pepper—might properly have given the FDA more credit for its campaign to restrain Laetrile. Hayes did believe that the agency "acted promptly" against "products that actually do or could harm users" but neglected those that deprived users of legitimate therapy and those posing hazard only to the purse. The overall task was too huge for the FDA alone; its staff power was woefully insufficient. The agency could afford only one or two prosecutions a year against the worst offenders and could "never hope to even stalemate the quacks with publicity." The regulatory agencies must cooperate. The Better Business Bureau might join with the medical and advertising professions to give quackery pitiless exposure.

A year later Commissioner Hayes congratulated the Pharmaceutical Advertising Council for acting on his cue and proposing plans for a joint public service campaign with the FDA, carried in a variety of media, focusing on quackery's flaws.[119] Internally, also, the FDA was rethinking its stance toward quackery, prompted by "concern and frustration" both at headquarters and in the field about the existing program.[120] This process was "agonizingly slow" because of conflicting opinions among agency

[117] *St. Petersburg Times*, July 29-August 1, 1984.

[118] Arthur Hull Hayes, Jr., "Remarks" to the Pharmaceutical Advertising Council, Inc., February 18, 1982.

[119] Hayes, "Remarks" to the Pharmaceutical Advertising Council, Inc., February 17, 1983.

[120] Associate Commissioner for Regulatory Affairs Joseph P. Hile to Policy Board, February 25, 1983.

personnel about what to do.[121] An effort at resolution occurred at a Policy Board Quackery Go-Away in March 1983, which determined to change the target name from "quackery" to "health fraud," arranged better internal coordination on health fraud matters, and agreed to allocate resources specifically for compliance in this field.[122]

More activity did occur. A pilot program, "Tipped Off or Ripped Off," aimed at medical devices whose promotion grossly deceived the public, even though no threat to health was involved.[123] The promoter of such a device would be warned of his sins and, unless changes were made within a month, the agency would publicize them. This plan was expanded to drugs, and a new standing committee on health fraud could decide on seizures, injunctions, or prosecutions to halt promotions dangerous to health.[124] Simultaneously, warning letters would go to firms marketing similar products. A Drugs and Biologic Fraud Branch was established for coordinating activities, initiating actions, and providing support to other federal regulatory agencies.[125] In the agency's *A Plan for Action*, issued in 1985 after Dr. Frank E. Young had become commissioner, health fraud became one of the FDA's top ten priorities, with the promise of "increased emphasis" on both enforcement and education.[126]

The climate for enforcement, however, was not propitious in the 1980s. Tight budgets and antiregulatory sentiment restrained the bureaucrat's hand. Decisions of a type the FDA had hitherto made on its own now might be overruled by officials in the Department of Health and Human Services or the Office of Management and Budget.[127] Prosecutions relating to quackery remained few and far between, and critics kept complaining.[128]

The arrival of a new, mysterious, frightening, infectious epidemic, when such contagions had been deemed on their way

[121] Arthur Hull Hayes, Jr., to author, August 26, 1982.
[122] Commissioner Hayes to Policy Board, April 5, 1983; notes taken at FDA Policy Board Quackery Go-Away.
[123] FDA Talk Paper, December 9, 1983.
[124] *Food Chemical News*, December 5, 1983, 3-4; *FDC Reports*, December 19, 1983, 10.
[125] FDA Talk Paper, October 15, 1984.
[126] FDA, *A Plan for Action* (Rockville, July 1985).
[127] *Food Chemical News*, June 17, 1985, 10-12.
[128] *Nutrition Forum* 4 (August 1987), 55; Stephen Budiansky, "New Snake Oil, Old Pitch," *U.S. News and World Report*, December 8, 1986, 68-70.

toward extinction, forced the Food and Drug Administration and other regulatory agencies into emergency action. "We stand nakedly in front of a very serious pandemic," stated the director-general of the World Health Organization, "as mortal as any pandemic has ever been."[129] Victims of acquired immunodeficiency syndrome, lacking approved medications that could cure or, for several years, even palliate their condition, turned desperately to rumored or fraudulently promoted treatments.[130] As gatekeeper for new medications, the FDA, when legitimate drugs seemed tardy in arriving, bore the brunt of AIDS activist organization wrath.[131] Many ordinary citizens, convinced the cause of AIDS was ubiquitous, panicked into purchasing falsely advertised "protective" devices.

Postal inspectors filed a complaint against an alleged air-purifying gadget called Viralaid—"The product of lightning harnessed for your use!"—to protect "bed linens, bath towels, even eating utensils."[132] The Environmental Protection Agency acted against antiseptics overpromising to safeguard home and office environments.[133] A plastic shield was vended to cover public telephones, to block the user from the breath and spit of previous mouths.[134]

Of those stricken with AIDS, or fearing this fate, a great many entered "a jungle of truly questionable and quack products."[135] Dr. John Renner of Kansas City tabulated over three hundred quack schemes and guessed there might be thousands more.[136] Victor Herbert pointed to one significant trend: "Every cancer scam has become an AIDS scam."[137] Robert Bradford and Mike

[129] Halfden Mahler cited in Loretta McLaughlin, "AIDS: An Overview," in *New England Journal of Public Policy* 4 (Winter-Spring 1988), 15.

[130] In this discussion of AIDS quackery, I follow my paper, "AIDS and Deceptive Therapies," given at the American Association for the History of Medicine convention in Birmingham, April 28, 1989.

[131] Eloise Salholz, "Acting Up to Fight AIDS," *Newsweek*, June 8, 1988, 42.

[132] U.S. Postal Service memorandum, March 1985.

[133] Environmental Protection Agency memorandum, February 9, 1988.

[134] Angelo J. Aponte speech, Food and Drug Administration audiovisual tape of excerpts from lectures at the National Health Fraud Conference, Kansas City, March 1988.

[135] Angelo J. Aponte lecture, National Association of Consumer Agency Administrators convention, June 12, 1987.

[136] John Renner cited in Janny Scott and Lynn Simross, "AIDS: Underground Options," *Los Angeles Times*, August 16, 1987.

[137] FDA press release, April 4, 1988.

Culbert, with headquarters in San Francisco and a treatment center in Tijuana, now covered AIDS as well as cancer.[138] Garlic pills, enemas, and meditation formed part of the regimen, but its central element, Culbert told a television interviewer, was "live cell therapy, the embryonic cellular extracts from calves, although sheep, goats will do just as well." In the Bahamas, Dr. Lawrence Burton, a zoologist, dispensed a blood serum treatment for cancer that possessed the potential of taking Laetrile's place as an American social movement built upon an unorthodox therapy.[139] Burton added AIDS to cancer as a disease that he claimed could be treated effectively by his therapy. With sad irony, it was later demonstrated that some samples of the serum had become contaminated, as shown by the presence of antibodies to the AIDS-causing human immunodeficiency virus. The FDA barred Burton's product from importation.

As the viral destruction of immunity became established and widely announced to be the genesis of AIDS, safeguarding immunity became a central doctrine in unorthodox therapy.[140] The health food industry eagerly latched on to this approach, and a variety of products surged into the marketplace with explicit or guarded claims for preventing or combating AIDS. The FDA took action against over-the-counter and mail-order medications using the immunity pitch if AIDS was named or obviously implied in the name or labeling. The agency sent regulatory letters to makers of whey-concentrate colostrum with names like Stimulac, and sought to stop the promotion of Prevention Plus and Resist-AIDS tablets.[141]

Another group of drugs presented the FDA with more difficult

[138] MacNeil/Lehrer News Hour, PBS, November 6, 1985.

[139] Stuart L. Nightingale, "Immunoaugmentative Therapy," *American Family Physician* 34 (December 1986), 159-60; "Isolation of Human T-Lymphotropic Virus Type III/Lymphadenopathy-Associated Virus from Serum Protein Given to Cancer Patients—Bahamas," Centers for Disease Control, *Morbidity and Mortality Weekly Report* 34 (1985), 489-91; FDA Import Alert, August 6, 1986. The FDA's Nightingale had earlier answered the question "Could there be another Laetrile?" with a reluctant affirmative. "Laetrile: The Regulatory Challenge of an Unproven Remedy," *Public Health Reports* 99 (1984), 333-38.

[140] FDA Health Fraud Bulletin 11, "Immune System Products," August 17, 1987; Stephen Barrett, "Strengthening the Immune System—A Growing Fad," *Nutrition Forum* 3 (1986), 24.

[141] FDA Health Fraud Bulletin 9, "Colostrum Products," January 15, 1987; Don Colburn, "AIDS and Desperation," *Washington Post Health*, January 6, 1987.

decisions. Unproven products, some made by American pharmaceutical firms, others derived from the science or folklore of foreign nations, had gained wide use in the guerrilla clinics of the AIDS underground.[142] A number of these drugs went into legitimate clinical trials, although too slowly to suit AIDS activists, a few to emerge with true therapeutic roles related to secondary afflictions to which AIDS patients were prone, others to prove ineffective or lethal.

Under the double pressure of the AIDS lobby and the Reagan administration's desire to reduce regulatory burdens, the FDA devised policies of earlier release for drugs showing some promise to treat life-threatening diseases.[143] Moreover, the agency did not interfere with individuals seeking the treatments dispensed at underground clinics, unless the marketers made illegal labeling claims.[144] The FDA further permitted people with AIDS to bring back from other countries, or to have mailed to them from abroad, limited supplies of any AIDS product that caught their fancy, except those on Import Alert.

The FDA's modifications of policy kept the agency in the middle of controversy, the changes seeming insufficient to the AIDS community, but to some health scientists threatening the integrity of the new drug introduction system and the control of quackery.[145] Commissioner Young gave a reporter this apologia for FDA policy: "I'd rather err on being compassionate. People with this dreaded disease have limited hope, and I don't want to rob them of it."[146]

With AIDS quackery as with other health fraud, FDA officials

[142] This subject was probed in *Therapeutic Drugs for AIDS: Development, Testing, and Availability*, Hearings before a Subcommittee of the Committee on Government Operations, House of Representatives, 100th Cong., 2d sess., April 28-29, 1988. Hereafter, April 1988 House Subcommittee Hearings.

[143] *Federal Register* 53 (October 21, 1988), 41516-24; Nancy Mattison, "The FDA's Treatment IND: Current Controversies," *Pharmaceutical Medicine* 3 (1988), 159-71.

[144] April 1988 House Subcommittee Hearings, 396.

[145] Ibid.; Mike King, "Ethics of FDA's Faster Drug Approval Process Questioned," *Atlanta Constitution*, January 4, 1988; Erich Stephen Berger, "FDA's AIDS 'Remedies': Misguided Compassion," *Los Angeles Times*, August 1, 1988, reprinted in *Priorities*, Winter 1989, 43-44; George J. Annas, "Faith (Healing), Hope and Charity at the FDA: The Politics of AIDS Drug Trials," *Villanova Law Review* 34 (1989), 771-97.

[146] Cited in Susan Okie, "AIDS Sufferers Buying Hope," *Washington Post*, April 3, 1988.

continued to assert that education had to play the leading role in the agency's counterattack. Its "big guns—regulatory actions and criminal prosecutions," would be fired off only occasionally, when the provocation seemed overwhelming.[147]

Intensive effort went into the FDA's educational campaign.[148] Cooperating with the Council of Better Business Bureaus, the FDA sought to secure tighter screening of advertising by all branches of the media and urged direct marketers to check more carefully their product claims. In a variety of ways, the agency and its allies also sought to jolt the broad public into greater awareness of health fraud hazards. The joint effort with the Pharmaceutical Advertising Council put spots on television and radio and public service announcements in newspapers, magazines, and medical publications, all warning of quackery. A consumer brochure produced by the Council, the FDA, the FTC, and the Postal Service received massive circulation. The FDA undertook special programs to increase sensitivity about health fraud among physicians, nurses, pharmacists, and pharmaceutical manufacturers. An Information Exchange Network was inaugurated with the National Association of Consumer Administrators, and Health Fraud Surveillance Teams were begun with the Association of Food and Drug Officials, thus strengthening federal and state cooperation in detecting and planning attacks on fraudulent ventures.

*FDA Consumer* published numerous articles on the health fraud theme, and the agency issued press releases on newsworthy developments. The FDA's Consumer Affairs Officers stressed health fraud in their numerous meetings with members of the public. Special programs were targeted at groups deemed especially vulnerable: the elderly, Hispanic citizens, arthritis sufferers, and people with AIDS.

The National Health Fraud Conferences of the 1960s were revived. The first of the new series, sponsored by the FDA, the FTC, and the Postal Service, met in Washington in September 1985.[149] Congressman Claude Pepper, on his eighty-fifth birth-

[147] Deputy Commissioner John Norris cited in *Food Chemical News*, March 21, 1988, 7-8.
[148] FDA Office of Consumer Affairs, "Health Fraud Activities Status Report," February 1987; ibid., 1989.
[149] Ibid.; *Consumer Newsweekly*, September 16, 1985.

AFTERWORD

day, came to bestow his blessing on the enterprise. Commissioner Young called health fraud "a disease, devouring, destroying and contagious," and quackery's most committed critics, among them Victor Herbert, Stephen Barrett, and Grace Powers Monaco, elaborated the grim details.

Regional conferences across the country and in Puerto Rico carried the message closer to the grass roots until the next National Health Fraud Conference, sponsored by the FDA and Trinity Lutheran Hospital, convened in Kansas City, Missouri, in March 1988.[150] Those who assembled seemed to accept some basic assumptions: that quackery was too deeply entrenched to be destroyed, but much could be done "to minimize the negative impact . . . upon society."[151] There were hopeful signs: a recent "substantial increase," despite low budgets, in federal enforcement[152] and a considerable improvement in networking among quackery's foes. The current masks worn by the illegitimate were vividly described. Much time at the conference went into considering the practical aspects of combating health fraud: how to gather evidence during an investigation; how to write accurately about the problem; how to avoid legal difficulties; how to improve education in the schools.

Another National Health Fraud Conference would meet in Kansas City in September 1990. This time the Food and Drug Administration would not be among the four official sponsors, while the American Medical Association would resume its 1960s role. The theme of the conference, according to the preliminary announcement, would be "Quackery, Health Fraud, and Misinformation: A Pandora's Box."

Quackery has always been Pandora's box, constantly reopened with hope, never releasing a genuine benefit, although sometimes the opener is fooled into believing so. The box has an infinite capacity. Old cheats like before-and-after pictures and the fake diagnostic test come out wrapped in new tinsel.[153] In one case, for a weight-loss scam, both pictures were taken on the

---

[150] *1988 National Health Fraud Conference Proceedings.*

[151] William Jarvis, ibid., 11.

[152] Victor Herbert, ibid., 31. FDA's greater regulatory activity also received comment in "FDA in Battle on Health Food Frauds," *New York Times*, June 1, 1989.

[153] *NCAHF Newsletter*, 9 (March/April 1986), 2; 8 (August 1985), 2.

same day of the same woman, the company president, who apparently donned a padded robe for "before" and a swimsuit for "after." In another instance, a Los Angeles lab claiming to test blood for allergies was itself put to the test. Federal investigators paid the required $350 fee, sending in blood from a vegetarian described as "overweight, irritable [and] constipated." The lab reported allergies to milk, blue cheese, and yogurt. The patient was a cow.

Pandora's box continues to be stuffed with a variety of brazen health deceptions beyond recounting, perhaps beyond reckoning. Despite increased efforts at education, the perennial proneness seems not to have diminished perceptibly. A national survey conducted by Louis Harris and Associates, which the FDA helped devise, found that more than a quarter of the American public reported using one or more questionable health care treatments.[154] At Kansas City, Deputy Commissioner Norris stated that the agency believed this figure "seriously underestimated the extent of the problem."[155] More than half of such users thought they had derived some benefit, certainly evidence of self-deception. The poor and sick seemed at special risk, but college education offered no protection against resort to questionable products.

Cancer quackery offers evidence of how both populist and elitist elements of the population have been preyed upon. James Patterson stressed the class nature of the phenomenon.[156] The poor have been vulnerable in both an economic and an educational sense, constituting a counterculture suspicious of expert knowledge, especially skeptical of orthodox medical opinion, trusting instead in folk tradition, home remedies, faith healing, and quackery. A survey conducted by Jon D. Miller of Northern Illinois University found that three-quarters of his respondents believed "there are good ways of treating sickness that medical science does not recognize."[157]

Remarks by Glen Rutherford at the Kansas City hearing on

---

[154] Louis Harris and Associates, "Executive Summary" of national health fraud survey, 1987; FDA, "Health Fraud Activities Status Report," 1989.

[155] *1988 National Health Fraud Conference Proceedings*, 3.

[156] Patterson, *The Dread Disease*.

[157] *San Francisco Chronicle*, February 15, 1986, cited in *NCAHF Newsletter*, 10 (July/August 1987), 2.

Laetrile conducted by the FDA catch the bitter feeling often expressed toward establishment medicine.[158] "You people in authority," the FDA's stubborn opponent said, "consider all the rest of us a bunch of dummies. . . . You set yourself up as God and Jesus Christ all rolled up into one. And we don't have any rights. . . . Patrick Henry said: 'Give me liberty, or give me death.' Glen Rutherford says, 'Let me choose the way I want to die. It is not your prerogative to tell me how. Only God can do that.' "

The educated also become seduced by cancer unorthodoxy. Revealing this truth again, Barrie Cassileth and her colleagues followed her terse answer to the question "After Laetrile, What?" with an empirical study, sampling the experience of patients in her Philadelphia region treated both in cancer centers and by unorthodox practitioners.[159] The researchers found that patients taking unorthodox treatment alone or in addition to conventional therapy tended to be better educated than those receiving only conventional treatment. The study reported that 54 percent of patients on conventional therapy also used unorthodox treatments, and that 40 percent of those so doing abandoned conventional care. Eight percent of the patients had received no conventional treatment at all. Perhaps the most surprising finding was that 60 percent of the dispensers of unorthodox treatment were physicians.

The principal unorthodoxies Cassileth and her associates discovered were those of the new wave, "metabolic therapy, diet therapies, megavitamins, mental imagery applied for anti-tumor effect, spiritual or faith healing, and 'immune' therapy." A "common perspective" gave unity to the diversity: "Cancer and other chronic illnesses tend to be viewed not as disease entities, but as symptoms of underlying dysfunction, disorder, or toxicity." As a consequence, therapy was aimed at enhancing the patient's physical and mental capacity to counteract what was deemed fundamentally wrong.

This pattern reveals that unorthodox cancer treatment had

[158] Rutherford, vol. 11, 308, 315-16, FDA Administrative Hearing, Laetrile, Docket 77N-0048.

[159] Barrie L. Cassileth, et al., "Contemporary Unorthodox Treatments in Cancer Medicine: A Study of Patients, Treatments, and Practitioners," *Annals of Internal Medicine* 101 (1984), 105-12.

moved to a considerable degree under the "alternative" or holistic umbrella. From this position the foes of scientific medicine not only condemn the medical/regulatory establishment and lobby against it in legislative bodies, but they also frame a counter-paradigm that they seek to persuade the public is intellectually more valid and therapeutically more effective than the system of science. "One of the major successes of pseudoscientific thinking," William Jarvis has written, "has been tacit acceptance of the word 'alternatives' into current health jargon."[160] "Holistic medicine," Clark Glymour and Douglas Stalker have argued, "is a pablum of common sense and nonsense offered by cranks and quacks and failed pedants who share an attachment to magic and an animosity toward reason. Too many people seem willing to swallow the rhetoric—even too many medical doctors—and the results will not be benign."[161] These two philosophers have edited a book in which scholarly specialists expose the illogic of major elements in the holistic movement.[162]

As a sociologist has observed, "the fate of medical social movements is not determined by the soundness of their theories or the effectiveness of their therapies, but by their ability to mobilize political and social resources effectively."[163] The civil war that Robert Bradford predicted over Laetrile is now being waged fiercely on a broader front, and it is too soon to say whether science or antiscience will win. At the peak of the Laetrile movement, scientist Thomas Jukes, a dedicated foe of quackery, asserted that public acceptance of unorthodox health practices had become "so well established, and [is] so little challenged that its impact will produce a decline of scientific medicine and its re-

[160] California Medical Association, *The Professional's Guide to Health & Nutrition Fraud* (San Francisco, 1987), 9.

[161] Clark Glymour and Douglas Stalker, "Engineers, Cranks, Physicians, Magicians," *New England Journal of Medicine* 308 (1983), 960-64.

[162] Stalker and Glymour, *Examining Holistic Medicine*. See also Gerald E. Markle and James C. Petersen, "Social Context of the Laetrile Phenomenon," in Markle and Petersen, *Politics, Science, and Cancer*, 151-73; Loretta Kopelman and John Moskop, "The Holistic Health Movement: A Survey and Critique," *Journal of Medicine and Philosophy* 6 (1981), 209-35; Denise Hatfield, "The Holes in Holistic Medicine," *ACSH News & Views* 6 (November-December 1985), 12-13.

[163] Marcine J. Cohen, "Medical Social Movements in the United States (1820-1982): The Case of Osteopathy" (University of California, San Diego, dissertation, 1983), xii.

placement by quackery."[164] Despite a decade of counterattack on pseudomedicine by the revived legions of regulators and quack-busters, Dr. Jukes commented early in 1990, "Unfortunately, I see no reason to retract my pessimistic opinion." Whatever the odds, the intense contest continues for the allegiance of the people. Those dedicated to the cause of science and reason need to take a committed stand.

[164] Thomas H. Jukes to author, August 11, 1978, and March 13, 1990.

# A NOTE ON THE SOURCES

RESEARCH for this book began—although I did not at the time yet realize it—on a warm summer evening in 1951 at Atlanta's Lakewood Park. The occasion was a Hadacol Caravan Show presented by Louisiana state senator Dudley J. LeBlanc. Would that all the research hours that were to follow might have proved equally beguiling.

The research problems for *The Medical Messiahs* turned out to be much different from those for *The Toadstool Millionaires*. For the earlier work, the task was to find whatever shreds of evidence many repositories might yield and hope that there would be enough to form a pattern. That book ended with an account of the passage of the Pure Food and Drugs Act of 1906. With regulation came records. So for this sequel, the basic task has been to decide how many and which of the thousands of cubic feet of records in governmental archives to survey. The indispensable material from which *The Medical Messiahs* is constructed comes from the archives of three regulatory agencies and two private organizations: the Food and Drug Administration, the Post Office Department, the Federal Trade Commission, the American Medical Association, and the National Better Business Bureau.

Enforcement of the 1906 act began in the Bureau of Chemistry of the Department of Agriculture. In 1927, still within this Department, the Food, Drug, and Insecticide Administration was created, the "Insecticide" being dropped from the name three years later. In 1940 the FDA left Agriculture to be part of the new Federal Security Agency, and in 1953 it became part of the new Department of Health, Education, and Welfare. I have used Bureau of Chemistry records, from Record Group 97 in the National Archives, and Department of Agriculture records, from Record Group 16. Especially helpful were files of the General Correspondence of the Office of the Secretary, and Solicitor's Office papers concerned with cases being worked up for trial. Food and Drug Administration records are found in Record Group 88 in the National Archives or its outlying record centers. More current records are housed in the FDA offices. Of the many types of FDA primary documents used, most central to my research were the extensive jackets concerned with adjudicated cases, papers accumulated from various bureaus and field offices in preparation for drafting FDA annual reports, and files of correspondence and clippings relating to the effort to secure stronger legislation during the 1930's. Also of importance were files of public addresses delivered by agency officials; press releases, starting in 1915; *Notices of Judgment,* the legal method of announcing terminated cases; and the *Food and Drug Review,* a house organ of restricted circulation which began in 1917 to keep employees of the agency and cooperating state and local food and drug officials informed. Printed annual reports of the FDA have been brought together conveniently by the Food Law Institute in *Federal Food, Drug, and Cosmetic Law, Administrative Reports, 1907-1949* (Chicago, 1951). Sage counsel as to how I might discover what would be most useful in the manuscript records came from the late John J. McCann, Jr., of FDA and from Helen T. Finneran, Jerome Finster, and Harold T. Pinkett of the National Archives.

Post Office Department medical fraud records form part of Record Group 28 in the National Archives; more recent records, of course, remain in the Department. Valuable for this study were the Fraud Order Case File, a terse summary of findings and action taken in each case; the Fraud Order Jackets, each a complete record of a case (although not all case jackets have been preserved); Transcripts of Hearings of Fraud Order Cases, verbatim testimony (again, the preservation process has been selective); and various docket books. The docket books reveal the logging in of complaints and record step by step the stages in each case's development until its resolution. As Post Office fraud machinery has been modified, docket book titles have changed: Fraud and Lottery Docket (1902-1951); Hearing Examiners' Docket (1951–     ); Solicitor's Docket (1951-1956); General Council's Docket (1956-1958); Post Office Department Docket (1958–     ). In the General Counsel's file room, there exists a card file covering Post Office fraud cases classified alphabetically by schemes for the period 1920 into the early 1950's. The annual reports of the

Postmaster General also proved of value. Arthur Hecht of the National Archives served as an expert guide through the intricacies of Post Office Department Records.

The Federal Trade Commission has published its *Decisions* from the date of its creation, the first volume appearing in 1920. The docket for each official case, containing all the legal papers, is available for public examination in the FTC's Docket Room. A number of such dockets were studied for this book. Addresses by commissioners and by members of the staff were found in the Speech File in the FTC Library. Press releases treat all aspects of the Commission's activity, and helpful annual reports are issued.

Beginning early in the century, the American Medical Association began to assemble information concerning nostrums and their proprietors, a task that still continues. Hundreds of folders, each containing a case history, are filled with thousands of items, the sources for numerous articles on quackery in the *Journal of the American Medical Association* and in *Today's Health* (and its predecessor, *Hygeia*), for scores of blue-bound pamphlets, and for the three useful *Nostrum and Quackery* volumes issued by the AMA in 1911, 1921, and 1936. Under the helpful guidance of Oliver Field and Juelma Williams, I used many of these folders, housed in the Department of Investigation at the AMA's Chicago headquarters. Also useful were the manuscript annual reports of this department.

The National Better Business Bureau in New York City retains a complete file of its bulletins and other publications, many of which concern questionable medical promotions. I was permitted to examine these sources, and also some data from case files, by Maye A. Russ and Dr. Irving Ladimer, successively in charge of food and drug matters for the Bureau.

The modes of operation employed by promoters of drugs and devices emerge with vivid clarity from the case files of these regulatory and private agencies. All files contain printed promotional material devised by proprietors in mounting their schemes.

Valuable material has been provided me, at the headquarters offices in New York and also through the mail, by Dr. Roald N. Grant and Irene L. Bartlett of the American Cancer

Society and by Dr. Ronald W. Lamont-Havers and James L. Curran of the Arthritis and Rheumatism Foundation. In 1964 this Foundation consolidated with other agencies in the field to form The Arthritis Foundation.

Judicial proceedings have provided source material of great importance. The transcripts of four trials in federal district courts were made available by the Office of the General Counsel in the Department of Health, Education, and Welfare: these transcripts concerned the Drown, Hohensee, Hoxsey, and Kaadt cases. Some checking was done in the Records of the District Courts of the United States, Record Group 21, Federal Record Center, Region 3, and in the case records of the United States Supreme Court. Court decisions were studied in the various legal volumes reporting them. With respect to cases involving food and drug law, these decisions have been helpfully assembled in a series of volumes. *Decisions of Courts in Cases under the Federal Food and Drugs Act* of 1906 was compiled by Mastin G. White and Otis H. Gates complete up to the date their volume appeared (Washington, 1934). Decisions under the 1938 law have been conveniently reprinted in a Food Law Institute Series, edited by Vincent A. Kleinfeld, Charles Wesley Dunn, and Alan H. Kaplan, each of the six volumes entitled *Federal Food, Drug and Cosmetic Act: Judicial and Administrative Record*, with the appropriate covering dates, from *1938-1949* (Chicago, 1949), through *1961-1964* (Chicago, 1965). The *1949-1950* volume contains significant cases decided under the 1906 law after the appearance of the White-Gates volume. These works also periodically bring up to date the reprinting of FDA annual reports, first assembled in a volume covering 1907-1949, as mentioned above, and reprint other Food and Drug Administration data.

Hearings and reports of Congressional committees and the *Congressional Record* have been of great value to me in preparing this book, especially in studying the background of the Food, Drug, and Cosmetic Act of 1938, the Durham-Humphrey Act of 1951, and the Kefauver-Harris Act of 1962. Charles Wesley Dunn assembled the pertinent passages from the *Congressional Record*, draft copies of the bills at various stages, committee reports, and excerpts from hearings in *Fed-*

*eral Food, Drug, and Cosmetic Act, A Statement of Its Legislative Record* (N.Y., 1938), and *Wheeler-Lea Act, A Statement of Its Legislative Record* (N.Y., 1938).

The Harvey W. Wiley Papers in the Manuscripts Division of the Library of Congress were examined for some aspects of Wiley's nostrum regulation while he was chief of the Bureau of Chemistry. An effort was made to determine President Roosevelt's role in the effort to secure stronger food and drug legislation during the New Deal by studying manuscripts in the Franklin D. Roosevelt Library at Hyde Park.

Interviews proved to be of inestimable value in acquiring new information, a clarification of printed records, and an achievement of more adequate perspective. It would be almost impossible to list all those helpful to me in this way. Of those at the Food and Drug Administration who now are or who were officials during the course of my research, I received significant aid from Dr. James L. Goddard, Gilbert S. Goldhammer, William W. Goodrich, Wallace F. Janssen, George P. Larrick, John J. McCann, Jr., Dr. Kenneth L. Milstead, Winton B. Rankin, John W. Sanders, and James L. Trawick. At the Post Office Department, I was helped in my research especially by T. N. Berdeen, William F. Callahan, Louis J. Doyle, Charles E. Dunbar, Richard S. Farr, Abraham Levine, and Ralph Manherz. At the Federal Trade Commission I profited from several interviews with Dr. Frederick W. Irish and Charles A. Sweeny. At the American Medical Association, Dr. W. W. Bauer, Oliver Field, and Juelma Williams gave me great assistance. At the National Better Business Bureau, Maye A. Russ and Dr. Irving Ladimer discussed interpretive problems helpfully. Among the many others who have provided me with information or insights are Dr. Walter Alvarez of Chicago; Dr. Oscar E. Anderson of NASA; Mrs. Ruth Lamb Atkinson of Brookline, Mass.; Dr. Harry F. Dowling of the University of Illinois College of Medicine; Dr. A. Hunter Dupree of the University of California at Berkeley; Dr. Morris Fishbein of Chicago; George Griffenhagen of the American Pharmaceutical Association; Boisfeuillet Jones, then of the Department of Health, Education, and Welfare; Justice Simon Sobeloff, then

Solicitor General of the United States; and Dr. Fredrick J. Stare of the Harvard University School of Public Health.

Newspapers and magazines have also provided information of value to me in fashioning this book, as the footnotes testify. A few journals deserve specific mention. *Standard Remedies* from 1915 into the 1930's reflected the perspective of the major proprietary drug manufacturers. The trade papers *Oil, Paint and Drug Reporter* and *Drug Trade News* covered all developments of significance with respect to drugs. With the advent of the 1938 law, an industry newsletter, *FDC Reports—Drugs and Cosmetics*, generally known as "The Pink Sheet," probed deeply into what was happening and likely to happen on the drug scene, presenting its facts and speculation with considerable historical perspective. Many articles of great importance, especially on the legal aspects of federal regulation, have appeared in the *Food Drug Cosmetic Law Journal*. The AMA journals, as mentioned above, the *American Journal of Public Health*, the *Journal of the American Pharmaceutical Association*, journals of opinion like the *Nation* and the *New Republic*, magazines expressing the consumer viewpoint like *Consumers' Research Bulletin* and *Consumer Reports*, have all provided me with useful information. Two issues of *Law and Contemporary Problems* (Dec. 1933 and Winter 1939) were devoted to the New Deal crusade to strengthen the food and drug law. *World Medical Journal* for Sep. 1962 considers quackery in a worldwide setting. The Sep. 1963 issue of the *Journal of the American Pharmaceutical Association* focuses upon quackery, and with the Sep. 1966 issue began a series on "Home Remedies in Review." A symposium on "The Government and the Consumer: Evolution of the Food and Drug Laws" appeared in the *Journal of Public Law*, 13 (1964), 189-221. The *Emory University Quarterly* Summer 1965 issue presented a symposium on "The American Drug Scene."

The *Proceedings* of two conferences, jointly sponsored by the AMA and the FDA, *National Congress on Medical Quackery* [Oct. 6-7, 1961] (Chicago, 1962), and *Second National Congress on Medical Quackery* [Oct. 25-26, 1963] (Chicago, 1964), reprint addresses by the leading figures from the ranks of government, medicine, and business concerned with regulating quackery or educating against it. Some of the addresses given at a third conference are included in *Third National Congress on Medical Quackery, October 7-8, 1966, Chicago, Illinois, Papers* (Chicago, 1967), which preceded the publication of the *Proceedings* of the Congress (Chicago, 1967).

A basic list of books concerned with quackery in the 20th century, or with the broader setting within which quackery operates, includes the following: American Cancer Society, *Unproven Methods of Cancer Treatment* (N.Y., 1966); Oscar E. Anderson, Jr., *The Health of a Nation, Harvey W. Wiley and the Fight for Pure Food* (Chicago, 1958); James G. Burrow, *AMA, Voice of American Medicine* (Baltimore, 1963); Gerald Carson, *The Roguish World of Doctor Brinkley* (N.Y., 1960); Stuart Chase and F. J. Schlink, *Your Money's Worth* (N.Y., 1927); Chase, *The Tragedy of Waste* (N.Y., 1925); Consumers Union, *The Medicine Show* (N.Y., 1961); James Cook, *Remedies and Rackets, The Truth about Patent Medicines Today* (N.Y., 1958); Ronald M. Deutsch, *The Nuts among the Berries* (N.Y., 1961); M.N.G. Dukes, *Patent Medicines and Autotherapy in Society* (The Hague, 1963) [mainly concerned with Britain and the Netherlands]; A. Hunter Dupree, *Science in the Federal Government, A History of Policies and Activities to 1940* (Cambridge, Mass., 1957); Morris Fishbein, *Fads and Quackery in Healing* (N.Y., 1932); Fishbein, *A History of the American Medical Association, 1847 to 1947* (Philadelphia, 1957); Fishbein, *The Medical Follies* (N.Y., 1925); Fishbein, *The New Medical Follies* (N.Y., 1927); Martin Gardner, *In the Name of Science* (N.Y., 1952); T. Swann Harding, *The Popular Practice of Fraud* (N.Y., 1935); Richard Harris, *The Real Voice* (N.Y., 1964); Richard J. Hopkins, "Medical Prescriptions and the Law: A Study of the Enactment of the Durham-Humphrey Amendment to the Federal Food, Drug, and Cosmetic Act" (Atlanta, 1965: unpublished Emory University M.A. thesis); Arthur Kallet and F. J. Schlink, *100,000,000 Guinea Pigs* (N.Y., 1933); Ruth deForest Lamb, *American Chamber of Horrors* (N.Y., 1936); Louis Lasagna, *The Doctors' Dilemmas* (N.Y., 1962); Elmer V. McCollum, *A History of Nutrition* (Boston, 1957); Morton Mintz,

*The Therapeutic Nightmare* (Boston, 1965); Otis Pease, *The Responsibilities of American Advertising, Private Control and Public Influence, 1920-1940* (New Haven, 1958); Frank Presbrey, *The History and Development of Advertising* (Garden City, 1929); Francis X. Quinn, ed., *Ethics, Advertising and Responsibility* (Westminster, Md., 1963); Richard H. Shryock, *The Development of Modern Medicine, An Interpretation of the Social and Scientific Factors Involved* (N.Y., 1947); Ralph Lee Smith, *The Health Hucksters* (N.Y., 1960); Bernard Sternsher, *Rexford Tugwell and the New Deal* (New Brunswick, N.J., 1964); Julius Stieglitz, ed., *Chemistry in Medicine* (N.Y., 1928); Paul Talalay, ed., *Drugs in Our Society* (Baltimore, 1964); Ruth Walrad, *The Misrepresentation of Arthritis Drugs and Devices in the United States* (N.Y., 1960); Gustavus A. Weber, *The Food, Drug, and Insecticide Administration, Its History, Activities and Organization* (Baltimore, 1928); Harvey W. Wiley, *An Autobiography* (Indianapolis, 1930); Wiley, *The History of a Crime against the Food Law* (Washington, 1929).

My own articles along the road to this volume are: "The Hadacol Phenomenon," *Emory University Quarterly*, 7 (June 1951), 72-86; "The 'Elixir Sulfanilamide' Disaster," *ibid.*, 14 (Dec. 1958), 230-37; "The 1938 Food, Drug, and Cosmetic Act," *Journal of Public Law*, 13 (1964), 197-204; "Social History of American Drug Legislation," in Talalay, ed., *Drugs in Our Society*, 217-29; and "Device Quackery in America," *Bulletin of the History of Medicine*, 39 (Mar.-Apr. 1965), 154-62.

# INDEX

abortifacients, 57, 64, 101, 194, 302
Abrams, Albert, 137-42, 244, 254, 258, 383
Abundavita, 340
"accompanying such article," 200-202
acetanilid, 4-12, 31, 36, 193, 195, 302-303, 319
Acuff, Roy, 323
Adams, Samuel Hopkins: on headache mixtures, 6; on Radol, 27; writes "The Great American Fraud," 30-32, 34; quoted, 41; on early impact of 1906 law, 44; resumes patent medicine criticism, 52, 55; articles reprinted by AMA, 130; mentioned, 163
Addiline, 116
"adequate directions for use," 194-200, 265-66, 275
Administrative Procedure Act of 1946, 284, 292
advertising: of old English patent medicines, 13-14; of early American patent medicines, 16-18; scope of 19th-century, 20-22; use of germ theory in, 26-27; and "red clause," 29-31; in JAMA, 30, 39; abuse of guaranty clause, 46; misuse of Wiley's name in, 47; need for control of, 55-56; Proprietary Association code, 57-58; relation to mail fraud, 68-69; for Interstate Remedy Co., 75-76; of pharmaceuticals criticized, 81; of venereal disease remedies, 84; indirect control by Bureau of Chemistry, 96; bills aimed at controlling, 97; of influenza remedies, 103; FTC asked to control, 114, 116; origin of self-regulation of, 114-16; early FTC regulation of, 116-17; William Humphrey on, 117-18; FTC 1920's campaign against deception in, 118-20; self-regulation through NBBB, 119-21; impact of depression on, 121-22, 128, 148-57; of Marmola, 123; Cramp's comments on, 134-35, 143; emotional appeals increase in, 144-47, 308-309; expansion during 1920's, 145, 147-49;

role of radio in, 149-50; self-regulation during depression, 151; criticized during depression, 152-57; and news coverage of food and drug law revision, 162-63; efforts to control in Tugwell bill, 165-66; contest over federal control of, 173-74, 180-84; Proprietary Association's code revision, 192; FDA control through "adequate directions for use" clause, 197-206; of over-the-counter drugs, 266; Wheeler-Lea Act provisions, 296-98; control of under Wheeler-Lea Act, 299-315; ways of avoiding FTC action, 306-308; expansion in volume, 308; criticized during 1950's, 309-10; criticized during 1960's, 314-15; of Hadacol, 317-25, 327-29; of "health foods," 336-37; restraint and taste in, 390; codes tightened, 396; of prescription drugs, 411-12; of prescription drugs brought under FDA control, 418-19; of self-medication drugs criticized, 419-20, 433
advertising agencies, 22, 146, 151
affirmative disclosure, 297, 303-304, 311
Alberty, Ada, 202, 303-304, 311
alcohol, 5, 7, 8, 24, 29, 31, 34, 36, 44, 58, 132, 177, 317, 325-26
Alexander, Dan Dale, 401
*Alice in Wonderland*, 133, 406
Alka-Seltzer, 302, 348
Allen, Eleanor, 253
Allen, Gracie, 323
Allison, Kathy, 385-86
Alsberg, Carl L.: on 1906 law's inadequacies, 54, 59; background, 59; views of his role, 60, 99; compared with Wiley, 60; testifies, 61-62; sets up project system, 98; mentioned, 66
aluminum cooking ware, 352
Alvarez, Walter, 140-41, 427
American Association of Advertising Agencies, 146, 151
American Association for Medico-Physical Research, 142, 382
American Association of University Women, 176

[ 481 ]

American Cancer Society, 373, 389, 391, 398-99, 401, 422
*American Chamber of Horrors*, 180
American College of Apothecaries, 277-78
American College of Physicians, 213
American Diabetes Association, 224
American Dietetic Association, 357
American Health Aids Co., 289-91
American Medical Association: issues *Nostrums and Quackery*, 27n; reforms *JAMA* advertising, 30; role in securing 1906 law, 35; raises standards, 39, 47; fights patent medicines during 1910's, 53, 64; criticized by Proprietary Association, 58-59; criticizes pharmaceutical advertising, 81; on weight-reducing craze, 123; on Marmola, 125; campaign against quackery, 129-43; establishes *Hygeia*, 136-37; Wine of Cardui libel suit, 142; criticized by Kallet and Schlink, 155; role in effort to revise food and drug law, 183; conspiracy with FDA charged, 214; investigates Kaadts, 219-20; investigates Drown, 246-47; helps Post Office Dept., 283, 402; criticizes advertising, 309-10; efforts to improve advertising, 312-13; investigates Hadacol, 327-28; asked about Hohensee, 341; criticizes nutritional promotions, 357-59; collaborates with NBBB, 359, 396; collaborates with FDA, 359, 402-403; investigates Hoxsey, 364-67, 374-75, 380, 382; intensifies anti-quackery campaign, 397; collaborates with FTC, 402; co-sponsors National Congresses on Medical Quackery, 402-407, 429; and Ribicoff, 409; mentioned, 154, 224, 281, 342, 356. *See also* Cramp, Arthur J.; Fishbein, Morris; *Journal of the American Medical Association*
American Naturopathic Association, 382
American Pharmaceutical Association, 57-58, 279
American Public Health Association, 357
American Rally, 382
American Revolution, 14, 16
American School of Magnetic Healing, 69-72

American Society for Pharmacology and Experimental Therapeutics, 81
AMHO-Whitehall, 314
aminopyrine, 193
amphetamines, 280
analgesics, 3-12, 31, 36, 45, 47, 54, 103, 193-95, 267, 268, 276, 279, 301-303, 307, 319
anemia, 260
antacids, 268, 311
antihistamines, 268, 303, 305, 395
antipyrine, 5
Anti-Saloon League, 132
antiseptics, 101, 102, 155, 165, 189, 268
*Apostles of Discord*, 431
appendicitis, 95
apple growers, 187, 188
*Arthritis and Common Sense*, 401
Arthritis and Rheumatism Foundation, 391, 399-400, 419, 422, 427
arthritis remedies, 85, 206, 288, 301, 303, 311, 396, 399-401, 405, 422, 427-28
aspirin, 267, 268, 276, 279, 319
Associated Advertising Clubs of the World: asks FTC to control advertising, 114, 116; created as Associated Advertising Clubs of America, 115; name broadened, 115; sets up National Vigilance Committee, 115; work of committee, 116; committee becomes National Better Business Bureau, 119; aided by AMA, 132. *See also* National Better Business Bureau
Association of National Advertisers, 151
Atkinson, Brooks, 314
Atlanta city council, 326
Atwell, William, 374-75, 378-80
Aunt Fanny's Worm Candy, 23
Aycock, Charles, 86-87

B. & M. External Remedy: wins 1922 case, 88; therapeutic claims, 88, 90, 92; origin, 89; composition, 89; acquired by Rollins, 89-90; Massachusetts state action, 91; seizure action, 91-92; seizure uncontested, 105; Rollins contracts for research, 105-106; contested seizure action, 106-12; criminal case, 112; exhibit in "Chamber of Horrors," 169; mentioned, 113, 164, 183
*Babbitt*, 245

folk remedies marketed as patent medicines, 15-16
Folsom, James, 330
food: in relation to health mid-19th century, 20-21; adulteration in late 19th century, 28-29; early nutrition research, 39, 334; 1906 law restricts adulteration, 41; sold with health claims, 335-38. *See also* nutritional promotions
Food and Drug Administration: established, 98; and political climate of 1920's, 98-100; appropriations and staff, 100, 102, 156, 172, 191, 209-10, 216, 393, 405; key projects of 1920's, 101; depression policies, 102, 103; relations with Proprietary Association, 102, 264-65; collaborates with Post Office Dept., 103, 220-21, 283; collaborates with FTC, 103, 302-303, 433; criticized by industry, 103-104, 172; B. & M. case, 104-12; loss of major cases, 112; criticized by Kallet and Schlink, 156-57; and background of 1938 law, 158-88; Elixir Sulfanilamide case, 184-86; prepares to enforce 1938 law, 190; impact of World War II, 191, 194; voluntary compliance under 1938 law, 192; court cases interpreting 1938 law, 193-216; problems of promoters using speech, 204-208; Marmola case, 210-15; conspiracy with AMA charged, 214; Kaadt case, 227-38; Drown case, 242, 246-57; device cases, 245, 258-59; Micro-Dynameter case, 258-59; and new drugs, 261-62; policy on prescription vs. non-prescription drugs, 265-66, 269-71, 275-80; issues proprietary label warnings, 268; Sullivan case, 270-71, 275; prescription refill controversy, 271-77; given more control over dangerous drugs, 280n; given regulation of prescription drug advertising, 315, 419; and LeBlanc, 319, 321, 331; and cod liver oil, 335-36; cases against nutritional promotions, 336-37, 340, 356-58; "minimum daily requirements" for food nutrients, 338-39;

Hohensee case, 343-55; collaborates with AMA, 359, 402-403; collaborates with NBBB, 359, 402; Hoxsey litigation, 375-80, 386-89; Electronic Medical Foundation case, 383; criticized by National Health Federation, 383-84; criticized by Citizens Advisory Committees, 392-93, 414; regulatory victories ca. 1960, 400-401; co-sponsors National Congresses on Medical Quackery, 402-407, 429; control of prescription drugs, 411-12, 418-19; criticism of prescription drug regulation, 413-19; thalidomide case, 415-18; Krebiozen case, 420; court victories in 1960's, 421; handicaps in controlling quackery, 421; coordinates survey of "Susceptibility to Health Fallacies," 431-33; proposes regulations for special dietary products, 433; mentioned, 87, 124, 297, 305, 390, 391, 394. *See also* Bureau of Chemistry
*Food and Drug Review*, 63n
Food and Nutrition Board, 338-39
Food, Drug, and Cosmetic Act of 1938: Roosevelt authorizes effort to secure, 158-59; Tugwell bill drafted, 159-60; industry conferences, 160; effort to secure compared with that preceding 1906, 161-63; Copeland introduces, 164-66; Senate hearings, 166; bill criticized by industry, 166-69; Copeland revises bill, 170-72; new Senate hearings, 171-72; bill criticized by industry, 171; Copeland makes more revisions, 172-73; Roosevelt's message, 173; Senate debates and passes bill, 173-75; advertising control issue, 173-74, 180-82, 186-87; multiple seizure issue, 173-74, 178, 180, 187-88; reactions to bill, 175-76; House hearings, 177-79; House bill passes, 180-81; conference compromise rejected by House, 181-82; reactions to, 182-83; Elixir Sulfanilamide episode, 186; Roosevelt's position on, 186-87; regulations issue, 187; House passes new bill, 187-88; conference report, 188; bill passed

[ 495 ]